ENDOCRINE SECRETS

ENDOCRINE SECRETS

MICHAEL T. McDERMOTT, M.D.

Clinical Professor of Medicine
University of Colorado School of Medicine
Denver, Colorado
Chief, Endocrine Service
Fitzsimons Army Medical Center
Aurora, Colorado

HANLEY & BELFUS, INC./ Philadelphia
MOSBY/ St. Louis • Baltimore • Boston • Chicago
London • Philadelphia • Sydney • Toronto

Publisher: HANLEY & BELFUS, INC.
                    210 S. 13th Street
                    Philadelphia, PA 19107
                    (215) 546-7293

North American and worldwide sales and distribution:

                    MOSBY
                    11830 Westline Industrial Drive
                    St. Louis, MO 63146

In Canada: Times Mirror Professional Publishing, Ltd.
                    130 Flaska Drive
                    Markham, Ontario L6G 1B8
                    Canada

Library of Congress Cataloging-in-Publication Data

McDermott, Michael T., 1952–
     Endocrinology secrets / Michael T. McDermott.
         p.   cm.
     Includes bibliographical references and index.
     ISBN 1-56053-116-9 : $28.95
     1. Endocrinology—Miscellanea.   I. Title.
     [DNLM: 1. Endocrine Diseases—physiopathology.   WK 100 M78e 1994]
     RC649.M36 1994
     616.4—dc20
     DNLM/DLC
     for Library of Congress   94-31930
                                                              CIP

Disclaimer: The opinions or assertions contained in this book are the private views of the authors and are not to be construed as reflecting the views of the Department of the Army of the Department of Defense.

ENDOCRINE SECRETS   ISBN 1-56053-116-9

Last digit is the print number: 9   8   7   6   5   4   3   2   1

CONTENTS

IV. ADRENAL DISORDERS

V. THYROID DISORDERS

VI. REPRODUCTIVE ENDOCRINOLOGY

VII. MISCELLANEOUS

Contents

CONTRIBUTORS

Nadine H. Alex, M.D.
Endocrine Service, Fitzsimons Army Medical Center, Aurora, Colorado

Arnold A. Asp, M.D., FACP
Endocrine Service, Fitzsimons Army Medical Center, Aurora, Colorado

Brenda K. Bell, M.D.
Endocrine Service, Fitzsimons Army Medical Center, Aurora, Colorado

Daniel H. Bessesen, M.D.
Associate Professor of Medicine, Department of Medicine, Division of Endocrinology, Metabolism and Diabetes, University of Colorado School of Medicine, Denver, Colorado

Kenneth P. Burman, M.D.
Professor of Medicine, Uniformed Services University of the Health Sciences, Bethesda, Maryland; Director, Section of Endocrinology, Washington Hospital Center, Washington, D.C.

Barrett L. Chapin, M.D.
Assistant Chief, Endocrinology Service, Department of Medicine, William Beaumont Army Medical Center, El Paso, Texas

Reed S. Christensen, M.D.
Fellow, Endocrine Service, Department of Medicine, Fitzsimons Army Medical Center, Aurora, Colorado

Stephen C. Clement, M.D., MAJ, MC
Assistant Professor of Medicine, Uniformed Services University of the Health Sciences, Bethesda, Maryland

William E. Duncan M.D.
Endocrinology Service, Walter Reed Army Medical Center, Washington, D.C.

James E. Fitzpatrick, MD., COL, MC
Chief, Dermatology Service, Fitzsimons Army Medical Center, Aurora, Colorado; Clinical Assistant Professor, Department of Dermatology, University of Colorado School of Medicine, Denver, Colorado

Robert H. Gates, M.D.
Assistant Chief, Department of Medicine, Fitzsimons Army Medical Center, Aurora, Colorado; Assistant Clinical Professor of Medicine, University of Colorado School of Medicine, Denver, Colorado

William J. Georgitis, M.D.
Assistant Chief, Endocrine Service, Fitzsimons Army Medical Center, Aurora, Colorado; Associate Clinical Professor of Medicine, University of Colorado School of Medicine, Denver, Colorado

Allan R. Glass, M.D.
Professor of Medicine, Uniformed Services University of the Health Sciences, Bethesda, Maryland; Assistant Chief, Endocrinology, Walter Reed Army Medical Center, Washington, D.C.

Bryan R. Haugen, M.D.
Assistant Professor of Medicine, Division of Endocrinology, Metabolism and Diabetes, University of Colorado School of Medicine, Denver, Colorado

Fred D. Hofeldt, M.D.
Professor of Medicine, University of Colorado School of Medicine, Denver, Colorado

Robert E. Jones, M.D., FACP
Chief, Endocrinology Service, Madigan Army Medical Center, Tacoma, Washingon; Associate Professor of Medicine, Uniformed Services University of the Health Sciences, Bethesda, Maryland

William J. Lasswell, Jr., M.D., Ph.D.
Department of Medicine, Womack Army Medical Center, Fort Bragg, North Carolina

Michael T. McDermott, M.D.
Clinical Professor of Medicine, University of Colorado School of Medicine, Denver; Chief, Endocrine Service, Fitzsimons Army Medical Center, Aurora, Colorado

John A. Merenich, M.D.
Assistant Professor of Medicine, Division of Endocrinology, Metabolism and Diabetes, University of Colorado School of Medicine, Denver, Colorado

Jane E. B. Reusch, M.D.
Assistant Professor, Department of Medicine, Division of Endocrinology, Metabolism and Diabetes, University of Colorado School of Medicine, Denver, Colorado

E. Chester Ridgway, M.D.
Professor of Medicine, and Chief, Division of Endocrinology, Metabolism and Diabetes, University of Colorado School of Medicine, Denver, Colorado

Julie I. Rifkin, M.D.
Clinical Assistant Professor of Medicine, University of Colorado School of Medicine, Denver, Colorado

Mary H. Samuels, M.D.
Assistant Professor of Medicine, Division of Endocrinology, Diabetes and Clinical Nutrition, Oregon Health Sciences University, Portland, Oregon

Leonard R. Sanders, M.D., FACP
Clinical Associate Professor, Department of Medicine, University of Texas Health Sciences Center, San Antonio, Texas; Attending Physician, Fitzsimons Army Medical Center, Aurora and Denver Veterans Administration Medical Center, Denver, Colorado

Virginia Sarapura, M.D.
Assistant Professor of Medicine, Division of Endocrinology, Metabolism and Diabetes, University of Colorado School of Medicine, Denver, Colorado

Kenneth J. Simcic, M.D.
Chief, Endocrinology Service, William Beaumont Army Medical Center, El Paso, Texas; Assistant Professor of Medicine, Texas Tech University Health Sciences Center School of Medicine, El Paso, Texas

Robert H. Slover, M.D.
Assistant Professor of Pediatrics, University of Colorado School of Medicine, Denver, Colorado

Robert C. Smallridge, M.D.
Director, Division of Medicine, Walter Reed Army Institute of Research, Washington, D.C.; Professor of Medicine, Uniformed Services University of the Health Sciences, Bethesda, Maryland

Javier I. Torrens, M.D., CPT, MC
Fellow, Endocrine-Metabolic Service, Walter Reed Army Medical Center, Washington, D.C.

PREFACE

The education of a physician requires the combined efforts of many people. It is my hope that this book will be one small but significant contribution. Thanks must first go to those who so generously donated their time and efforts to the writing of these chapters. They shared not only their knowledge and experience but also their humanity and humor. It is all greatly appreciated. Thanks and congratulations also go to the students who diligently seek the knowledge, skills and humanitarian ideals necessary to be complete physicians. Finally, thanks must go to all our patients, who are our best teachers. Through their suffering and forbearance, our minds are able to expand and our hearts to develop genuine compassion. It is ultimately for them that we make this effort.

Michael T. McDermott, M.D.
Aurora, Colorado

I. Fuel Metabolism

1. DIABETES MELLITUS

Stephen Clement, M.D.

1. What is diabetes mellitus?

Diabetes mellitus is a chronic disorder characterized by the abnormal metabolism of fuels, particularly glucose and fat. By tradition, the diagnosis of diabetes rests on the demonstration of an abnormality in glucose tolerance. The array of entities called diabetes mellitus is linked by the common abnormality of glucose intolerance and the potential for developing complications from altered glucose and lipid metabolism. The various types of diabetes and glucose intolerance are listed in the following tables:

Types of Diabetes Mellitus and Other Categories of Glucose Intolerance

CLINICAL CLASSES	DISTINGUISHING CHARACTERISTICS
Diabetes mellitus (DM) Insulin-dependent diabetes mellitus (IDDM) type I	Patients may be of any age, are usually thin, and usually have abrupt onset of signs and symptoms with insulinopenia before age 30. These patients often have strongly positive urine ketone tests in conjunction with hyperglycemia and are dependent on insulin therapy to prevent ketoacidosis and to sustain life.
Non-insulin-dependent diabetes mellitus (NIDDM) type II (obese or nonobese)	Patients usually are older than 30 years at diagnosis, obese, and have relatively few classic symptoms. They are not prone to ketoacidosis except during periods of stress. Although not dependent on exogenous insulin for survival, they may require it for adequate control of hyperglycemia.
Other types of diabetes mellitus	Patients with other types of diabetes mellitus have certain associated conditions or syndromes (see next table).
Impaired glucose tolerance (IGT) (obese or nonobese)	Patients with impaired glucose tolerance have plasma glucose levels that are higher than normal but not diagnostic for diabetes mellitus.
Other types of impaired glucose tolerance	Patients with other types of impaired glucose tolerance have certain associated conditions or syndromes (see next table).
Gestational diabetes mellitus (GDM)	Patients with gestational diabetes mellitus have onset or discovery of glucose intolerance during pregnancy.
STATISTICAL RISK CLASSES*	
Previous abnormality of glucose tolerance (PreAGT)	Patients in this category have normal glucose tolerance and a history of transient diabetes mellitus or impaired glucose tolerance.
Potential abnormality of glucose tolerance (PotAGT)	Patients in this category have never experienced abnormal glucose tolerance but have a greater than normal risk of developing diabetes mellitus or impaired glucose tolerance.

*Used for epidemiologic and research purposes.
From American Diabetes Association: Physician's Guide to Non-Insulin-Dependent (Type II) Diabetes: Diagnosis and Treatment, 2nd ed. Alexandria, VA, American Diabetes Association, 1988, with permission.

Other Types of Diabetes Mellitus and Impaired Glucose Tolerance

Secondary to:	
Pancreatic disease	**Examples:** pancreatectomy, hemochromatosis, cystic fibrosis, chronic pancreatitis
Endocrinopathies	**Examples:** acromegaly, pheochromocytoma, Cushing's syndrome, primary aldosteronism, glucagonoma
Drugs and chemical agents	**Examples:** certain antihypertensive drugs, thiazide diuretics, glucocorticoids, estrogen-containing preparations, psychoactive agents, catecholamines
Associated with:	
Insulin-receptor abnormalities	**Example:** acanthosis nigricans
Genetic syndromes	**Examples:** hyperlipidemia, muscular dystrophies, Huntington's chorea
Miscellaneous conditions	**Example:** malnutrition ("tropical diabetes")

For a more complete list, see National Diabetes Data Group: Classification and diagnosis of diabetes mellitus and other categories of glucose tolerance. Diabetes 28:1039–57, 1979.
From American Diabetes Association: Physician's Guide to Non-Insulin-Dependent (Type II) Diabetes: Diagnosis and Treatment, 2nd ed. Alexandria, VA, American Diabetes Association, 1988, with permission.

2. How is diabetes diagnosed?

The diagnosis of diabetes rests on the demonstration of elevated blood glucose levels. Normal fasting plasma glucose levels are less than 115 mg/dl. After a meal or after a glucose tolerance test (ingestion of 75 gm of oral glucose), the normal plasma glucose level remains below 200 mg/dl from 30–90 minutes after ingestion and is less than 140 mg/dl two hours after ingestion. The criteria for establishing the diagnosis of diabetes are listed in the table below.

Diagnostic Criteria for Diabetes Mellitus, Impaired Glucose Tolerance, and Gestational Diabetes

NONPREGNANT ADULTS

Criteria for Diabetes Mellitus. Diagnosis of diabetes mellitus in nonpregnant adults should be restricted to those who have *one* of the following:
- random plasma glucose level of 200 mg/dl or greater *plus* classic signs and symptoms of diabetes mellitus including polydipsia, polyuria, polyphagia, and weight loss;
- fasting plasma glucose level of 140 mg/dl or greater on at least 2 occasions; or
- fasting plasma glucose level less than 140 mg/dl *plus* sustained elevated plasma glucose levels during at least 2 oral glucose tolerance tests. The 2-hour sample and at least one other between 0 and 2 hours after 75-gram glucose dose should be 200 mg/dl or greater. Oral glucose tolerance testing is not necessary if patient has fasting plasma glucose level of 140 mg/dl or greater.

Criteria for Impaired Glucose Tolerance. Diagnosis of impaired glucose tolerance in nonpregnant adults should be restricted to those who have *all* of the following:
- fasting plasma glucose of less than 140 mg/dl;
- 2-hour oral glucose tolerance test plasma glucose level between 140 and 200 mg/dl; and
- intervening oral glucose tolerance test plasma glucose level of 200 mg/dl or greater.

PREGNANT WOMEN

Criteria for Gestational Diabetes. After an oral glucose load of 100 grams, diagnosis of gestational diabetes may be made if 2 plasma glucose values equal or exceed (in mg/dl)

Fasting	1 Hour	2 Hour	3 Hour
105	190	165	145

CHILDREN

Criteria for Diabetes Mellitus. Diagnosis of diabetes mellitus in children should be restricted to those who have *one* of the following:
- random plasma glucose level of 200 mg/dl or greater *plus* classic signs and symptoms of diabetes mellitus, including polyuria, polydipsia, ketonuria, and rapid weight loss; or
- fasting plasma glucose level of 140 mg/dl or greater on at least 2 occasions *and* sustained elevated plasma glucose levels during at least 2 oral glucose tolerance tests. Both the 2-hour plasma glucose and at least one other between 0 and 2 hours after glucose dose (1.75 g/kg ideal body weight up to 75 grams) should be 200 mg/dl or greater.

Criteria for Impaired Glucose Tolerance. Diagnosis of impaired glucose tolerance in children should be restricted to those who have *both* of the following:
- fasting plasma glucose concentration of less than 140 mg/dl; and
- 2-hour oral glucose tolerance test plasma glucose level of greater than 140 mg/dl.

From American Diabetes Association: Physician's Guide to Non-Insulin-Dependent (Type II) Diabetes: Diagnosis and Treatment, 2nd ed. Alexandria, VA, American Diabetes Association, 1988, with permission.

3. What effect does genetics have on type I diabetes?

The interplay between genetics and environment in diabetes is complex and still not well understood. For type I (insulin-dependent) diabetes, the cumulative risk for siblings of diabetic patients is 6–10% versus 0.6% for the general population. Regarding the effect of parental genes, the offspring of women with type I diabetes have a lower risk of disease (2.1%) than the offspring of men with type 1 diabetes (6.1%). The reason for this disparity is unknown. Monozygotic twins have a 20–50% concordance for type I diabetes. The susceptibility for type I diabetes is associated with the genetic expression of certain proteins coded by the HLA region of the major histocompatibility complex. These proteins are present on the surface of lymphocytes and macrophages and are considered essential for triggering the autoimmune destruction of the beta cells. Although all the genetic markers (HLA and others) for type I diabetes are not known, future progress in this field will allow for population screening for genetic susceptibilty.

4. What is the role of genetics in the development of type II diabetes?

The familial clustering of type II (non–insulin-dependent) diabetes suggests a strong genetic component to the disease. Monozygotic twins have a 60–90% concordance for type II diabetes. The cumulative risk for type II diabetes in siblings of diabetic patients is 10–33% versus 5% for the general population. Offspring of women with type II diabetes have a twofold to threefold greater risk for developing diabetes than offspring of men with the disease. The exact mode of inheritance for type II diabetes is not known, but is thought to be polygenic. Specific mutations that code for type II diabetes have been identified in a small percentage of patients. For the

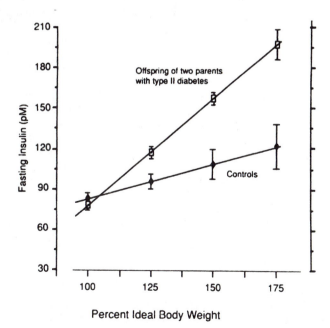

From Warram JH, Martin BC, Krolewski AS, et al: Slow glucose removal rate and hyperinsulinemia precede the development of type II diabetes with the offspring of diabetic parents. Ann Intern Med 113:909–915, 1990, with permission.

majority of patients, however, a specific gene has not yet been identified. The interplay between genetic and environmental influences is seen by the demonstration of higher fasting insulin levels for every weight category in offspring of two parents with type II diabetes compared with controls (see figure on p. 3). High insulin levels are a marker for insulin resistance and are predictive of progression to type II diabetes.

5. What is the pathogenesis of diabetes?

For type I diabetes, the primary pathogenic step is the activation of host T-lymphocytes against specific antigens present on the patient's beta cells. These activated T-cells orchestrate a slow destruction of the beta cells via the recruitment of T- and B-lymphocytes, macrophages, and cytokines. Morphologic study of the pancreases of children who died at the onset of diabetes have shown an inflammatory infiltrate of mononuclear cells confined to the islets—called **insulitis.** The final result is total destruction of the beta cells over a span of years. The finding of high-titer islet-cell autoantibodies (ICAs) in the serum of a child is highly predictive for progression to type I diabetes. Various antigens that are expressed by the beta cell have been implicated as the target for the autoimmune attack. Candidate antigens include insulin itself and a 64 kilo-dalton protein (now recognized as glutamic acid decarboxylase, or GAD). The triggering event for T-cell activation against these autoantigens is unknown, but may involve the exposure to some environmental substance that is antigenically similar to the autoantigen. The T-cells that are activated against this environmental antigen can then cross-react with the antigen on the beta cells—a process called **molecular mimicry.** Suspected environmental triggers for type I diabetes are viruses, toxins, and foods. For example, exposure to cow's milk in the first 6 weeks of life has been implicated in the development of type I diabetes in genetically susceptible children. Viruses may trigger type I diabetes via molecular mimicry or by direct alteration of the beta cell, causing abnormal expression of autoantigens, or by direct destruction of the beta cells.

6. What is the pathogenesis of type II diabetes?

The pathogenesis of type II diabetes is unclear but appears to be multifactorial. The earliest defect that can be detected is insulin resistance, manifested as elevated plasma insulin levels—either fasting or after an oral or intravenous glucose tolerance test. This abnormality can be seen as early as late adolescence and may precede the development of diabetes by one or two decades. In this early stage, insulin resistance is seen even in the absence of obesity. Prospective studies indicate that the inheritance of this insulin resistance trait is necessary but not sufficient for the development of diabetes. The development of diabetes does not occur in genetically susceptible individuals who maintain close to ideal body weight. Only genetically susceptible persons who become obese are affected. Obesity, particularly truncal obesity, is associated with insulin resistance and is postulated to place an increased demand on the beta cells.

The figure at the top of page 5 shows the relationship between waist circumference (measure of truncal obesity) and insulin sensitivity in women with various degrees of glucose tolerance. Women with the smallest waist measurements were the most insulin sensitive compared to women with the largest waist measurements. An identical relationship was demonstrated for men.

For persons genetically susceptible to type II diabetes, the beta cells are able to compensate, to a point, for the insulin resistance. However, over years, the beta cells lose this ability. This point of beta cell failure is often when clinical diabetes is diagnosed. This progression from insulin resistance to beta-cell failure has been clearly demonstrated in humans. Similarly, animal models for type II diabetes progress in a predictable fashion through various stages of insulin resistance and insulin deficiency.

7. What causes beta-cell failure?

The cause for the failure of the beta cells to "keep up" with the increased demand in type II diabetes is unclear. Subtle defects in beta-cell function have been described early in the course of the disease. One provocative theory is that glucose itself, once above the normal range, may actually be "toxic" to the beta cells. This theory is supported by a number of animal studies which demonstrate that beta cells fail to respond appropriately to glucose when ambient glucose

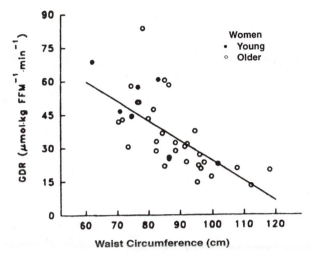

Relationship between insulin resistance measured by the euglycemic clamp technique and waist circumference in women with various degrees of glucose tolerance. GDR = glucose disposal rate. A high GDR = insulin sensitive. A low GDR = insulin resistant. r = −.71, P<0.01 for women; r = −.65, P<0.01 for men (graph not shown). (From Kohrt WM, Kirwan JP, Staten MA, et al: Insulin resistance in aging is related to abdominal obesity. Diabetes 42:273, 1993, with permission.)

levels are maintained above ≈120 mg/dl. The studies suggest that glucose itself may contribute to a vicious cycle of increasing blood glucose levels and decreasing beta-cell function. This acquired defect in beta-cell function appears to be reversible, once the glucose levels are normalized.

Other causes for beta-cell dysfunction have been implicated in type II diabetes, including genetically determined reduced beta cell mass and the accumulation of amyloid-like fibrils in the beta cells (amylin). The relative contribution of these factors is not known. Over the course of the disease, beta-cell function in type II diabetes diminishes and can eventually progress to an entity similar to type I diabetes, manifested by profound insulin deficiency and a predisposition to ketosis (see figure below).

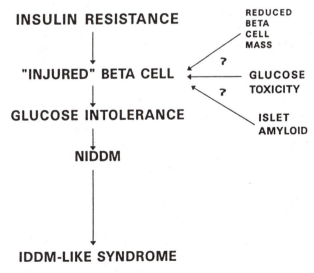

Natural history of NIDDM.

8. How does the liver contribute to sustaining fasting hyperglycemia in type II diabetes?
The fasting glucose level is determined by the balance between glucose utilization by peripheral tissues and hepatic glucose production. In the nondiabetic state, the basal fasting insulin level is sufficient to suppress hepatic glucose production and maintain glucose levels in the normal range. However, in type II diabetes, the circulating insulin level is not sufficient to suppress hepatic glucose production, which increases in the late phases of diabetes progression and becomes the major contributor to fasting hyperglycemia. So in the advanced stages in the development of type II diabetes, insulin resistance, insulin deficiency, and increased hepatic glucose production all play a role in sustaining hyperglycemia. A comparison of the known pathogenic factors for type I and type II diabetes is provided below.

Comparison of Known Pathogenic Factors for Types I and II Diabetes

PATHOGENIC FACTOR	TYPE I (INSULIN-DEPENDENT)	TYPE II (NON–INSULIN-DEPENDENT)
Genetic	Disease risk associated with specific HLA haplotypes	Strong familial clustering, but a specific gene marker not identified
Environmental	? Viral-triggered autoimmunity ? Ingested antigens (i.e., cow's milk)	Sedentary lifestyle, obesity ? Drugs
Autoimmunity	Yes	No
Other	?	? Reduced beta cell mass ? Amylin ? Glucose "toxicity"

Adapted from a lecture by Michael Bush, M.D., unpublished.

9. What other metabolic abnormalities are seen with diabetes?
Diabetes is characterized by an abnormality in metabolism of fuels, of which glucose is the most obvious. In addition, persons with diabetes have abnormal metabolism of free fatty acids (FFA) and amino acids. Insulin promotes clearance of FFA and is a potent inhibitor of lipolysis. In states of insulin deficiency or insulin resistance, this antilipolytic effect of insulin is impaired, leading to elevated FFA and triglyceride levels.

Reaven coined the term "Syndrome X" to describe the constellation of abnormalities often seen together: hyperinsulinemia, impaired glucose tolerance, hypertension, increased plasma triglycerides, and decreased high-density lipoprotein cholesterol concentrations. A sixth feature that is closely associated with the syndrome is truncal obesity. This clustering of abnormalities often occurs in patients at risk for or with previously diagnosed type II diabetes and suggests a single etiologic factor. Although a genetic marker for the syndrome has not been determined, tissue resistance to glucose uptake is universally found. Implications of Syndrome X are that patients with even mild glucose intolerance are at increased risk for atherosclerotic disease due to associated lipid and blood pressure abnormalities. Correction of these disorders should be addressed at the etiologic level of the syndrome, namely insulin resistance.

10. What constitutes optimal treatment for type I diabetes?
The treatment strategies for type I diabetes have changed dramatically over the last decade. Prior to 1980, standard insulin therapy consisted of a fixed dose of one or two injections of a mixture of regular and NPH insulin, a fixed diet and exercise regimen, and urine glucose testing. The availability of self-monitoring blood glucose testing (SMBG), the use of multiple-dose insulin regimens, and the evolution of the diabetes treatment team have allowed for a marked improvement of glycemic control in the motivated patient. Interest in implementing more intensive treatment regimens using this approach has been greatly enhanced by the recent results of the Diabetes Control and Complications Trial (DCCT).

11. Describe the DCCT model for type I diabetes management.
The Diabetes Control and Complications Trial (DCCT) showed a 34–76% reduction in clinically meaningful retinopathy in type I diabetic patients using intensive diabetes therapy compared to

Syndrome X

Solid arrows signify proven relations and open arrows signify unproven but probable relations.

patients randomized to standard diabetes therapy. Marked reductions in albuminuria and neuropathy were also seen. An adverse effect of intensive therapy is a three-fold increase in severe hypoglycemia. The implementation of intensive therapy requires that the patient monitor his or her blood glucose 4–8 times per day and use a multiple-dose (three or more injections) insulin regimen or an insulin infusion pump. The patient must count the exact amount of carbohydrate ingested or use the diabetic exchange system in order to make rational decisions on insulin adjustment.

Intensive therapy is best managed by a specialized team consisting of a certified diabetes educator (CDE), nurse, dietitian, behavioral medicine specialist, and physician with special training in intensive therapy (usually an endocrinologist). Patient contact with the team is frequent, consisting of monthly clinic visits and often weekly telephone contacts for review of SMBG results. Computer modem or FAX are now frequently used to transmit SMBG results. Frequent adjustments are made in the insulin, food, and exercise regimen (see the sample forms provided).

Based on the DCCT results, the American Diabetes Association recommends that "patients should aim for the best level of glucose control they can achieve without placing themselves at undue risk for hypoglycemia or other hazards associated with tight control."[1]

INSULIN PUMP SETTINGS FOR

1. BASAL RATE
1ST BASAL RATE 12 MIDNIGHT TO _____ : _____/HR
2ND BASAL RATE _____ TO _____ : _____/HR
3RD BASAL RATE _____ TO _____ : _____/HR

2. MEAL PLAN/INSULIN BOLUS   INSULIN BOLUS

Breakfast	__ BR	__ Fruit	__ Milk	(__g CHO)	__ units
Lunch	__ BR	__ Fruit	__ Milk	(__g CHO)	__ units
Dinner	__ BR	__ Fruit	__ Milk	(__g CHO)	__ units
Snack	__ BR	__ Fruit	__ Milk	(__g CHO)	__ units

ONE UNIT OF INSULIN WILL COVER *APPROXIMATELY* _____ GRAMS CHO.

3. SUPPLEMENTAL INSULIN
Give one extra unit bolus for every _____ points your BG is above __
Give supplemental insulin only after waiting at least four hours since last insulin bolus.

4. TIMING
If BG is 80–150, give bolus 30 min. prior to meal.
If BG is >150, give bolus 45 min. prior to meal.
If BG is <80, give bolus and eat immediately.

5. HYPOGLYCEMIA
Treat hypoglycemia with ___ grams fast-acting CHO, then 15 grams bread exchange or 1 milk.

6. EXERCISE
Reduce meal bolus by ___ units prior to exercise.
For prolonged exercise, reduce basal rate to ___/hr during and _____ hours after exercise.

7. BG GOALS
Fasting _____, 2 hr post meal _____, 3AM > 60.

* * * *

Insulin Dosages for (insert name below):

_____

NORMAL INSULIN DOSE

MORNING	PRE-DINNER	BEFORE BED
_____ NPH	_____ NPH	_____ NPH
_____ REG	_____ REG	
WITH INCREASED FOOD, ADD	_____ REG TO ABOVE DOSE	

WITH INCREASED ACTIVITY *LESS* INSULIN IS NEEDED

TAKE ____ REG, ____ NPH IN THE AM WITH DAY-TIME ACTIVITY
TAKE ____ REG IN THE PM WITH EVENING ACTIVITY

SUPPLEMENTAL INSULIN—*ADD* TO YOUR USUAL DOSAGE IF YOUR SUGAR IS HIGH:
IF > 200, ADD ____ UNITS REGULAR
IF > 250, ADD ____ UNITS REGULAR

TIMING—IF BG IN NORMAL RANGE, TAKE INSULIN 30 MIN PRIOR TO EATING
—IF BG LOW, TAKE INSULIN AND EAT IMMEDIATELY
—IF BG HIGH, TAKE INSULIN ONE HOUR PRIOR TO EATING

12. Is intensive diabetes therapy cost-effective?
Analyses of the cost-effectiveness suggest that the potential reduction in cost for treating diabetic complications (laser photocoagulation, dialysis, hospitalization for amputations and rehabilitation) justifies the cost of personnel and supplies to support intensive diabetes therapy. The risk-benefit ratio for intensive therapy may be less favorable for prepubertal children, patients with far advanced complications, and patients with coronary or cerebral vascular disease.

13. Can glycemic control be improved without resorting to intensive therapy?
The DCCT model for type I diabetes management is considered the gold standard. However, various simple alterations in insulin management may yield improvements in glycemic control as well. In our experience, simply splitting the evening insulin dose so that the regular insulin is taken before dinner and the NPH is taken before bed stabilizes nocturnal glycemic control. The rationale is that the NPH insulin taken before bed does not peak until 5–6 AM. For persons with a prominent dawn phenomenon (increased insulin requirements due to counterregulatory hormones), this regimen covers this increased requirement and minimizes the chance of nocturnal hypoglycemia. The evening NPH can then be adjusted more easily to control the fasting glucose level.

14. What is the approach to the patient with a labile blood glucose profile?
A careful history, searching for causes of glucose variability, is essential for optimizing a diabetes regimen. The presence and cause of hypoglycemic reactions are crucial information because

WHEN IS YOUR INSULIN WORKING?

REG: ONSET 45 MIN
PEAK 2 HOURS
DURATION 6 HOURS

NPH: ONSET 3 HRS
PEAK 6-7 HRS
DURATION 13 HRS

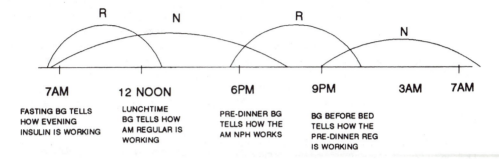

| 7AM | 12 NOON | 6PM | 9PM | 3AM 7AM |

FASTING BG TELLS
HOW EVENING
INSULIN IS WORKING

LUNCHTIME
BG TELLS HOW
AM REGULAR IS
WORKING

PRE-DINNER BG
TELLS HOW THE
AM NPH WORKS

BG BEFORE BED
TELLS HOW THE
PRE-DINNER REG
IS WORKING

hypoglycemia often leads to overtreatment with carbohydrate, causing hyperglycemia. Hypoglycemia may also blunt the patient's ability to respond to subsequent hypoglycemic episodes in the ensuing 24 hours (see chapter 2). A common strategy for optimizing a diabetes regimen is as follows:

- Address and abolish causes of hypoglycemia.
- Optimize the fasting glucose.
- "Fine tune" the regimen to optimize the pre- and postprandial glucose readings.
- Address special situations (increased exercise, dining out, travel, infections, intercurrent illnesses).
- Use hemoglobin Alc (glycohemoglobin) levels to follow progress.

Some of the causes of glucose variability are listed in the table below.

Troubleshooting an Insulin Regimen

- Check accuracy of SMBG
- Pharmacokinetics:
  Insulin drawing and mixing (be careful with reg/lente mix)
  Injection sites (abdomen > arms > thighs)
  ? Injecting into "active" limbs
  Potency of insulin (storage)
  Timing of regular insulin (? 30 min. prior to meals)
- Fasting hyperglycemia: Somogyi vs. dawn phenomenon
- Nutrition:
  Timing of meals
  ? Food "binges"
  ? Consider gastroparesis
- Exercise:
  Acute hypoglycemia
  Delayed hypoglycemia (especially with prolonged exercise)
- Alcohol: delayed hypoglycemia
- Drugs: e.g., corticosteroids
- Stress
- Illness
- Hormonal: e.g., menses (insulin requirements may increase at mid-cycle and decrease on first day of menses)

15. What is the optimal treatment for type II diabetes?

Because type II diabetes is a heterogeneous disorder and patients may have other comorbid illnesses, treatment must be individualized. The most common mistake in management is to label type II diabetes as "borderline" or to neglect treatment completely. Patients with fasting glucose levels > 140 mg/dl or postprandial glucose levels > 200 mg/dl, even though asymptomatic, are at risk for diabetic complications. Questions regarding whether intensive diabetes management will prevent diabetic complications in type II patients have been addressed in recent reviews (see reference 7).

The optimal treatment strategy for type II diabetes is one that normalizes blood glucose levels by increasing insulin sensitivity. Unfortunately, there are no medications available in the United States today that directly improve insulin sensitivity. The lifestyle interventions of diet and exercise can dramatically enhance insulin sensitivity in sufficiently motivated patients. The initial intervention should include providing a specific prescription for an aerobic exercise program. Insulin sensitivity can be enhanced with a program as simple as brisk walking for 20 minutes daily. The exercise program should fit the patient's lifestyle and schedule. An optimal program is one in which the patient can be part of a supervised exercise group. Dietary intervention should include an initial evaluation by a dietitian and personalized follow-up visits or classes. The goal should be modest but steady weight loss (if appropriate).

16. Can glycemic levels be controlled by diet and exercise?

Diet and exercise alone often are not sufficient for achieving optimal glycemic goals. Oral hypoglycemic agents—primarily sulfonylureas—have been used extensively for the treatment of type II diabetes. Their main mechanism of action is enhancement of beta-cell sensitivity to glucose, so that the beta cell releases more insulin at every glucose level. Patients with fasting blood glucose levels less than 250 mg/dl are best candidates for sulfonylureas.

The common therapeutic dilemma is how to treat the type II diabetic patient who has failed to achieve treatment goals with diet, exercise, and a sulfonylurea. Reasons for failure of sulfonylurea therapy include noncompliance with the diet and exercise regimen, failure to lose weight, or diminished insulin secretory capacity. Regardless of the cause, administration of insulin may be required for optimal glycemic control. Some of the strategies for patients failing therapy with oral hypoglycemic agents are listed in the table below.

Strategies for Patients Failing Oral Hypoglycemic Agents

- "Short course" of insulin therapy
- Inpatient weight loss and behavior modification
- Intensive outpatient program (weekly visits)
- Bedtime insulin, daytime sulfonylurea (BIDS therapy)

The type II diabetic patient may fall anywhere on the spectrum of insulin resistance or insulin deficiency. For example, the patient with new-onset diabetes who is near ideal body weight (nonobese) may in fact have latent type I diabetes, even without ketosis. In these patients, despite the absence of islet cell antibodies in the serum, it may be prudent therapy to initiate insulin therapy at the time of diagnosis. This may preserve residual beta-cell function and enhance control in the future. Finally, an extensive list of medications may impair glucose tolerance, many of which are used in diabetic patients to treat other conditions. Care must be taken to orchestrate the treatment regimen so that these medications achieve the best therapeutic goal with the least adverse effects. In summary, the pharmacologic therapy for type II diabetes is a balancing act of optimizing glycemic control while simultaneously trying to improve insulin sensitivity through lifestyle changes. The author's priorities are listed in the following table.

Priorities for Treatment in NIDDM

- Control the blood glucose (fasting <120, postprandial <200 mg/dl)
- Minimize the dose of medication
- Control the hypertension and lipids with agents that are "friendly" to glucose tolerance

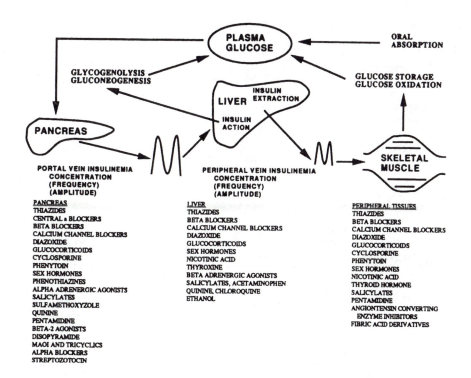

Potential sites of action for drugs influencing glucose metabolism. (From Pandit MK, Burke J, Gustafson AB, et al: Drug-induced disorders of glucose intolerance. Ann Intern Med 118:529, 1993, with permission.)

17. What is BIDS therapy?

The addition of a dose of bedtime NPH insulin to the current regimen of sulfonylurea is called bedtime insulin, daytime sulfonylurea (BIDS) therapy. The rationale is that bedtime insulin is a potent inhibitor of hepatic glucose production—the cause of fasting hyperglycemia (see pathogenesis of type II diabetes). By titrating the NPH dose upward, the fasting glucose level can often be safely normalized with only minimal risk of hypoglycemia. With a normal fasting glucose, the day-time sulfonylurea is often then able to control the glucose level during the day. The technique of BIDS therapy can be learned quickly in the outpatient setting with the help of a diabetes nurse educator. A popular initial treatment dose is 6–10 units NPH before bedtime. The dose can be increased every 3–4 days by two units until the fasting blood glucose is in the 80–120 mg/dl range. Once this level is achieved, efficacy of the program can be monitored by having the patient test his or her blood glucose before breakfast and the evening meal. If the fasting A.M. blood glucose is normalized but the evening glucose level is elevated, then traditional twice-a-day insulin therapy is indicated.

18. Are there established standards for the medical care of patients with diabetes mellitus?

Yes. The American Diabetes Association publishes minimum standards of care.[4] These standards are based on the literature by health care providers from diverse fields of expertise. For example, the standards state that patients should have a complete history and physical examination at the initial visit. Laboratory testing should include a fasting lipid profile and glycosylated hemoglobin

(HbA1c) level. Surveillance for complications should include an annual physical exam, ophthalmologic exam, and urinalysis (see also chapter 3). Laboratory follow-up should include a glycosylated hemoglobin test at least semiannually in all patients and quarterly in insulin-treated patients and patients with poorly controlled type II diabetes.

19. What is the role of diabetes education in the management of diabetic patients?
Few chronic diseases require the patient to participate in his or her care as much as is required for diabetes. The quality and intensiveness of diabetes education often determine success or failure in diabetes management. Diabetes education is provided by all health care providers. However, active input by a diabetes nurse educator and dietitian is considered essential for optimal care. These professionals not only can enhance adherence to the treatment regimen, but they can address barriers to compliance and resolve obstacles that may not be obvious to the physician (for review, see reference 12).

BIBLIOGRAPHY

1. American Diabetes Association: Implications of the diabetes control and complications trial. Diabetes Care 16:1517–1520, 1993.
2. American Diabetes Association: Physician's Guide to Insulin-Dependent (Type I) Diabetes: Diagnosis and Treatment, 2nd ed. Medical management of type I diabetes. Alexandria, VA, American Diabetes Association, 1994.
3. American Diabetes Association: Physician's Guide to Non-Insulin-Dependent (Type II) Diabetes: Diagnosis and Treatment, 3rd ed. Medical management of type II diabetes. Alexandria, VA, American Diabetes Association, 1994.
4. American Diabetes Association: Standards for medical care for patients with diabetes mellitus. Diabetes Care 17:616–623, 1994.
5. Bogardus C: Insulin resistance in the pathogenesis of NIDDM in Pima Indians. Diabetes Care 16(Supplement 1):228–233, 1993.
6. Diabetes Control and Complications Trial Research Group: The effect of intensive diabetes treatment on the development and progression of long-term complications in insulin-dependent diabetes mellitus. N Engl J Med 329:977–986, 1993.
7. Eastman RC, Siebert CW, Harris M, Gorden P: Implications of the diabetes control and complications trial. J Clin Endocrinol Metab 77:1105–1107, 1993
8. Gerich JE: Oral hypoglycemic agents. N Engl J Med 321:1231–1245, 1989.
9. Hirsch IB, Farkas-Hirsch Ruth, Skyler JS: Intensive insulin therapy for treatment of type I diabetes. Diabetes Care 13:1265–83, 1990.
10. Immunology and diabetes. Diabetes Rev 1 (entire volume), 1993.
11. Leahy JL, Bonner-Weir S, Weir GC: B-Cell dysfunction induced by chronic hyperglycemia. Diabetes Care 15:442–455, 1992.
12. Muhlhauser I, Berger M: Diabetes education and insulin therapy: when will they ever learn? J Intern Med 233:321–326, 1993.
13. Pandit MK, Burke J, Gustafson AB, et al: Drug-induced disorders of glucose tolerance. Ann Intern Med 118:529–539, 1993.
14. Reaven G: Role of insulin resistance in human disease. Diabetes 37:1595—1607, 1988.
15. Soneru IL, Agrawal L, Murphy JC, et al: Comparison of morning or bedtime insulin with and without glyburide in secondary sulfonylurea failure. Diabetes Care 16:896–901, 1993.
16. Taylor SI, Accili D, Imai Y: Insulin resistance or insulin deficiency: which is the primary cause of NIDDM? Diabetes 43:735–740, 1994.
17. Warram JH, Martin BC, Krolewski AS, et al: Slow glucose removal rate and hyperinsulinemia precede the development of type II diabetes in the offspring of diabetic parents. Ann Intern Med 113:909–915, 1990.

2. ACUTE COMPLICATIONS OF DIABETES MELLITUS

Stephen Clement, M.D., MAJ, MC, and Javier Ivan Torrens, M.D., CPT, MC

1. What are the most common acute complications of diabetes?

Acute complications of diabetes are a direct result of abnormalities in the plasma glucose level: hyperglycemia or hypoglycemia. Initial symptoms of hyperglycemia are increased thirst (polydipsia), increased urination (polyuria), fatigue, or blurry vision. If uncorrected, hyperglycemia eventually may lead to diabetic ketoacidosis (DKA) or nonketotic hyperosmolar coma. DKA and hyperosmolar coma have traditionally been considered separate entities. In actuality, they represent parts of a spectrum of a disease process characterized by varying degrees of insulin deficiency, overproduction of counterregulatory hormones, and dehydration. In some situations, features of DKA and hyperosmolar coma may be present concurrently.

Hypoglycemia, another acute complication of diabetes, results from an imbalance between the medication for diabetes treatment (insulin or sulfonylurea) and the patient's food intake or exercise. Because the brain depends almost entirely on glucose for normal function, a dramatic fall in circulating glucose can lead to confusion, stupor, or coma.

2. What is diabetic ketoacidosis (DKA)?

DKA is a state of uncontrolled catabolism triggered by a relative or absolute deficiency in circulating insulin. The triad of DKA is metabolic acidosis (pH < 7.35), hyperglycemia (blood glucose level usually > 250 mg/dl), and positive ketones in the urine or blood. The relative or absolute deficiency of insulin is accompanied by a reciprocal elevation in counterregulatory hormones (glucagon, epinephrine, growth hormone, and cortisol), causing increased glucose production by the liver (gluconeogenesis) and catabolism of fat (lipolysis). Lipolysis provides the substrate (free fatty acids) for the uncontrolled production of ketones by the liver. The production of ketones leads to acidosis and elevation of the anion gap, which almost always occur in DKA.

3. What causes DKA?

Any disorder that alters the balance between insulin and counterregulatory hormones can precipitate DKA. A minority of cases of DKA occur in persons (generally older persons) previously not diagnosed with diabetes. Most cases (up to 80%) of DKA, however, occur in persons with previously diagnosed diabetes owing to **inadequate insulin** or **intercurrent illness.**

Many patients with recurrent episodes of DKA are found to have deficient knowledge about their insulin regimen or have not been taught how to test their urine for ketones or how to handle their diabetes during times of illness. These are deficiencies in diabetes education.

The most common·intercurrent illnesses that may trigger DKA are infection and myocardial infarction. Even local infections such as urinary tract infections or prostatitis have precipitated DKA. Other triggering events include severe emotional stress, trauma, and exogenous medications (i.e., corticosteroids, pentamidine), or hormonal changes (i.e., pre-ovulation) in women. DKA is most often associated with type I (insulin-dependent) diabetes. However, it also may occur in the older patient with type II (non–insulin-dependent) diabetes, particularly when associated with a major intercurrent illness.

4. How is DKA diagnosed?

Prompt diagnosis is essential because delays may lead to increased morbidity and mortality. Levels of serum electrolytes and glucose should be determined prior to initiating intravenous fluids in any patient who appears to be dehydrated. Dehydrated patients should routinely be asked if they have any symptoms suggestive of diabetes.

Signs and symptoms suggestive of DKA are rapid or Kussmaul respirations, an acetone odor on the breath, nausea or vomiting, or diffuse abdominal pain (seen in 30% of patients). Other important features of the history are symptoms of infection, ischemic heart disease, other possible precipitating factors, and pattern of insulin use.

The diagnosis should be suspected if the patient presents with marked hyperglycemia (glucose >300 mg/dl) and metabolic acidosis. An elevated anion gap (>13 mEq/L) is usually, but not always, present. The finding of elevated ketones in the blood or urine in the above setting confirms the diagnosis.

If blood or urine ketones are negative and DKA is strongly suspected, treatment with fluids and insulin should still be initiated. During the course of treatment, the blood and urine ketone tests will become positive. This "delay" in positivity for measured ketones is due to a limitation of the laboratory test for ketones, which detects only acetoacetate. The predominant ketone in untreated DKA is betahydroxybutyrate. As DKA is treated, acetoacetate becomes the predominant ketone, causing the test for ketones to turn positive.

5. How is DKA treated?
First Hour

1. Obtain baseline electrolytes, BUN, creatinine, glucose, urinalysis, urine/blood ketone measurements, ECG.

2. Obtain an arterial blood gas if the patient appears ill or tachypneic, or if the serum bicarbonate is very low (< 10 mEq/L).

3. Start a flow sheet for recording fluid intake, output, and laboratory data (see sample flow sheet provided).

4. Fluids: Normal saline, 15 cc/kg/hour (≈1 L/hr for 70 kg).

5. Potassium: Look at the T waves on the ECG. If the T waves are peaked or normal, no potassium is necessary initially. If T waves are low or if U waves are present (denoting hypokalemia), add 40 mEq of KCL to each liter of IV fluids.

6. Insulin: Bolus with 10–20 units IV followed by a continuous infusion of 5–10 units per hour (.1 unit/kg/hr). The insulin drip is mixed by adding 500 units of regular insulin to 1 liter of normal saline (concentration: .5 units/ml). Run the first 50 ml through the IV tubing into the sink prior to hooking up to the patient. Use **only** regular insulin.

7. Look for a precipitating event for DKA (such as infection, myocardial infarction, etc).

DIABETIC KETOACIDOSIS FLOW SHEET

Hour	Blood Pressure	Pulse	Resp Rate	Blood Glucose	Blood Ketones	Na	K	Cl	HCO₃	Anion Gap	Blood Gas pH	Insulin	IV Fluid Type	Amount	KCL (mEq)	Urine Output	Neuro Exam

Second Hour

1. Assess the patient's breathing, vital signs, alertness, level of hydration, urine output.
2. Obtain repeat electrolytes, glucose, urine/blood ketones.
3. Fluids: Continue normal saline at approximately 1 L/hr.
4. Potassium: adjust KCL supplement in fluids to maintain the serum potassium at 4–5 mEq/L. Anticipate a need for 40 mEq replacement per hour as therapy continues.
5. Insulin: Continue the insulin infusion. If the serum glucose is less than 250 mg/dl, change fluids to 5–10% dextrose with saline. The insulin infusion rate may be doubled if the serum glucose does not decline. The optimal rate of glucose decline is 100 mg/dl/hr. The serum glucose level should not be allowed to fall to less than 250 mg/dl during the first 4–5 hours of treatment.

Third and Subsequent Hours

1. Assess the patient as above.
2. Repeat lab tests as above.
3. Fluids: Adjust infusion rate based on the patient's state of hydration. Consider changing to .45% saline if the patient is euvolemic and hypernatremic.
4. Potassium: Adjust supplement in fluids as noted above.
5. Insulin: Continue infusion as long as acidosis is present. Supplement with dextrose as needed. Follow the anion gap. Once the anion gap corrects to normal, the pH is ≥ 7.3, or the serum bicarbonate is ≥ 18 mEq/L, the patient can be given a **subcutaneous** dose of regular insulin to cover a meal. The insulin infusion can be discontinued **30 minutes** after the insulin dose. If the patient is unable to eat, give 5 units of regular insulin, continue the dextrose solution, and give supplemental regular insulin every 4 hours based on the blood glucose level (e.g., 5–15 units every 4 hours).

Other Interventions

1. Consider replacing phosphate as potassium phosphate, 10–20 mEq/hr in the IV fluids if the initial serum phosphorus is less than 1.0 mg/dl.
2. Sodium bicarbonate replacement is not recommended unless other causes of severe acidosis are present (such as sepsis or lactic acidosis) or the arterial pH is very low (pH < 6.9). If used, dilute in IV fluids and give over 1 hour.
3. New-onset diabetes and young age are risk factors for cerebral edema. If the patient suddenly develops a headache or becomes confused during therapy, give mannitol, 1 gm/kg **immediately.**

6. What is the prognosis for persons with DKA?

In the young person with no intercurrent illnesses and when DKA is adequately managed, the prognosis is excellent. However, when the acidosis is severe, when the patient is elderly, or when the intercurrent illness is significant (such as sepsis or myocardial infarction), there is significant mortality. The presence of coma or hypothermia is a particularly poor prognostic sign. Careful monitoring of fluids and electrolytes and treatment of intercurrent illnesses are crucial for optimizing outcome.

7. What is nonketotic hyperosmolar coma?

In 1957 Sument and Schwarts described a syndrome of marked diabetic stupor with hyperglycemia and hyperosmolarity in the absence of ketosis. Since their description, the syndrome has been given a number of names, including nonketotic hyperosmolar coma, diabetic hyperosmolar state, and hyperosmolar nonacidotic diabetes. All these terms refer to the same entity:

- marked hyperglycemia (serum glucose ≥ 600 mg/dl)
- hyperosmolarity (serum > 320 mOsm/L)
- arterial pH ≥ 7.3

The syndrome occurs primarily in elderly patients with or without a history of type II diabetes and is always associated with severe dehydration. Polyuria and polydipsia often occur days to weeks prior to presentation of the syndrome. Elderly persons are predisposed to the syndrome because they have a higher prevalence of impaired thirst perception. Another compounding problem, impaired renal function (commonly seen in the elderly), prevents clearance of excess glucose in the urine. Both factors contribute to dehydration and marked hyperglycemia. The absence of metabolic acidosis is due to the presence of circulating insulin and/or lower levels of counterregulatory hormones. These two factors prevent lipolysis and ketone production. Hyperglycemia, once triggered, leads to glycosuria, osmotic diuresis, hyperosmolarity, cellular dehydration, hypovolemia, shock, coma, and, if untreated, death.

8. What are the signs, symptoms, and laboratory findings of hyperosmolar coma?

Altered mental status is the most common reason patients are brought to the hospital. An effective osmolarity of > 340 mOsm/L is required for coma to be attributed to the syndrome. To calculate the effective osmolarity, the following equation is used:

$$Effective \ osmolarity = 2(Na + K) + glucose/18$$

The serum Na and K are in mEq/L. The serum glucose is in mg/dl. "Effective osmolarity" refers to the true osmolarity seen by the cell. Because urea is freely permeable through membranes, it does not contribute to this condition and is not used in the equation. If the patient's mental status is out of proportion to the effective osmolarity, another etiology for impaired mental state should be sought. For other causes of altered mental state, keep in mind the mnemonic **AEIOU TIPSS**:

A	=	Alcohol	**T**	=	Trauma
E	=	Encephalopathy	**I**	=	Insulin
I	=	Infection	**P**	=	Psychosis
O	=	Overdose	**S**	=	Syncope
U	=	Uremia	**S**	=	Seizures

Other neurologic signs that may be present include bilateral or unilateral hypo- or hyperreflexia, seizures, hemiparesis, aphasia, positive Babinski sign, hemianopsia, nystagmus, visual hallucinations, acute quadriplegia, and dysphagia. Fever is *not* part of the syndrome and, if present, should suggest an infectious component to the illness. Other physical features are those of profound dehydration. The physical exam and other tests should be performed to search for possible precipitating factors, such as infection, myocardial infarction, cerebrovascular events, pancreatitis, gastrointestinal hemorrhage, or exogenous medications.

The hallmark laboratory finding is marked hyperglycemia (often > 1000 mg/dl). The serum sodium is often factitiously low due to hyperglycemia. To correct for this, the following formula is used:

$$Corrected \ Na = serum \ Na + 1.6 \ \frac{(serum \ glucose - 100)}{100}$$

Other laboratory abnormalities include an elevated BUN, creatinine, hypertriglyceridemia, and leukocytosis.

9. What is the treatment of hyperosmolar coma?

After the diagnosis is made, attention should be directed to replacing the patient's fluid deficit. The fluid deficit is usually severe, ranging from 9–12 L. The most critical issue in fluid replacement is having an accurate means of monitoring the patient's level of hydration and response to therapy. In the presence of renal insufficiency or cardiac disease, monitoring may require central venous line access. In the patient with an altered mental state, an indwelling urinary catheter is also usually required. Although there is controversy about whether to use isotonic or hypotonic fluids, the present authors recommend using isotonic (.9%) saline at a rate of approximately 1–2 L over the first hour until the blood pressure normalizes. After the first hour, the fluids may be changed based on the measured serum sodium level. If the serum sodium is between 145 and 165 mEq/L, a change to half normal saline should be considered to replace the free water deficit. If the serum sodium is lower or higher than 145–165 mEq/L, then isotonic saline should be continued. Replacement of one half of the calculated fluid deficit over the initial 5–12 hours is recommended, with the balance of the deficit replaced over the subsequent 12 hours. The use of a continuous intravenous insulin infusion, as described for DKA, has been found to be useful for reducing the glucose levels at a predictable rate. Care must be taken not to induce hypoglycemia. The replacement of other electrolytes, including potassium, is identical to the protocol for DKA.

10. What are the potential complications of hyperosmolar coma?

Estimates of mortality vary from 20% to 80%. This high mortality rate has been attributed to the high prevalence of underlying disease or to delay in diagnosis or treatment. Patients with initially normal lung exams and normal chest radiographs have been reported to develop adult respiratory distress syndrome or distinct lung infiltrates during fluid resuscitation. The cause for these findings is unknown, but may be an underlying infection that was not initially apparent in the severely dehydrated state. For this reason repeat physical exam, and, when indicated, chest radiographs should be considered as therapy progresses. Other reported complications are coagulopathy, pancreatitis, and venous or arterial thrombosis.

11. What are the causes of hypoglycemia in diabetes mellitus?

For diabetic patients on sulfonylureas or insulin, hypoglycemia is an "occupational hazard" of the therapy. Particularly in type I diabetes, it is impossible to mimic the peaks and troughs of a normal insulin secretory pattern with intermittent subcutaneous insulin injections. Even a perfectly designed insulin regimen can lead to hypoglycemia when the patient even slightly decreases food intake, delays a meal, or exercises slightly more than usual. Menstruating women can experience hypoglycemia at the time of menses due to a rapid fall in estrogen and progesterone. Elderly patients given a sulfonylurea for the first time may respond with severe hypoglycemia. In addition to "misadventures" in therapy, patients with diabetes may develop hypoglycemia as a result of a number of other contributing disorders, which are summarized below.

Causes of Postabsorptive (Fasting) Hypoglycemia

---

1. Drugs: Especially insulin, sulfonylureas or alcohol
2. Critical organ failure: Renal, hepatic or cardiac failure; sepsis; inanition
3. Hormonal deficiencies: Cortisol, growth hormone, or both; glucagon + epinephrine
4. Non-β-cell tumor
5. Endogenous hyperinsulinism: β-cell tumor (insulinoma); functional β-cell hypersecretion; autoimmune hypoglycemia; ? ectopic insulin secretion
6. Hypoglycemias of infancy and childhood

From Cryer PE, Gerich JE: Hypoglycemia in insulin dependent diabetes mellitus: Insulin excess and defective glucose counterregulation. In Rifkin H, Porte D; (eds): Ellenberg and Rifkin's Diabetes Mellitus: Theory and Practice, 4th ed. New York, Elsevier, 1990, pp. 526–546, with permission.

12. Are some diabetic patients more susceptible to hypoglycemia than others?

Yes. It has been established that some type I diabetic patients have a defect in glucose counterregulation. When the blood glucose is lowered experimentally, counterregulatory hormones (glucagon and epinephrine, among others) normally are released. These hormones stimulate glycogenolysis and gluconeogenesis by the liver, resulting in a reversal of hypoglycemia. In some patients with type I diabetes, this hormone release is blunted, leading to severe hypoglycemia or delayed recovery from hypoglycemia. This defective counterregulation is often associated with "hypoglycemic unawareness." This term describes the situation in which the patient reports having none of the typical neurogenic warning symptoms of hypoglycemia (see table below). In contrast, the predominant signs and symptoms are due to decreased delivery of glucose to the brain—so-called neuroglycopenic symptoms. The cognitive impairment associated with neuroglycopenia may prevent the patient from responding appropriately to self-treat the hypoglycemia. The result may be a traumatic automobile accident, seizure, coma, or death.

Clinical Manifestations of Hypoglycemia

NEUROGENIC	NEUROGLYCOPENIC
Diaphoresis	Cognitive impairment
Palpitations	Fatigue
Tremor	Dizziness/faintness
Arousal/anxiety	Visual changes
Pallor	Paresthesias
Hypertension	Hunger
	Inappropriate behavior
	Focal neurologic deficits
	Seizures
	Loss of consciousness
	Death

From Cryer PE, Gerich JE: Hypoglycemia in insulin dependent diabetes mellitus: Insulin excess and defective glucose counterregulation. In Rifkin H, Porte D; (eds): Ellenberg and Rifkin's Diabetes Mellitus: Theory and Practice, 4th ed. New York, Elsevier, 1990, pp. 526–546, with permission.

It was previously thought that the development of hypoglycemic unawareness or defective counterregulation was an unpreventable manifestation of autonomic neuropathy from the diabetes. However, recent studies suggest that this disorder may be the body's maladaptation to previous episodes of hypoglycemia. A single episode of hypoglycemia has been shown to reduce autonomic and symptomatic responses to hypoglycemia the following day in normal subjects and patients with type I diabetes. In contrast, meticulous prevention of hypoglycemia has been shown to reverse the defective counterregulation and reestablish the neurogenic symptoms after 3 months. So initial studies suggest that meticulous attention to **prevent** hypoglycemia in patients without established autonomic neuropathy may be very beneficial in reversing hypoglycemic unawareness.

13. How is hypoglycemia treated?
Once detected, hypoglycemia is easily self-treated by the patient. For mild hypoglycemia (blood glucose 50–60 mg/dl), 15 gm of simple carbohydrate such as 4 oz of unsweetened fruit juice or nondietetic soft drink is sufficient. For more profound symptoms of hypoglycemia, 15–20 gm of simple carbohydrate should be ingested quickly and followed by 15–20 gm of a complex carbohydrate, such as crackers or bread. Patients who are unconscious should never be given liquids. In this situation, more viscous sources of sugar (honey, glucose gels, cake icing in a tube) can be carefully placed inside the cheek or under the tongue. Alternatively, 1 mg of glucagon may be injected intramuscularly. Glucagon indirectly causes the blood glucose level to increase via its effect on the liver. In the hospital setting, IV dextrose (D-50) is probably more accessible than glucagon and results in a prompt return of consciousness.

Instruction on the use of glucose gels and glucagon should be an essential part of training for persons living with insulin-treated diabetic patients. Patients and family members should be instructed not to overtreat hypoglycemia, particularly if it is mild. Overtreatment leads to subsequent hyperglycemia. Patients should also be instructed to test their blood glucose level when symptoms occur to confirm hypoglycemia whenever feasible. If testing is not possible, it is best to treat first. Patients on medication should be instructed to test their blood glucose level prior to driving a vehicle. If the glucose level is lower than a pre-set level (e.g., less than 125 mg/dl), the patient should be instructed to ingest a small source of carbohydrate prior to driving.

14. Is hypoglycemia a risk of intensive diabetes management?
Yes. Patients in the intensive therapy arm of the Diabetes Control and Complications Trial experienced a three-fold increased incidence of severe hypoglycemic episodes compared with the standard therapy group. This potential risk of hypoglycemia must be weighed against the proven benefit of intensive therapy in reducing the risk of microvascular complications. The risk for hypoglycemia can be reduced by frequent blood glucose monitoring, self-adjustment of insulin

dosing, and self-adjustment of food and exercise. This requires intensive training in diabetes self-management. The risk for hypoglycemia associated with intensive diabetes therapy may outweigh the potential benefit in patients with established autonomic neuropathy, the elderly, or in patients unable to perform frequent blood glucose monitoring.

BIBLIOGRAPHY

1. Amiel SA, Tamborlane WV, Simonson DC, Sherwin RS: Defective glucose counterregulation after strict glycemic control of insulin-dependent diabetes mellitus. N Engl J Med 316:1376–1383, 1987.
2. Cryer PE: Hypoglycemia begets hypoglycemia in IDDM. Diabetes 42:1691–93, 1993
3. Cryer PE: Hypoglycemia unawareness in IDDM. Diabetes Care 16 (Suppl 3):40–47, 1993.
4. Cryer PE, Gerich JE: Hypoglycemia in insulin dependent diabetes mellitus: Insulin excess and defective glucose counterregulation. In Rifkin H, Porte D (eds): Ellenberg and Rifkin's Diabetes Mellitus: Theory and Practice, 4th ed. New York, Elsevier, 1990, pp 526–546.
5. Fanelli CG, Epifano L, Rambotti AM, et al: Meticulous prevention of hypoglycemia normalizes the glycemic thresholds and magnitude of most of neuroendocrine responses to, symptoms of, and cognitive function during hypoglycemia in intensively treated patients with short-term IDDM. Diabetes 42:1683–1689, 1993
6. Kitabchi AE, Murphy MB: Diabetic ketoacidosis and hyperosmolar hyperglycemic nonketotic coma. Med Clin North Am 72:1545–63, 1988.
7. Kriesberg RA: Diabetic ketoacidosis. In Rifkin H, Porte D (eds): Ellenberg and Rifkin's Diabetes Mellitus: Theory and Practice, 4th ed. New York, Elsevier, 1990, pp 591–603.
8. Pope DW, Dansky D: Hyperosmolar hyperglycemic nonketotic coma. Emerg Med Clin North Am 7:849–57, 1989.
9. Siperstein MD: Diabetic ketoacidosis and hyperosmolar coma. Endocrinol Metab Clin North Am 21:415–431, 1992.
10. Stagnaro-Green A: Diabetic ketoacidosis: In search of zero mortality. Mt Sinai J Med 57:3–8, 1990.

3. CHRONIC COMPLICATIONS OF DIABETES MELLITUS

Stephen Clement, M.D.

1. What are the common long-term complications of diabetes mellitus?

Although patients with diabetes are susceptible to an extensive array of medical complications, most of these problems can be attributed to particular susceptibility to damage to the eye (retinopathy), the kidney (nephropathy), the peripheral nerves (neuropathy), and the blood vessels (atherosclerosis). The first three categories of complications are relatively specific for diabetes and are characterized by pathologic endothelial changes, such as basement membrane thickening and increased vascular permeability. For this reason retinopathy, nephropathy, and neuropathy have been categorized as **microvascular complications** of diabetes. The increased susceptibility to atherosclerosis and its ensuing complications are categorized as **macrovascular complications.**

2. What mechanism(s) underlie the development of long-term diabetic complications?

The pathophysiology of diabetic complications is far from clear. Chronically elevated glucose levels appear to be a necessary component for the development of complications. The results of the Diabetes Control and Complications Trial (DCCT) (see chapter 1), as well as extensive animal data, have proved that fact. However, the mechanism(s) of how increased glucose levels predispose to such varied pathologic findings is only recently being unraveled. Cerami, Vlassara, Brownlee, and others have demonstrated that glucose nonenzymatically attaches to proteins. The initial reaction forms an intermediate compound called an Amadori product (see figure).

GLUCOSE   PROTEIN   SCHIFF BASE   AMADORI PRODUCT   GLUCOSE-DERIVED CROSS-LINK (FFI)

The chemical structure is known for glucose-protein Schiff bases and Amadori products. Workers have yet to learn the structure of most AGE's and AGE-derived cross-links, but one link has been identified: 2-furanyl-4(5)-(2-furanyl)-1*H*-imidazole, or FFI. (From Cerami A, Vlassara H, Brownlee M: Glucose and Aging. Sci Am 256:90–96, 1987, with permission.)

The Amadori product remains in equilibrium with the native protein and glucose. After weeks to years, the Amadori product undergoes a slow and irreversible conversion and cross-linkage to form complex compounds known as advanced glycosylation end-products (AGEs). These products have been found in the connective tissue of blood vessels, the matrix of the renal glomerulus, and the phospholipid component of low-density lipoproteins (LDLs), and as a component of thickened basement membranes. These structural alterations are associated with altered function such as increased vascular permeability, loss of vascular elasticity, altered enzyme function, and reduced clearance of lipoprotein particles. AGEs in the circulation appear to be efficiently cleared by the normal kidney. In diabetic nephropathy, however, the level of circulating AGEs is dramatically elevated. Because these particles may be atherogenic, the buildup of AGEs in the circulation may be a primary contributor to the accelerated atherosclerosis and death seen with diabetic nephropathy. A postulated mechanism for diabetic neuropathy is the accumulation of sorbitol and depletion of myoinositol in the supporting Schwann cells of the nerves. These abnormalities are associated with altered nerve function, demyelinization, and axonal damage. Similar alterations have been described in the capillaries of the retina.

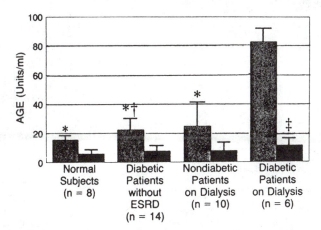

Mean serum levels of AGEs. (From Makita Z, Radoff S, Rayfield EJ, et al: Advanced glycosylation end products in patients with diabetic nephropathy. N Engl J Med 325:836–842, 1991, with permission.)

3. What is the cost burden for treating diabetic complications?

The cost burden for the treatment of diabetic complications is significant. A recent analysis by Rubin et al. estimated that approximately one in seven U.S. health care dollars is spent on a person with diabetes. Age-adjusted direct health care costs for diabetic patients is 2.47-fold higher than the costs for nondiabetic patients. The majority of this increased cost is currently for the treatment of diabetic complications, namely for surgery, diagnostic and therapeutic procedures, and inpatient care.

4. What is the most common type of diabetic neuropathy?

The clinical manifestations of diabetic neuropathy are extremely diverse. The most common entity, distal symmetric polyneuropathy, is usually discovered on routine physical exam by the finding of loss of vibration sense in the toes and loss of ankle reflexes. Light touch and pinprick sensation are subsequently lost. Common associated symptoms are numbness and paresthesias of the feet, especially at night. The paresthesias may evolve to severe knifelike or burning pain, which can be quite disabling. Sensory loss or pain in the hands may also occur from axonal degeneration, but more commonly is a manifestation of entrapment neuropathy, such as carpal tunnel syndrome. Entrapment neuropathies are common in patients with diabetes and may result from increased susceptibility of these nerves to external pressure. Loss of nerve fibers for proprioception can result in an abnormal gait, leading to "pressure spots" on the foot that are signaled by the presence of a thick callus. If untreated, the callus may ulcerate and become infected. Neuropathy, vascular disease, and predisposition to infection are the primary pathogenic components for the increased incidence of foot injury and amputation in patients with diabetes.

5. What other peripheral neuropathies are common in diabetics?

A number of other distinct neuropathic syndromes are associated with diabetes. Mononeuropathies may affect the third, fourth, sixth, and seventh cranial nerves. Most mononeuropathies are of

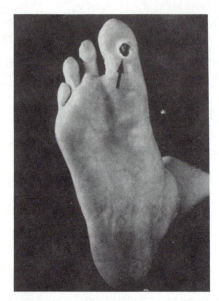 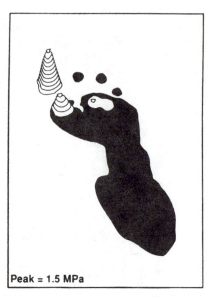

Peak = 1.5 MPa

Left, Photograph from a patient with loss of protective sensation and a neuropathic ulcer under the great toe. *Right,* Computer-generated diagram depicting the peak plantar pressures during the late support phase of gait for the same patient when stepping on a pressure-sensitive plate. Each contour interval depicts an increase above basal pressure. (From Sims DS, Cavanagh PR, Ulbrecht JS: Risk factors in the diabetic foot: Recognition and management. Phys Ther 68:1887, 1988, with permission.)

sudden onset and resolve spontaneously over weeks to months. Third nerve palsy may be preceded by a prickling dysesthesia on the upper lid or retro-orbital pain. Third nerve palsy is usually complete, with lateral deviation of the affected eye and ptosis. Pupillary function is usually spared, which may be the only distinguishing feature between diabetic third nerve palsy and a leaking cerebral aneurysm. The pathogenesis of diabetic mononeuropathies is unknown, but the sudden nature of the complication suggests infarction of the nerve fibers. Neuropathy of the T4-12 nerves, often referred to as intercostal radiculopathy or truncal neuropathy, may be manifested as pain in the chest or abdomen. The pain may follow a specific dermatome or may cover several dermatomes and be confused with pain from a gastrointestinal or cardiac source. Characteristics of pain suggestive of neuropathy include constant, unrelenting nature, worsening at night, and a normal abdominal and chest exam. The diagnosis can be confirmed by nerve conduction studies.

6. What other neuropathies are associated with diabetes?

Diabetes is associated with an autonomic neuropathy that is manifested by the impairment of both sympathetic and parasympathetic nerves. Classic signs are resting tachycardia and postural hypotension. A lack of R-R variation on the electrocardiogram with deep breathing, Valsalva maneuver, or squatting is used to confirm the diagnosis. A common symptom of cardiovascular autonomic neuropathy is postural dizziness. Gastrointestinal symptoms from autonomic neuropathy are secondary to a lack of peristalsis in the stomach (gastroparesis) or intestine. Symptoms include early satiety, bloating, nausea, belching, abdominal distention, constipation, or diarrhea. Urinary bladder dysfunction causing incontinence or urinary retention may be seen. Impotence is a common manifestation of autonomic neuropathy in men with diabetes.

7. What systemic manifestations may be associated with diabetic neuropathies?

Diabetic neuropathic cachexia and diabetic amyotrophy are terms that refer to a poorly understood syndrome of painful neuropathy associated with profound weight loss and, often, depression and anorexia. Physical signs invariably include a distal symmetric sensory polyneuropathy and may reveal wasting of the quadriceps muscles. The pathogenesis of the syndrome is unclear, and most patients undergo an extensive work-up to rule out a possible malignancy. With supportive care, the symptoms slowly resolve and most patients begin to regain weight after 6–12 months.

8. What are the characteristics of diabetic retinopathy?

The progression of significant diabetic retinopathy may occur without symptoms. The initial visible lesions are microaneurysms that form on the terminal capillaries of the retina. Increased permeability of the capillaries is manifested by the leaking of proteinaceous fluid, causing hard exudates. Dot and blot hemorrhages occur from the leaking of red blood cells. These findings by themselves do not lead to visual loss and are categorized as nonproliferative retinopathy (see table). Proliferative retinopathy, by contrast, develops when the retinal vessels are further damaged, causing retinal ischemia. The ischemia triggers new, fragile vessels to develop, a process termed neovascularization. These vessels may grow into the vitreous cavity and may bleed into the preretinal area or vitreous, causing significant vision loss. Loss of vision also may result from retinal detachment secondary to the contraction of fibrous tissue, which often accompanies neovascularization.

Clinical Manifestations of Eye Disease

Nonproliferative Diabetic Retinopathy
Nonproliferative Diabetic Retinopathy
- Retinal microaneurysms
- Occasional blot hemorrhages
- Hard exudates
- One or two soft exudates

Preproliferative Diabetic Retinopathy
- Presence of venous beading
- Significant areas of large retinal blot hemorrhages
- Multiple cotton wool spots (nerve fiber infarcts)
- Multiple intraretinal microvascular abnormalities

Proliferative Diabetic Retinopathy
- New vessels on the disc (NVD)
- New vessels elsewhere on the retina (NVE)
- Preretinal or vitreous hemorrhage
- Fibrous tissue proliferation.

High-risk Proliferative Diabetic Retinopathy
- NVD with or without preretinal or vitreous hemorrhage
- NVE with preretinal or vitreous hemorrhage

Diabetic Macular Edema
- Any thickening of retina <2 disc diameters from center of macula
- Any hard exudate <2 disc diameters from center of macula with associated thickening of the retina
- Any nonperfused retina inside the temporal vessel arcades
- Any combination of the above

From Centers for Disease Control: The prevention and treatment of complications of diabetes mellitus. Department of Health and Human Services, Division of Diabetes Translation, Atlanta, GA, 1991, with permission.

Diabetic macular edema occurs when fluid from abnormal vessels leaks into the macula. It is detected with indirect fundoscopy by the finding of a thickened retina near the macula and is commonly associated with the presence of hard exudates. Over a lifetime, up to 70% of patients with type I diabetes may develop proliferative retinopathy. In type II diabetes, 2% of patients may have significant nonproliferative and even proliferative retinopathy or macular edema at the time of diagnosis of diabetes. This may be due to the long asymptomatic (and undiagnosed) period of hyperglycemia that often occurs in subjects with type II diabetes. Risk factors for the development of retinopathy are duration of diabetes, level of glycemic control, and possibly hypertension. Diabetic nephropathy is strongly associated with proliferative retinopathy in type I and insulin-treated type II diabetes. Other ophthalmologic complications of diabetes are cataracts and open-angle glaucoma.

9. What are the characteristics of diabetic nephropathy?
Diabetic nephropathy is currently the leading cause of end-stage renal disease in the U.S. The onset and progression of disease follow a relatively predictable pattern. Stage 1 is characterized by renal hypertrophy and an increase in glomerular filtration rate (GFR). Patients with a sustained GFR 125 cc/min are at particularly high risk for progression of disease. Stage 2 nephropathy is defined by demonstration of histologic changes in the glomerulus, which are distinctive for diabetes. Stage 3 is marked by mildly elevated urinary albumin excretion (microalbuminuria) on a 24-hour or timed urine collection. Normal urinary albumin is less than 30 mg/day. Microalbuminuria is defined as the excretion of 30-300 mg /day. Patients with microalbuminuria are at markedly increased risk for progression to clinical nephropathy. Hypertension is commonly present at this stage, particularly in patients with type II diabetes. Stage 4 is defined by Dipstix-positive proteinuria, as measured by routine urinalysis. The urinary albumin excretion in this stage is > 300 mg/day or total protein > 500 mg/day. Hypertension is invariably present. During this stage proteinuria increases and GFR declines slowly but steadily. Stage 5 nephropathy is end-stage renal disease.

10. What is the risk that a diabetic person will develop nephropathy?
Patients with type I diabetes are at highest risk for nephropathy, which affects approximately 30%. The risk of nephropathy is approximately 10 times less for type II patients, but because of the overwhelming prevalence of type II diabetes, this group currently outnumbers type I patients with end-stage renal disease. In addition to glycemic control, genetics appears to play a key role in determining the risk for diabetic nephropathy. Genes that code for essential hypertension are suspected to increase risk. Known risk factors for diabetic nephropathy with the accompanying risk ratios (RR) are:

1. A family history of hypertension (RR = 3.7)
2. Sibling with diabetic nephropathy (RR > 4.0)
3. Black race (RR = 2.6 *vs* whites)
4. History of smoking (RR = 2.0)
5. History of poor glycemic control (RR = 1.3–2.0)

11. What is the most common cause of death in persons with diabetic nephropathy?
Diabetic nephropathy places the patient at a markedly increased risk for cardiovascular disease. For example, the cardiovascular and overall mortality for type II diabetic Pima Indians with proteinuria is 3.5 times greater than for the same group without proteinuria. Although the cause for this association is not clear, the nephropathy augments any genetic tendency for hypertension and lipid abnormalities. As stated earlier, nephropathy prevents clearance of AGEs, which may be directly atherogenic. Other mechanisms are clearly involved but require further research.

12. What are the characteristics of macrovascular disease in diabetes?
Patients with diabetes are at twofold to fourfold increased risk for both cardiovascular disease (CVD) and peripheral vascular disease (PVD) compared with the nondiabetic population. Women with diabetes have as high a risk for CVD as men. The commonly identified risk factors for CVD—smoking, hypercholesterolemia, and hypertension—adversely affect CVD risk in diabetic persons (see figure).

The increased risk for CVD from diabetes is due to risk factors that may be specific for diabetes. For example, the blood in diabetic patients has been found to have increased platelet aggregation, decreased red cell deformability, and reduced fibrinolytic activity. The glycation of lipoproteins may lead to decreased clearance by the liver and increased atherosclerosis. The blood vessels themselves have distinct abnormalities. Long-standing diabetes predisposes the arteries to calcification. In the lower extremity, diabetes is associated with atherosclerotic disease below the

*Progression of Renal Disease in Insulin-dependent Diabetes**

STAGE	ONSET	FUNCTIONAL ABNORMALITIES	STRUCTURAL ABNORMALITIES	RISK FACTORS FOR PROGRESSION TO NEXT STAGE	% PROGRESSING TO NEXT STAGE
1 Early hypertrophy and hyperfunction	Present at time of diagnosis	↑ GFR ↑ Glomerular capillary pressure	↑ Kidney size ↑ Glomerular volume ↑ Capillary filtration surface area	Hyperglycemia	100
2 Renal lesions, no clinical signs	By 2–3 y after diagnosis	↑ GFR ↑ Glomerular capillary pressure	↑ Thickness of glomerular and tubular capillary basement membrane ↑ Mesangial volume Glomerulosclerosis	Hyperglycemia Glomerular capillary pressure Genetic factors (eg, family history of hypertension) ? Systemic hypertension ? High-protein diet	35–40
3 Incipient nephropathy	7–15 y after diagnosis	↑ UAE, 0.03–0.3 g/d GFR normal to slightly ↑, but beginning to decline	Further glomerulosclerosis	Systemic hypertension ? Hyperglycemia ? High-protein diet	80–100
4 Clinical diabetic nephropathy	10–30 y after diagnosis	UAE, >0.3 g/d GFR normal to slightly ↓, declines steadily	Widespread glomerulosclerosis	Systemic hypertension ? High-protein diet	75–100
5 End-stage renal disease	20–40 y after diagnosis	GFR, <10 mL/min Serum creatinine, ≥884 µmol/L			

*From Selby JV, FitzSimmons SC, Newman JM, et al: The natural history and epidemiology of diabetic nephropathy: Implications for prevention and control. JAMA 263:1954–1959, 1990, with permission.
†GFR indicates glomerular filtration rate; and UAE, urinary albumin excretion rate.

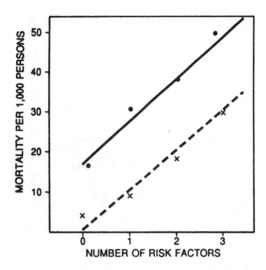

Effects of three major risk factors (hypercholesterolemia, smoking, and diastolic hypertension) on age-standardized cardiovascular disease mortality in 5245 diabetic subjects (solid line) and 350,977 nondiabetic subjects (broken line) between ages 35 and 57 years and free of myocardial infarction at baseline. Follow-up was in 6 years. Abscissa, number of risk factors present. (From Diabetes Care 16(Suppl 2):73, 1993, with permission.)

knee, but often sparing the foot. This unusual anatomy is often used by the vascular surgeon. Revascularization of the foot using distally placed in-situ saphenous bypass grafts often results in healing of limb-threatening foot infections or gangrene.

13. What are the clinical manifestations of ischemic heart disease in diabetic patients?

The symptoms for ischemic heart disease in diabetic patients may be more subtle than in nondiabetic patients. Diabetic patients have been shown to have an increased incidence of "silent" ischemia. Often the patient may experience only some of the autonomic symptoms of ischemia—nausea or sweating—without pain. Diabetic patients have a higher incidence of congestive heart failure and mortality after myocardial infarction than does the nondiabetic population.

14. Describe the treatment for diabetic retinopathy.

Early detection is essential for successful treatment of diabetic complications. For retinopathy, this requires annual examination (including dilation of the fundus) by a trained specialist, usually an ophthalmologist. If pre-proliferative or proliferative retinopathy or significant macular edema is detected, laser therapy may be indicated and can prevent significant vision loss. Vitrectomy or retinal surgery may be required for restoration of vision loss due to vitreous hemorrhage or retinal detachment.

15. How is diabetic nephropathy managed?

The progression of diabetic nephropathy can be slowed by aggressive treatment of hypertension. The use of captopril was recently shown to be particularly beneficial in reducing progression to renal failure in 50% in type I diabetic patients with stage 4 nephropathy. Smaller studies have shown a reduction of proteinuria with enalapril. The question of whether early use of an angiotensin-converting enzyme inhibitor, prior to the onset of hypertension (such as in stage 2 or 3), can prevent or slow the progression of renal disease is not definitively answered. Some, but not all, studies have shown reduced progression of renal disease in patients treated with a low-protein diet (<.6 gm/kg/day).

16. What treatments are effective for diabetic neuropathy?

There is no known treatment for sensory loss from diabetic neuropathy. Educational programs addressing proper foot care and prevention of foot injury have been shown to reduce the incidence of serious foot lesions. Routine foot examination and early referral to a podiatrist or vascular surgeon for patients with foot lesions are considered essential to prevent limb loss. Various medications have been tried with mixed success for the treatment of painful neuropathy. These medications include nonsteroidal anti-inflammatory drugs, tricyclic antidepressants, anticonvulsant medications and mexiletine (for review, see reference 15). A new topical agent, capsaicin, has been shown to provide temporary relief from painful neuropathy in a subset of patients. Postural hypotension from autonomic neuropathy is improved by the use of supportive stockings to prevent venous pooling in the legs. Fludrocortisone is effective but must be used cautiously to prevent worsening of hypertension or edema. Other drugs that have demonstrated benefit include clonidine, octreotide, and midodrine. The symptoms from diabetic gastroparesis can be improved by reducing fiber and fat in the diet, by decreasing meal size, and by increasing exercise. Metoclopramide, and more recently, cisapride, have been shown to increase gastrointestinal motility and reduce symptoms. Cisapride may be preferred because it is not associated with the extrapyramidal system side effects that may accompany metoclopramide.

17. How can macrovascular disease be prevented in the diabetic population?

Treatment of the macrovascular complications in diabetic patients is similar to that for the nondiabetic population. Aggressive reduction of cardiovascular risk factors (hypertension, dyslipidemia, smoking, inactivity) should be started at the initial clinic visit. Antihypertensive medications that have unfavorable effects on lipids or insulin sensitivity should be avoided.

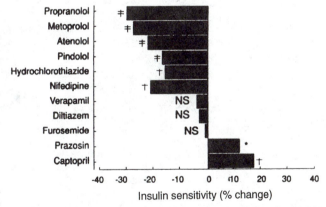

Effect of various antihypertensive drugs on insulin sensitivity. (From Berne C, Pollare T, Lithell H: Effects of antihypertensive treatment on insulin sensitivity with special reference to ACE inhibitors. Diabetes Care 14(Suppl 4): 39, 1991, with permission.)

For hyperlipidemia, improving glycemia often causes a dramatic reduction in the triglyceride level and a modest reduction in LDL cholesterol. If goals for lipids are not achieved through glycemic control, diet, and exercise, then anti-lipid drug therapy should be considered.

In general, drug therapy for dyslipidemia works well in diabetic patients. Niacin, although effective, may worsen glycemic control and must be used with caution. Estrogen replacement therapy for postmenopausal women should be strongly considered for its potential protective effect against cardiovascular disease. For the type II diabetic patients, strategies for reducing insulin resistance through life-style changes (e.g., reduced fat/calorie intake, increased exercise) should be emphasized. The physician should maintain a low threshold for working up a patient for possible ischemic heart disease, since it often is asymptomatic.

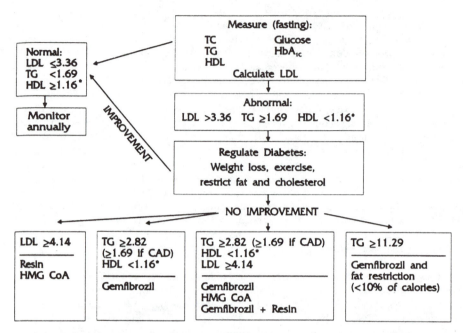

*Higher levels recommended for women.
All measurements expressed in mmol/L.

Approaches to the diabetic patient with dyslipidemia. (From Garber AJ, Vinik AI, Crespin SR: Detection and management of lipid disorders in diabetic patients: A commentary for clinicians. Diabetes Care 15:1071, 1992, with permission.)

BIBLIOGRAPHY

1. Centers for Disease Control: The prevention and treatment of complications of diabetes mellitus. Department of Health and Human Services, Division of Diabetes Translation, Atlanta, GA, 1991
2. Cerami A, Vlassara H, Brownlee M: Glucose and Aging. Sci Am 256:90–96, 1987.
3. Cowie CC, Port FK, Wolfe RA, et al: Disparities in incidence of diabetic end-stage renal disease according to race and type of diabetes. N Engl J Med 321:1074–1079, 1989.
4. Davis M: Diabetic retinopathy—A clinical overview. Diabetes Care 15:1844–1874, 1992.
5. Garber AJ, Vinik AJ, Crespin SR: Detection and management of lipid disorders in diabetic patients. Diabetes Care 15:1068–1073, 1992.
6. Klein R, Klein BE, Moss SE: Epidemiology of proliferative diabetic retinopathy. Diabetes Care 15:1875–1891, 1992.
7. Klein R, Klein BE, Moss SE: Incidence of gross proteinuria in older-onset diabetes. Diabetes 42:381–389, 1993.
8. Krolewski AS, Canessa M, Warram JH, et al: Predisposition to hypertension and susceptibility to renal disease in insulin-dependent diabetes mellitus. N Engl J Med 318:140–145, 1988.
9. Lewis EJ, Hunsicker LG, Bain RP, et al: The effect of angiotensin-converting enzyme inhibition on diabetic nephropathy. N Engl J Med 329:1456–1462, 1993.
10. Makita Z, Radoff S, Rayfield E, et al: Advanced glycosylation end products in patients with diabetic nephropathy. N Engl J Med 325:836–842, 1991.
11. Nathan DM: Long-term complications of diabetes mellitus. N Engl J Med 328:1676–1685, 1993.
12. Nelson RG, Pettit DJ, Carraher MJ, et al: Effect of proteinuria on mortality in NIDDM. Diabetes 37:1499–1504, 1988.
13. Selby JV, Fitzsimmons SC, Newman JM, et al: The natural history and epidemiology of diabetic nephropathy. JAMA 263:1954–1959, 1990.
14. Sims D, Cavanagh PR, Ulbrecht JS: Risk factors in the diabetic foot. Phys Ther 68:1887–1902, 1988.
15. Vinik AI, Holland MT, Le Beau JM, et al: Diabetic neuropathies. Diabetes Care 15:1926–1975, 1992.
16. Zeller K, Whittaker E, Sullivan L, et al: Effect of restricting dietary protein on the progression of renal failure in patients with insulin-dependent diabetes mellitus. N Engl J Med 324:78–84, 1991.

4. DIABETES IN PREGNANCY

Jane E-B. Reusch, M.D.

1. What are the changes in fuel metabolism during normal pregnancy?

Pregnancy is a complex metabolic state that involves dramatic alterations in the hormonal milieu (increases in cortisol, progesterone, prolactin, estrogen, human chorionic gonadotropin and human placental lactogen) as well as an increasing burden of fuel utilization from the conceptus. Increased insulin sensitivity during the first trimester is believed to be secondary to relaxin. From 20 weeks onward, insulin resistance is noted, primarily in the skeletal muscle. In fact, the sensitivity of adipose tissue to insulin is unchanged. In normal pregnancy, maternal secretion of insulin increases in the late second and full third trimester to compensate for the insulin resistance. Women usually have lower fasting levels of plasma glucose and an exaggerated periprandial glucose excursion. Glucose is not the only fuel altered in normal pregnancy; amino acids are decreased, whereas triglycerides, cholesterol, and free fatty acids are increased.

2. How do fuel changes in pregnancy affect the management of diabetes in the first, second, and third trimesters?

Diabetes optimally should be under tight control before conception. During the first trimester, nausea and increased insulin sensitivity may place the mother at risk for hypoglycemia. Hypoglycemia poses a great risk to the 2–4-week embryo, which depends entirely on glycolysis for energy. Often during the first trimester, glycemic control just above the normal range may be safer than "normal" and may decrease the risk of fetal hypoglycemia. From 20 weeks onward, peripheral insulin resistance increases insulin requirements. Frequent monitoring—once weekly after a meal—allows appropriate adjustment of dose. The maintenance of normal glucose control is the key to prevention of complications such as macrosomia and those listed below. Achievement of tight control in the face of pregnancy-induced insulin resistance often requires insulin with each meal.

3. What is the most important aspect of preconception counseling of individuals with diabetes?

The answer is control. Before the recent publication of the Diabetes Control and Complications Trial, the only long-standing indications for tight metabolic control in diabetes were preconception and pregnancy. The incidence of congenital abnormalities in offspring of diabetic mothers in the early era of insulin use was 33%. In the 1970s, 6.5% of offspring had birth defects. Over the past decade, with the advent of home blood glucose monitoring and more rigid objectives, this percentage has fallen to 1.6–2% of offspring. Epidemiologic and prospective studies have shown that the level of HgbA$_1$C in the 6 months before conception and during the first trimester correlates with outcome. Mothers with normal HgbA$_1$C have an incidence of neonatal abnormalities similar to normal pregnancy. Given these data, preconception counseling is one of the top priorities in diabetes management for girls and women of reproductive age.

4. What are the goals of glucose control for pregnant women with diabetes?

The goals of blood glucose control during pregnancy are rigorous. Optimally premeal glucose should be less than 100 mg/dl, with the 2-hour postbrandial value not exceeding 130 mg/dl. To achieve these goals, patients frequently need to contact the doctor or support personnel multiple times each week and to use 3–4 injections/day or an insulin pump. Home glucose monitoring should be done 4 times/day (before meals and at bed time). Once a week it should be done also after meals. The physician must have a low threshold for bringing the expectant mother into the hospital to optimize education and glycemic control. Failure to achieve optimal control in early pregnancy may have teratogenic effects (especially hypoglycemia) or lead to early fetal loss.

Ultrasound at 7–14 weeks of gestation assesses crown-rump length and assists in the detection of early embryopathy. Later in the pregnancy, poor control predisposes to macrosomia and other complications listed below.

5. What is the risk of diabetic ketoacidosis (DKA) in pregnancy?

Women with insulin-dependent diabetes are at risk for developing DKA during pregnancy. There is a single case report of DKA in a woman with gestational diabetes mellitus. Two recent studies (involving 7 patients in Great Britain and 20 patients in the United States) reported a risk of fetal loss ranging from 22–35%. Fetal loss frequently occurred before presentation at the hospital. Once the patient was hospitalized and treated, the risk of fetal loss declined dramatically. Risk factors for fetal loss included third-trimester; glucose > 800 mg/dl; BUN > 21 mg/dl; osmolality > 300 mmol/L; high insulin requirements; and longer duration until resolution of DKA. Causes of DKA were similar to those among the general diabetic population: infection, initial presentation (6 of 20), and poor compliance. Neither series reported increased mortality of the mothers. Prenatal care attuned to the signs and symptoms of new-onset diabetes and good metabolic control may allow prevention in most cases.

6. What happens to retinopathy during the diabetic pregnancy?

The worsening of retinopathy during pregnancy is reproducible and well documented. This phenomenon is most prevalent in women with high-risk diabetic eye disease and severe preproliferative or proliferative retinopathy. In light of recent data about rapid institution of tight control and progression of retinopathy, it is unclear whether the tight control during pregnancy or the changes of pregnancy per se lead to progression of retinopathy. Given this uncertainty, it is best to intensify glycemic control and to stabilize retinopathy before conception. Women with low-risk eye disease should be followed by an ophthalmologist during pregnancy, but significant vision-threatening progression of retinopathy is rare.

7. What is gestational diabetes? How is it diagnosed?

Gestational diabetes mellitus (GDM) is a glucose-intolerant state first diagnosed in pregnancy and limited to pregnancy. The criteria for diagnosis in the United States are outlined in the table.

Screening and Diagnostic Criteria for Gestational Diabetes Mellitus

Screening
1. By glucose measurement in plasma
2. 50-g oral glucose load administered between the 24th and 28th wk and without regard to the time of day or time of last meal to all pregnant women who have not been identified as having glucose intolerance before the 24th wk
3. Venous plasma glucose measured 1 h later
4. A value of ≥7.8 mM in venous plasma indicates the need for a full diagnostic glucose tolerance test

Diagnosis
1. 100-g oral glucose load administered in the morning after overnight fast for at least 8 h but not more than 14 h and after at least 3 days of unrestricted diet (≥150 g carbohydrate) and physical activity
2. Venous plasma glucose is measured fasting and at 1, 2, and 3 h; subject should remain seated and not smoke throughout the test
3. Two or more of the following venous plasma concentrations must be met or exceeded for positive diagnosis
   Fasting, 5.8 mM
   1 h, 10.6 mM
   2 h, 9.2 mM
   3 h, 8.1 mM

From Kalkhoff RK: Diabetes 40(Suppl 2):198, 1991, with permission.

The incidence of GDM ranges from 2–8% of pregnancies throughout the world. In the United States, most studies suggest that 2–3% of pregnancies are complicated by GDM. Because of the common nature of the problem and the risks to offspring, the screening of pregnant women between 24 and 28 weeks of gestation with 50 gm of oral glucose is routine. Women with a 1-hour venous glucose > 140 mg/dl should proceed to the formal 100-gm, 3-hour, oral glucose tolerance test (OGTT). The O'Sullivan criteria for diagnosis of GDM are used in the United States; that is, if any two values on the 3-hour OGTT are abnormal, therapy is instituted.

8. What are the risks to the mother with GDM?

The immediate risks to the mother with GDM is an increased incidence of cesarean section, hypertension without proteinuria, and preeclampsia. Studies have failed to show any change in the incidence of pyelonephritis, polyhydramnios, birth trauma, or preterm labor in appropriately managed cases of GDM.

The long-term risk to the mother is related to recurrent GDM pregnancies and the increased incidence of developing non–insulin-dependent diabetes mellitus (NIDDM). Counseling with regard to diet, weight loss, exercise, medications, and contraception (especially use of oral contraceptive pills) is often instituted. No long-term study has established that appropriate changes in lifestyle delay or prevent the onset of NIDDM (such studies are currently being planned).

9. What are the risks to the infant of a mother with GDM?

Even with the advent of screening and aggressive management of GDM, the incidence of neonatal complications ranges from 12–28%. The most common complications are macrosomia, hyper-bilirubinemia, and polycythemia. Other complications include hypoglycemia, hypocalcemia, thrombocytopenia, and miscellaneous abnormalities. A new ultrasound technique, called humeral soft-tissue thickness, is a highly sensitive and specific predictor of the large-for-gestational-age infant and may assist with obstetric decision making.

The long-term sequelae of GDM for offspring are much more ambiguous. Reports of increased adolescent obesity and increased NIDDM are compelling. Fewer data are available to support animal models that suggest abnormalities in neurobehavioral development.

10. What causes glucose intolerance in pregnancy?

The main cause of glucose intolerance during pregnancy is hormonally induced peripheral insulin resistance. During the course of pregnancy, circulating levels of prolactin (PRL), estrogen, corticosteroids, human chorionic gonadotropin (HCG), human placental lactogen (HPL), and progestins (PG) increase. Corticosteroids, PRL, and/or PG have been shown to decrease insulin-receptor (IR) binding. Estrogen may actually increase IR binding. HCG and HPL have no effect on IR binding but decrease postreceptor effects of insulin (glucose oxidation and glycogen synthase activity).

In all women (with and without GDM), fasting insulin levels and the insulin secretory response to a meal or an intravenous glucose load is increased in late pregnancy. The resistance to insulin in pregnancy is similar in women with and without GDM. This was demonstrated by assessing insulin effect on a muscle biopsy obtained at the time of cesarean section in women with and without GDM. A diminished beta-cell responsiveness leads to a loss of first-phase insulin secretion and inadequate secretion to maintain normoglycemia.

11. What is the best therapy for women with GDM? Specify the role of insulin and oral agents.

The best therapy for GDM depends entirely on the mother's response and the extent of the glucose intolerance. Oral agents are not used at all in pregnancy. In class A1 GDM, in which fasting blood glucose is < 105 mg/dl, dietary therapy alone is sufficient. If fasting blood glucose is > 130 mg/dl (class B GDM), institution of insulin therapy is necessary. Recent data from the Netherlands suggest that fasting blood glucose between 105 and 130 mg/dl (class A2 GDM) still carries an increased risk of macrosomia. Such patients should be followed aggressively, and insulin should be instituted if diet fails. Most authors have shown that dietary therapy within the recent guidelines of the National Science Foundation for pregnancy or mild calorie restriction is the cornerstone of management. A relatively high (35–45%) carbohydrate content is desirable. Even with strict dietary compliance, glucose monitoring is necessary to confirm adequate control.

12. Is exercise standard therapy for GDM?

No. Exercise is an interesting therapeutic option for anyone with insulin resistance and glucose intolerance. Exercise, even moderate, has been shown to improve insulin sensitivity, lipid profiles, and overall well-being as well as to lower blood glucose and blood pressure. The use of exercise in GDM has recently been evaluated for safety. Upper-extremity exercise in one study and non–weight-bearing exercise in another study were shown to be safe in pregnancy. In each study, exercise decreased or negated the need for insulin; thus it is an attractive option. Exercise is not routine, and each program needs to be individually designed and monitored.

13. How do diabetes and GDM lead to increased fetal size?

Many theories have been generated over the years to explain the macrosomia associated with diabetes in pregnancy. Overall, the theory of excessive flux in maternal fuel to the conceptus holds the most credence and has the most supportive data. The accompanying figure outlines the hypothesis of Freinkel, recently expanded by many authors. Diabetes in pregnancy is associated with increased delivery of glucose and amino acid to the fetus via the maternal circulation. These fuels lead to increased fetal insulinemia and growth. Other maternal substrates (e.g., free fatty acids, triglycerides) add to the excessive supply of fetal substrate to support excessive growth. It is, therefore, the goal of management of pregnancies complicated by diabetes to normalize the above parameters with good metabolic control.

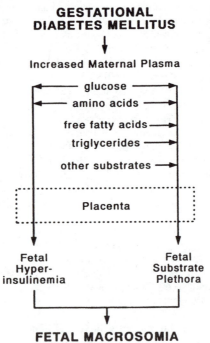

Proposed scheme for development of fetal macrosomia in gestational diabetes mellitus. (From Kalkhoff RK: Impact of maternal fuels and nutritional state on fetal growth. Diabetes 40:18–24, 1991, with permission; adapted from Freinkel.[4])

14. Explain newborn hypoglycemia. Why does it happen and how should these newborns be followed and treated if necessary?

Approximately 20–25% of infants of diabetic mothers (IDM) experience neonatal hypoglycemia during the first 4–6 hours of life (glucose < 40 mg/dl). IDM have hyperplastic or hyperfunctioning pancreatic islets secondary to intrauterine glucose and amino acid excess, and, as such, have a brisk insulin response to glucose. Normal infants have an early glucagon and catecholamine surge, with relatively low insulin secretion that favors endogenous glucose production to maintain normoglycemia. IDM should be monitored hourly until the first full feeding for hypoglycemia. Asymptomatic hypoglycemia can be treated with oral feedings. Symptomatic hypoglycemia can be treated with 300 μg/kg glucagon IV or IM followed by a glucose infusion with a 10% dextrose solution. Use of a 50% dextrose solution could increase insulin secretion and exacerbate the problem. Note that glucose reagent strips are not accurate in the low glucose range and thus all abnormal values need to be confirmed by the laboratory.

BIBLIOGRAPHY

1. Cousins L: Insulin sensitivity in pregnancy. Diabetes 40:39–43, 1991.
2. Coustan DR: Diagnosis of gestational diabetes—what are our objectives? Diabetes 40:14–17, 1991.
3. Freinkel N, Ogata E, Metzger BE: The offspring of the mother with diabetes. In Rifkin H, Porte D (eds): Diabetes Mellitus: Theory and Practice, 4th ed. New York, Elsevier, 1990, pp 651–660.
4. Freinkel N, Phelps RL, Metzger BE: The mother in pregnancies complicated by diabetes. In Rifkin H, Porte D (eds): Diabetes Mellitus: Theory and Practice, 4th ed. New York, Elsevier, 1990, pp 634–650.
5. Hod M, Merlob P, Friedman S, et al: Gestational diabetes mellitus—A survey of perinatal complications in the 1980's. Diabetes 40:74–79, 1991.
6. Kalkhoff RK: Impact of maternal fuels and nutritional state on fetal growth. Diabetes 40:61–65, 1991.
7. King JC: New National Academy of Sciences Guidelines for nutrition during pregnancy. Diabetes 40:151–156, 1991.
8. Kuhl C: Insulin secretion and insulin resistance in pregnancy and GDM—Implications for diagnosis and management. Diabetes 40:18–24, 1991.
9. Langer O, Berkus M, Brustman L, et al: Rationale for insulin management in gestational diabetes mellitus. Diabetes 40:186–190, 1991.
10. Metzger BE and Organizing Committee: Summary and recommendations of the Third International Workshop–Conference on Gestational Diabetes Mellitus. Diabetes 40:197–201, 1991.
11. Montoro MN, Myers VP, Mestman JH, et al. Outcome of pregnancy in diabetic ketoacidosis. Am J Perinatol 10:17–20, 1993.
12. Schwatz R: Neonatal hypoglycemia: Back to basics in diagnosis and treatment. Diabetes 40:71–73, 1991.

5. INFECTIONS IN DIABETIC PERSONS

Robert H. Gates, M.D.

1. Are diabetic persons more likely to have infection?

The short answer is yes. The medical literature is replete with possible associations with particular organisms and specific infectious disease syndromes. Examples of such associations include urinary tract infections and rhinocerebral mucormycosis. Infection is usually not due to elevated serum glucose or the presence of serum ketoacidosis alone. Infections are more likely related to other effects of diabetes, including the effect on target end-organs, as exemplified by decreased white-cell function and a propensity to vaginal candidiasis. Other associations include peripheral neuropathy and foot ulcerations, incomplete cell basement membrane and bacterial myositis, and decreased intestinal motility and salmonella infections as well as atherosclerosis and pulmonary aspiration.

2. Why do diabetic persons have more infections?

The propensity of diabetic pesons to have more infections has been attributed to two broad categories. The first involves abnormal host defenses. Typically this is described as abnormal white-cell function, as shown by diminished ability of polymorphonuclear white cells to perform chemotaxis, a reduced ability to release degranulation products, decreased production of free oxygen radicals, and impaired intracellular killing of organisms such as *Candida* sp. Less well-defined defects in cell mediated immunity also contribute to the propensity for cryptococcal infection. In addition, poor control of diabetes may lead to malnutrition, which further impairs the function of the cell-mediated immune system.

The second category is end-organ dysfunction secondary to diabetes. This is best exemplified by the presence of neuropathy and vasculopathy, which are discussed more fully later. Other organ systems also have been found to have diabetes-related defects. The propensity of diabetics to have staphylococcal and streptococcal infections of the muscles may be due to incomplete cell membrane linings.

3. Which infecting organisms are more common or prevalent in diabetes?

The most likely organisms causing infections in diabetics are usually related to the specific clinical circumstances. For example, in bacteremia associated with soft-tissue infection, staphylococci and streptococci are predominant. In urinary tract infections, *Klebsiella* sp. is often found. Vaginitis is usually associated with *Candida* sp. Myositis is usually due to Group B streptococci and staphylococci. A mixed aerobic and anaerobic infection is often found in necrotizing soft-tissue infections such as cellulitis or fasciitis.

4. Name the organisms and related infections associated with diabetes mellitus.

Infections and Organisms Associated with Diabetes

ORGANISMS	INFECTIONS
Group B streptococci	Pyomyositis, cellulitis
Staphylococci	Arthritis, pyomyositis, sternal wound infection after coronary artery bypass grafting
	Tunnel catheter infection in continuous ambulatory peritoneal dialysis
Mucormycoses	Rhinocerebral mucormycosis
Salmonella enteritidis	Gastroenteritis
Clostridium septicum	Necrotizing cellulitis and necrotizing fasciitis
Mixed gram-negative aerobes and anaerobes	

Table continued on following page.

Infections and Organisms Associated with Diabetes (Continued)

ORGANISMS	INFECTIONS
Klebsiella sp.	Postoperative urinary tract infection
Candida sp.	Vaginitis
Cryptococcus sp.	Meningitis
Facultative gas-producing aerobes and anaerobes	Emphysematous cystitis and pyelonephritis

5. Name the postoperative infections that diabetic persons are most prone to develop.

The most common is urinary tract infection. However, the best studied postoperative infections in diabetic persons are sternal wound infections after coronary artery bypass grafting with internal mammary artery grafts. Data from these reports are conflicting, but it appears that bilateral internal mammary artery grafts are associated with an increase in sternal infections. Review of prosthetic hip replacement revealed a slightly increased risk of urinary tract infections but not an increased risk of infection of the prosthetic device itself. Several reports have documented the increased risk of infection of the tunnel of catheters place for chronic ambulatory peritoneal dialysis.

6. What should diabetic persons be told about the risk of blood-borne pathogens?

Education to prevent the transmission of blood-borne infection is necessary for all persons with diabetes. The risk of transmission of hepatitis B or human immunodeficiency virus (HIV) from a lancet needle, insulin syringe, or finger guard is not well studied but certainly exists. Syringes, platforms, and lancets should be considered medical waste and disposed of properly. Sharps disposal containers should be readily available in the homes of all HIV-infected diabetic patients who require invasive glucose monitoring or insulin therapy. More detailed recommendations are available in the guidelines from the American Association of Dental Examiners.

7. Vascular insufficiency is the most common cause of diabetic foot infection. True or false?

False. Neuropathy is by far the most common underlying reason for foot ulcerations leading to infection. The proposed pathogenesis goes as follows: uneven distribution of pressure on the plantar surface of the foot, perhaps aggravated somewhat by decreased fat within the foot, leads to microtrauma to the tissues, which serves as a portal of entry for bacteria that initially colonize the breaks. Superficial fungal infections likewise may serve as a portal of entry. The patient has no pain response to the initial trauma because of the underlying neuropathy; thus the trauma continues with associated tissue necrosis. Eventually the motion of the structures within the foot promotes deeper bacterial colonization and spread, with secondary infection leading to increased local inflammation, release of inflammatory mediators, and further compromise in the ability to contain the initial infection. These events result in deep soft-tissue and/or bone infection with associated necrosis that ultimately may lead to loss of the lower extremity, with or without associated bacteremia and sepsis.

8. What is the best way to culture a diabetic foot ulcer?

Despite controversy in the medical literature, it is fair to say that the organisms that cause disease in early infection are relatively few in number and often single, with staphylococci predominating. As infection progresses and further tissue necrosis occurs, the likelihood increases dramatically of multiple aerobic organisms and concurrent infection by anaerobic organisms. Swabs of ulcers on diabetic feet are basically worthless. Aspiration by needle through uninvolved tissue has been in vogue from time to time in recent years. The gold standard, of course, is deep biopsy of the involved tissue through uninvolved tissues, with particular emphasis on obtaining bone for culture. A more recent proposal is initial debridement with gauze. Immediately after debridement of the overlying tissue, curettage of the base of the ulcer is performed and the material promptly submitted for culture. Curettage has shown the best correlation with deep biopsy. As a guide to interpretation of the culture, the specimen also should be submitted for Gram stain.

9. What infection in diabetes causes the most morbidity?

In case you have not guessed by now, the answer is foot infection. Infections of the feet and their sequelae are most likely to lead to hospitalization. Approximately 1 of 5 diabetic patients admitted to the hospital has a foot infection. The estimated annual cost for such hospitalizations is greater than 200 million dollars. Approximately one-fourth of the 11 million Americans with diabetes will have foot problems during the course of their disease. Roughly 1 in 15 of such patients will require a limb amputation for ultimate control. The annual rate of amputation is approximately 59.7 per 10,000 diabetics. Indeed, diabetes accounts for approximately one-half of the 120,000 nontraumatic amputations performed in the United States each year. These numbers would impress Carl Sagan.

10. Which tests or techniques are the most useful in defining the extent of disease in diabetic foot infections?

The successful management of diabetic foot infections depends on early detection and prompt attention to infection and occult sources of infection that may need to be drained or debrided, such as necrotic tissue, soft-tissue abscesses, and particularly bony involvement. Attention also should be directed to the exclusion of marovascular disease (present in only a minority of cases), which may be amenable to immediate corrective therapy with various techniques, such as percutaneous angioplasty, atherectomy, laser-guided atherectomy, and bypass surgery.

Defining the extent of disease plays a key role in duration of therapy and in surgical intervention. Plain radiographs may show abnormalities suggesting involvement of bone with infection; these changes, however, are often difficult to distinguish from those secondary to diabetic osteonecrosis. Bone scans are extremely sensitive for detecting the presence of infection; however, they are highly nonspecific in the setting of possible trauma and diabetic bony involvement. The specificity of bone scans is improved by coupling them with either a gallium scan or an [111]indium white-blood-cell scan. However, the spatial resolution of the scans is not good enough to allow precise definition of the involved structures. CT scan has proved to be useful for better resolution of the anatomy and associated soft-tissue infection but not optimal for the delineation of the extent of bony involvement with infection. In the past several years, MRI has emerged as a key tool for defining the extent of disease. The MRI scan is as sensitive as the bone scan for detecting the presence of disease and at least as specific as the combination of bone and gallium or white-blood-cell scanning. MRI has the added advantage of not exposing the patient to the additional radiation required by a CT scan. The literature is full of reports of previously unsuspected bony or soft-tissue involvement, the surgical correction of which led to enhanced resolution of the underlying infection.

11. How can diabetic persons decrease their risk of infection?

The National Diabetes Advisory Board has suggested that more than 50% of lower-extremity amputations can be avoided if careful attention is given to general principles. Patients should maintain good glucose control to maximize the function of the body's immune system. They also must practice good preventive foot care on a daily basis, be particularly wary of foreign bodies in their shoes, and be especially careful when breaking in a new pair of shoes. Diabetics need to pay close attention to health maintenance, with particular emphasis on available vaccinations to prevent pneumococcal and influenza pneumonia. A multidisciplinary approach to prevention and to management of problems when they occur is the key to success.

12. Does the presence of diabetes change the management of infection?

The presence of diabetes should raise the suspicion of comorbid conditions, such as underlying neuropathy, which may mask the signs and symptoms of disease; accelerated atherosclerotic changes, which may lead to vascular problems; and diminished renal function, which may require monitoring and change in antibiotic therapy. The presence of diabetes also should enhance awareness of the possibility of specific disease presentations, as exemplified by rhinocerebral mucormycosis in diabetic ketoacidosis.

13. Does the presence of infection change diabetes?

In addition to the propensity of infections to increase serum glucose levels, there may be persistent and resistant serum ketoacidosis, even in the presence of adequate glucose control. Control of the ketoacidosis usually requires adequate treatment of the underlying infection; in addition to appropriate antibiotics, management may require debridement of involved tissues and/or associated soft-tissue abscesses. Infection that causes ketoacidosis is a leading cause of death in diabetes.

14. How can rational decisions be made regarding antibiotic therapy?

The general principles of selection of antibiotic therapy still hold. The setting always should be considered, even though it may be nonproductive. A history of an animal bite may alert the practitioner to the presence of organisms such as *Pasteurella* sp. A history of water exposure may suggest infection with *Aeromonas* sp. A puncture wound through a tennis shoe may lead to early consideration of anti-*Pseudomonas* therapy. The timing of presentation is also important. Early infection is more likely to have a solitary bacterial cause, whereas late disease with extensive necrosis suggests the presence of multiple organisms. The patient's allergies must be considered, along with route of administration of the drug. There is nothing magical about how the drug is delivered, whether it be intravenously or orally, as long as adequate serum levels are achieved with subsequently adequate tissue levels. Renal function should be assessed, because it may require dose modification or antibiotic change. Specific organisms should be considered; for example, with gram-positive organisms, staphylococcal and streptococcal coverage in the diabetic patient with soft-tissue-associated bacteremia leads to use of an antistaphylococcal agent. Urinary tract infection in the diabetic raises the prospect of multiple gram-negative organisms, particularly *Klebsiella* sp. Anaerobes should be covered in association with tissue necrosis.

In addition, the "zebras" listed in question 4 should be considered. Rhinocerebral mucormycosis should be considered in patients with ketoacidosis who present with an eschar in the nose. The patient with relatively subtle signs of meningitis and a negative routine culture may have infection with cryptococci. Emphysematous cystitis or pyelonephritis may be a clue to the presence of anaerobic organisms, such as *Clostridia* sp. or facultative gas-forming, gram-negative aerobes. Multiple antibiotics are available with adequate coverage if appropriate empirical therapy is based on the clinical setting.

BIBLIOGRAPHY

1. Bessman AN, Sapico FL: Infections in the diabetic patient: The role of immune dysfunction and pathogen virulence factors. J Diabetic Complications 6:258–262, 1992.
2. Brodsky JW, Schneidler C: Diabetic foot infections. Orthop Clin North Am 22:473–489, 1991.
3. Grunfeld C: Diabetic foot ulcers: Etiology, treatment and prevention. Adv Intern Med 37:103–132, 1991.
4. Isselbacher KJ, Braunwald E, Wilson JD, et al (eds): Harrison's Principles of Internal Medicine, 13th ed. New York, McGraw-Hill, 1994.
5. Lipsky BA, Pecoraro RE, Wheat LJ: The diabetic foot: Soft tissue and bone infection. Infect Dis Clin North Am 4:409–429, 1990.
6. Mandell GL, Douglas RG, Bennett JE (eds): Principles and Practice of Infectious Disease, 3rd ed. New York, Churchill Livingstone, 1990.
7. Nelson KE, Vlahov D, Cohn S, et al: Human immunodeficiency virus infection and diabetic intravenous drug users. JAMA 266:2259–2261, 1991.
8. Schwartz B, Schuchat A, Oxtoby MJ, et al: Invasive Group B streptococcal disease in adults. JAMA 266:1112–1114, 1991.
9. Wachtel TJ, Tetu-Mouradjian LM, Goldman DL, et al: Hyperosmolality and acidosis in diabetes mellitus. J Gen Intern Med 6:495–502, 1991.
10. Weinstein D, Wang A, Chambers R, et al: Evaluation of magnetic resonance imaging in the diagnosis of osteomyelitis in diabetic foot infections. Foot Ankle 14:18–22, 1993.

6. HYPOGLYCEMIA

Fred D. Hofeldt, M.D.

1. Define hypoglycemia.
Hypoglycemia was defined by the Third International Symposium on Hypoglycemia as a blood glucose value of less than 50 mg/dl (2.8 mmol/L).

2. In diagnosing hypoglycemia, what are the important clinical features?
The timely occurrence of symptoms in the fasting or postprandial state helps to distinguish among the various etiologies. Serious life-threatening conditions are classified under the **fasting hypoglycemic** disorders. Less serious and frequently diet-modifiable conditions occur under the **postprandial states** (reactive hypoglycemia). Frequently, the symptoms associated with fasting hypoglycemia are those of neuroglycopenia, which presents with altered mental status or neuropsychiatric manifestations. The postprandial disorders (reactive hypoglycemias) are associated with a rapid decline in plasma glucose values as occurs during an insulin reaction. The symptoms are those of a catecholamine-mediated response, such as increased sweating, palpitations, apprehension, anxiety, headache, blurring of vision, and occasionally progression to neuroglycopenia and mental confusion. Although this separation is important for clinical classification, some patients may have mixed-component symptomatology.

3. What are the causes of fasting hypoglycemia?
Pancreatic disorders
  Islet beta-cell hyperfunction (adenoma, carcinoma, hyperplasia)
  Islet alpha-cell hypofunction or deficiency
Hepatic disorders
  Severe liver disease (cirrhosis, hepatitis, carcinomatosis, circulatory failure, ascending infectious cholangitis)
  Enzyme defects (glycogen-storage disease, galactosemia, hereditary fructose intolerance, familial galactose and fructose intolerance, fructose 1-6 diphosphatase deficiency)
Pituitary–adrenal disorders (hypopituitarism, Addison's disease, adrenogenital syndrome)
Central nervous system disease (hypothalamus or brain stem)
Muscle (hypoalaninemia?)
Nonpancreatic neoplasms
  Mesodermal (spindle-cell fibrosarcoma, leiomyosarcoma, mesothelioma, rhabdomyosarcoma, liposarcoma, neurofibroma, reticulum-cell sarcoma)
  Adenocarcinoma (hepatoma, cholangiocarcinoma, gastric carcinoma, adrenocorticocarcinoma, cecal carcinoma)
Unclassified
  Excessive loss or utilization of glucose and/or deficient substrate (prolonged or strenuous exercise, fever, lactation, pregnancy, renal glycosuria, diarrheal states, chronic starvation)
  Ketotic hypoglycemia of childhood (idiopathic hypoglycemia of childhood)
Exogenous causes
  Iatrogenic (related to treatment with insulin or oral hypoglycemic agents)
  Factitious (seen especially in paramedical personnel)
  Pharmacologic (Ackee nut, salicylates, antihistamines, monoamine-oxidase inhibitors, propranolol, phenylbutazone, pentamidine, phenotolamine, alcohol, ACE inhibitors)

4. What are the causes of postprandial or reactive hypoglycemia?

Reactive to refined carbohydrate (glucose, sucrose)

Reactive hypoglycemia

Alimentary hypoglycemia (includes patients with previous gastrointestinal surgery, peptic-ulcer disease, disordered gastrointestinal motility syndromes, and functional gastrointestinal disease)

Early type II diabetes mellitus

Hormonal (includes hyperthyroidism and deficient reserve syndromes of cortisol, epinephrine, glucagon, thyroid hormone, and growth hormone)

Idiopathic

Other conditions

Deficient early hepatic gluconeogenesis (fructose-1,6-diphosphatase deficiency)

Drugs (alcohol [gin plus tonic], lithium)

Insulinoma

Insulin or insulin-receptor autoantibodies

Reactive to other substrate (fructose, leucine, galactose)

5. What are the artifactual causes of hypoglycemia?

A pseudohypoglycemia occurs in certain chronic leukemias when the leukocyte counts are markedly elevated. This artifactual hypoglycemia reflects utilization of glucose by leukocytes after the blood sample has been drawn. Such a hypoglycemic condition, therefore, is not associated with symptoms. Other artifactual hypoglycemias may be seen with improper sample collection or storage, errors in analytic methodology, or confusion between whole blood and plasma glucose values. The plasma glucose is about 15% higher than corresponding whole-blood glucose values.

6. When hypoglycemia occurs, what counterregulatory events occur to spare glucose for brain metabolism?

Glucagon and epinephrine are the dominant counterregulatory hormones. Other hormones that respond to hypoglycemic stress are norepinephrine, cortisol, and growth hormone, but their effects are delayed. The metabolic effects of glucagon and epinephrine are immediate; stimulation of hepatic glycogenolysis and later gluconeogenesis results in increased production of hepatic glucose. Glucagon appears to be the most important counterregulatory hormone during acute hypoglycemia. When glucagon secretion is intact, recovery from hypoglycemia occurs promptly. If glucagon secretion is decreased or absent, catecholamines serve as a principal counterregulatory hormone with immediate effects.

7. Which laboratory tests assist in the evaluation of fasting hypoglycemia?

Initially simultaneous measurement of fasting blood glucose and fasting insulin values is helpful. Hypoglycemia with inappropriate hyperinsulinemia suggests conditions of autonomous insulin secretion, such as those seen in the spectrum of patients with insulinoma (carcinoma, adenoma, and hyperplasia) or in the factitious use of insulin or hypoglycemic agents. When the hypoglycemia occurs with correspondingly suppressed values of insulin, the non–insulin-mediated causes of fasting hypoglycemia need to be evaluated.

8. Which laboratory tests assist in evaluating patients suspected of having an insulinoma?

In patients with pancreatic insulinomas, inappropriate secretion results in excessive insulin despite the presence of hypoglycemia. During symptomatic hypoglycemia, patients have high insulin values and an increased ratio of insulin to glucose. Such a hormone profile also may be seen in patients who have ingested an oral sulfonylurea; a drug screen separates the two entities. The fasting ratio of insulin to plasma glucose is normally less than 0.33. Normally, proinsulin is less than 10–20% of total fasting insulin immunoreactivity; this proportion is increased in patients with insulinoma but not in patients with an overdosage of oral sulfonylurea.

9. Which tests distinguish factitious insulin administration from insulinoma?

In addition to the above laboratory tests for evaluation of insulinoma, the measurement of C-peptide during the hypoglycemic episode helps to distinguish between the two conditions. Patients with insulinoma have evidence of excessive insulin secretion as characterized by high values of insulin, proinsulin, and C-peptide during hypoglycemia. Patients who are self-administering insulin, on the other hand, have suppressed function of endogenous beta islet cells, and C-peptide levels are low during hypoglycemia, whereas insulin values are elevated. A suppressed C-peptide value is less than 0.5 mg/ml. Of note, patients who are inadvertently or factitiously taking oral sulfonylureas have laboratory results similar to those of the patient with insulinoma, such as an elevated C-peptide value; their proinsulin level, however, is normal.

10. When suspicion of insulinoma is high but the work-up is inconclusive, what additional studies may be performed?

Stimulation and suppression tests are not helpful, and the results are frequently misleading. A prolonged 72-hour fast with measurements of glucose and insulin every 6 hours will unmask the hypoglycemia in most patients with insulinoma. Hypoglycemia is usually evident within 24 hours of fasting. It is important to obtain blood samples when the patient becomes symptomatic. If the patient remains asymptomatic at 72 hours, he or she should exercise to evoke the hypoglycemia seen in patients with insulinoma.

11. Which conditions cause beta-cell hyperinsulinemia?

In 75–85% of cases, the major cause of the insulinoma syndrome is a pancreatic islet-cell adenoma. In about 10% of the cases, there are multiple adenomas (adenomatosis). In 5–6% of cases, carcinoma is present, and an additional 5–10% have islet-cell hyperplasia.

12. If other family members have pancreatic tumors, what condition(s) is suggested?

Multiple endocrine neoplasia (MEN-1) occurs as an autosomal dominant tumor in family members who present with functioning and nonfunctioning pituitary tumors, parathyroid adenomas or hyperplasia, and islet-cell tumors, any of which may include insulinoma and gastrinoma (Zollinger-Ellision syndrome). Such pancreatic tumors may secrete many other polypeptides, including glucagon, pancreatic polypeptide, somatostatin, adrenocorticotropic hormone (ACTH), melanocyte-stimulating hormone (MSH), serotonin, or growth hormone-releasing factor. When this condition is suspected, multiple family members need to be screened for the components of polyglandular tumor disorder.

13. What is nesidioblastosis?

Nesidioblastosis is a type of islet-cell hyperplasia in which primordial pancreatic ductal cells remain undifferentiated islet cells capable of polyhormonal secretion (gastrin, pancreatic polypeptide, insulin, and glucagon). It is the leading cause of hyperinsulinemic hypoglycemia in newborns and infants but also may cause hypoglycemia in adolescents and adults.

14. After a diagnosis of pancreatic islet-cell hyperinsulinemia is established, what procedures are helpful to localize the tumor?

Procedures such as ultrasound, celiac angiography, aortography, and abdominal CT scan are frequently insensitive and localize only about 60% of insulinomas. Some insulinomas are extremely small (less than a few millimeters) and easily escape detection. Endoscopic ultrasonography may be useful. Transhepatic percutaneous venous sampling may be useful to localize occult tumors and to distinguish between an isolated solitary insulinoma and diffuse disease (adenomatosis, hyperplasia, or nesidioblastosis). Intraoperative ultrasound is most helpful for localizing such pancreatic tumors.

15. If surgical resection is not possible or the patient has metastatic or inoperable carcinoma, adenomatosis, hyperplasia, or nesidioblastosis, what medications may control the hypoglycemia?

The most commonly used medications in this setting are diazoxide, long-acting somatostatin analog, or streptozocin. Diet with frequent feeding and snacks is the cornerstone of medical management. Adjunctive therapy with other drugs is usually ineffective but may be tried in difficult cases. Possible choices include calcium channel blockers, propranolol, phenytoin, glucocorticoids, glucagon, and chlorpromazine. Other agents for cancer chemotherapy include mithramycin, adriamycin, fluorouracil, floxuridine, carmustine, mitomycin-C, L-asparaginase, doxorubicin or chlorozotocin.

16. What are the causes of childhood hypoglycemia?

The occurrence of hypoinsulinemic hypoglycemia in infants and young children suggests the inherited disorders of intermediary metabolism, such as the glycogen storage diseases, gluconeogenic disorders (deficiencies of fructose-1,6 diphosphatase, pyruvate carboxylase, and phosphoenolpyruvate carboxykinase), galactosemia, hereditary fructose intolerance, maple syrup urine disease, carnitine deficiency, and ketotic hypoglycemia. Hormonal deficiencies (glucagon, growth hormone, thyroid and adrenal hormones) may also cause hypoglycemia. Furthermore, children are very susceptible to accidental drug overdose, especially with salicylates and alcohol. As previously mentioned, children with hyperinsulinemic hypoglycemia may have nesidioblastosis or diffuse islet-cell hyperplasia.

17. What are the most common drugs that cause hypoglycemia in adults?

In adults the most common causes of drug-induced hypoglycemia include the diabetic oral agents (sulfonylureas), insulin, ethanol, propranolol, and pentamidine. A complete list of drugs associated with hypoglycemia in 1,418 cases is presented by Seltzer.[20]

18. How does alcohol cause hypoglycemia?

Ethanol may produce hypoglycemia in normal, healthy volunteers after a short 36–72 hour fast. Modest ingestions of alcohol (about 100 gm) may produce the effect. Alcohol induces hypoglycemia when associated with poor food intake or starvation which reduce hepatic glycogen stores. Alcohol causes hypoglycemia in these situations by disrupting the gluconeogenic pathway through alterations of the cytosol $NADH_2/NAD$ ratio. In addition to intracellular processes, ethanol also depresses the uptake of lactate, alanine, and glycerol by the liver, all of which ordinarily contribute as gluconeogenic substrate to production of hepatic glucose. Ethanol also acutely lowers circulating levels of alanine by inhibiting its efflux from muscle.

19. On occasion hypoglycemia is caused by non–islet-cell tumors. Which tumors are implicated, and what is the mechanism of the hypoglycemia?

Various mesenchymal tumors (mesothelioma, fibrosarcoma, rhabdomyosarcoma, leiomyosarcoma, liposarcoma, and hemangiopericytoma) and organ-specific carcinomas (hepatic, adrenocortical, genitourinary, and mammary) may be associated with hypoglycemia. Hypoglycemia may occur with pheochromocytoma and with carcinoid and hematologic malignancies (leukemias, lymphomas, and myeloma). The mechanism varies according to the type of tumor, but in many cases hypoglycemia is associated with tumor-related malnutrition and weight loss due to fat, muscle, and tissue wasting that impairs hepatic gluconeogenesis. In some cases, utilization of glucose by exceptionally large tumors may cause hypoglycemia. Tumors may also secrete hypoglycemic factors, such as nonsuppressible insulinlike activity (NSILA) and insulinlike growth factors (IGFs), most notably IGF-II. By binding to hepatic insulin receptors, IGF-II inhibits production of hepatic glucose and promote hypoglycemia. Also suspect are tumor cytokines, particularly tumor necrosis factor (cachectin). Rarely does a tumor secrete extrapancreatic insulin.

20. What autoimmune syndromes may be associated with hypoglycemia?

Autoantibodies directed against insulin or its receptor may provoke hypoglycemia. Insulinomimetic antireceptor antibodies bind the receptor and mimic the action of insulin by increasing the uptake of glucose uptake in affected tissue. Autoantibodies that bind insulin may undergo dissociation at inappropriate times, usually during the early postprandial fasting period, and acutely raise serum free insulin levels, thus causing hypoglycemia. Such an autoimmune insulin syndrome is observed most often in Japanese patients and frequently occurs in the presence of other autoimmune diseases, such as Graves' disease, rheumatoid arthritis, systemic lupus erythematosus, and type 1 diabetes mellitus.

21. What endocrine conditions are associated with hypoglycemia?

In addition to islet-cell disorders, hypoglycemia may be seen in anterior pituitary insufficiency, in which secretion of growth hormone, ACTH, and thyroid-stimulating hormone (TSH) is deficient. In addition, primary adrenal insufficiency and primary hypothyroidism may be associated with either fasting or reactive hypoglycemia.

22. When is hypoglycemia attributed to renal failure?

The clinical setting of renal failure involves malnutrition with anorexia, vomiting, and poor dietary food intake. A reduction in renal mass may be a predisposing condition for hypoglycemia, because the kidney contributes to about one-third of overall gluconeogenesis during hypoglycemic stress. Renal failure results in alterations in drug metabolism, which may contribute to the hypoglycemia. Liver failure may coexist with far advanced renal insufficiency. Sepsis in patients with renal failure further promotes hypoglycemia. In some cases, dialysis has been linked to hypoglycemia. Diabetic patients on insulin who develop progressive renal failure may develop hypoglycemia, because the kidney is an important extrahepatic site for insulin degradation. With loss of renal mass, diabetic patients require decreased dosages of insulin.

23. What conditions cause reactive hypoglycemia?

The vast majority of patients with reactive hypoglycemia have idiopathic reactive hypoglycemia, inasmuch as they have not been defined as having underlying disease of the gastrointestinal tract (alimentary reactive hypoglycemia), hormone deficiency, or diabetic reactive hypoglycemia. Most patients with idiopathic reactive hypoglycemia have a delayed discharge of insulin (dysinsulinism) that occurs inappropriately in conjunction with falling levels of plasma glucose; a few of them have postprandial hyperinsulinemia. Occasionally, the patient with insulinoma may present with hypoglycemia that appears to be reactive, because it occurs during the postprandial state. Patients with insulin autoantibodies may have a dissociation of insulin from antibody binding in the postprandial state. Reactive hypoglycemia has been noted in patients who consume gin-and-tonic cocktails and in some patients who take prescribed lithium.

24. What conditions should be considered in the patient self-diagnosed with reactive hypoglycemia?

Most patients that complain of postprandial spells do not have reactive hypoglycemia; instead they may have any one of a number of conditions that manifest as vague episodic symptoms, usually of an adrenergic nature.

Differential Diagnosis of Spells

Cardiovascular disease	Endocrine–metabolic disorders
Arrhythmias (sinus arrest, asystole, tachycardia, atrial fibrillation-flutter, tachybradycardial syndromes, including sick sinus syndrome, atrial-ventricular dissociation, and Stokes-Adams attacks)	Hyperthyroidism
	Hypothyroidism
	Reactive hypoglycemia
	Fasting hypoglycemia
	Pheochromocytoma
Pulmonary emboli and/or microemboli	Carcinoid syndrome
Orthostatic hypotension syndromes	Hereditary angioneurotic edema
DaCosta syndromes (beta-adrenergic hyperresponsive state)	Urticaria pigmentosa
	Hyperbradykinism
Mitral valve or apparatus dysfunction	Addison's disease
Congestive heart failure	Hypopituitarism

Table continued on following page.

Differential Diagnosis of Spells (Continued)

Psychoneurologic disease
  Seizure disorders
  Autonomic insufficiency
  Diencephalic epilepsy (autonomic epilepsy)
  Hyperventilation syndrome
  Cataplexy
  Anxiety neurosis
  Hysteria
  Migraine
  Syncope
  Psychophysiologic reaction
  Conversion hysteria
Gastrointestinal disorders
  Dumping syndrome after GI surgery
  Postprandial physiologic dumping without prior
    GI surgery
  Chinese-restaurant syndrome
  Irritable colon syndrome
  Food intolerance

Endocrine-metabolic disorders
  Hypothalamic–pituitary dysfunction
  Menopause
  Diabetes mellitus
  Diabetes insipidus
Miscellaneous disease
  Sepsis
  Anemia
  Cachexia
  Hypovolemia (dehydration)
  Diuretic abuse
  Clonidine withdrawal
  Monoamine oxidase inhibitors plus tyramine
    (cheese, wine)
  Asthma
  Idiopathic postprandial syndrome

25. How is reactive hypoglycemia diagnosed and treated?

Reactive hypoglycemia is a diagnosis made by exclusion, after most of the conditions that cause "spells" have been eliminated. In bona fide reactive hypoglycemia, the patient's condition is related to feeding; most likely the patient is ingesting an excessive amount of refined carbohydrates or food of a high glycemic index. The low blood glucose is a consequence of postprandial hyperinsulinism or dysinsulinism. Oral glucose tolerance testing demonstrates this refined carbohydrate sensitivity. Excessive intake of refined carbohydrates or foods of a high glycemic index may be evaluated by dietary recall. Restricting refined carbohydrates to 8–10% of total dietary intake cures the syndrome in patients with bona fide disease. Frequently, underlying neuropsychiatric disease, anxiety, or situational stress reactions are the real culprits of the episodic spells, which the patient characterizes or self-diagnoses as reactive hypoglycemia. True reactive hypoglycemia is rare.

BIBLIOGRAPHY

1. Archambeaud-Moaveraux F, Hac MC, Nadolon S, et al: Autoimmune-insulin syndrome. Biomed Pharmacother 43:581–586, 1989.
2. Arem R: Hypoglycemia associated with renal failures. Endocrinol Metab Clin North Am 18:103–121, 1989.
3. Arky RA: Hypoglycemia associated with liver disease and ethanol. Endocrinol Metab Clin North Am 118:75–90, 1989.
4. Burch HB, Clement S, Sokol MS, et al: Reactive hypoglycemia coma due to insulin autoimmune syndrome. Am J Med 92:681–685, 1992.
5. Crapo DS, Scarlett JA, Koltermann OG, et al: The effects of oral fructose, sucrose, and glucose in subjects with reactive hypoglycemia. Diabetes Care 5:512–517, 1982.
6. Fajans SS, Vinik AI: Insulin-producing islet cell tumors. Endocrinol Metab Clin North Am 18:45–74, 1989.
7. Field JB: Hypoglycemia: Definitions, clinical presentation, classification and laboratory tests. Endocrinol Metab Clin North Am 18:27–44, 1989.
8. Gerich JE, Cryer PE, Rizza RA: Hormonal mediamisms in acute glucose counterregulation: The relative roles of glucagon, epinephrine, norepinephrine, growth hormone and cortisol. Metabolism 29:1165–1175, 1980.
9. Glaser B, Valtysson G, Vinik AI, et al: Gastrointestinal/pancreatic hormone concentrations in the portal venous system of nine patients with organic hyperinsulinemia. Metabolism 130:1001–1010, 1981.
10. Gorman B, Charboneau JW, James EM, et al: Benign pancreatic insulinoma: Preoperative and intraoperative sonographic localization. AJR 147:929–934, 1986.

11. Heitz PU, Klöppel G, Hacki WH, et al: Nesidioblastosis. Diabetes 26:632–642, 1977.
12. Hofeldt FD: Reactive hypoglycemia. Metabolism 24:1193–1208, 1975.
13. Hofeldt FD: Reactive hypoglycemia. Endocrinol Metab Clin North Am 18:185–201, 1989.
14. Haymond MW: Hypoglycemia in infants and children. Endocrinol Metab Clin North Am 18:211–252, 1989.
15. Lefebve PJ, Andreani D, Marks V, et al: Statement on "postprandial" reactive hypoglycemia. In Hypoglycemia, Serono Symposium. New York, Raven Press, 1987, p 79.
16. Moertel CG, Lefkopoulo M, Lipsitz S, et al: Streptozocin-doxorubicin, streptozocin-fluorouracil or chlorozotocin in treatment of advanced islet cell carcinoma. N Engl J Med 326:519–523, 1992.
17. Peitzman SJ, Agarwal BN: Spontaneous hypoglycemia in end-stage renal failure. Nephron 19:131–139, 1977.
18. Rösch T, Lightdale CJ, Botet JF, et al: Localization of pancreatic endocrine tumor by endoscopic ultrasonography. N Engl J Med 326:1726–1736, 1992.
19. Sanders LR, Hofeldt FD, Kirk MC, et al: Refined carbohydrate as a contributing factor in reactive hypoglycemia. South Med J 75:1072–1075, 1982.
20. Seltzer HS: Drug-induced hypoglycemia. Endocrinol Metab Clin North Am 18:163–183, 1989.
21. Service FJ, McMahon MM, O'Brien PC, et al: Functioning insulinoma—Incidence, recurrence and long term survival of patients. Mayo Clin Proc 66:711–719, 1991.
22. Shapiro ET, Bell GI, Polonsky KS, et al: Tumor hypoglycemia: Relationship to high molecular weight insulin-like growth factor II. J Clin Invest 85:1672–1679, 1990.
23. Skogseid BJ, Eriksson B, Lundquist G, et al: Multiple endocrine neoplasia type 1. J Clin Endocrinol 73:281–287, 1991.

7. LIPID DISORDERS

Michael T. McDermott, M.D.

1. What are the major lipids in the bloodstream?

Cholesterol and triglycerides are the major circulating lipids. Cholesterol is utilized all over the body for cell synthesis and repair and for production of steroid hormones. Triglycerides are used as a fuel source by muscle cells or stored as fat in adipose tissue.

2. What are lipoproteins?

Lipoproteins transport lipids in the blood from one site to another. They are spherical particles that envelop the water-insoluble lipids with a surface of water-soluble proteins and phospholipids.

3. What are the major lipoproteins in the bloodstream?

Chylomicrons, very low density lipoproteins (VLDL), low density lipoproteins (LDL), and high density lipoproteins (HDL) are the major circulating lipoproteins. Their functions are shown below.

Lipoprotein	Function
Chylomicron	Transport dietary triglycerides from the gut to muscle and adipose tissue
VLDL	Transport hepatic-synthesized triglycerides from liver to muscle and adipose tissue
LDL	Transport cholesterol from the liver to peripheral tissues
HDL	Transport cholesterol from peripheral tissues to the liver

4. What are the apoproteins?

Apoproteins are located on the surface of lipoproteins. They usually function as ligands for binding to receptors or as cofactors for enzymes. The major apoproteins are listed below.

Apoprotein	Function
Apo C-II	Cofactor for lipoprotein lipase, which removes triglycerides from chylomicrons and VLDL, leaving remnant particles
Apo E	Binds to hepatic receptors for remnant particles
Apo B	Binds to peripheral and hepatic receptors for LDL
Apo A	Binds to peripheral receptors for HDL

5. How do lipoproteins promote atherosclerosis?

Excessive LDL is oxidized and engulfed by scavenger arterial subendothelial macrophages, which thus initiate the development of atherosclerotic plaque. HDL protects against atherosclerosis by transporting excessive cholesterol back to the liver.

6. Are triglycerides harmful?

Serum triglyceride levels exceeding 250 mg/dl appear to be associated with atherosclerosis. It is unclear, however, whether this association is due to triglycerides or to decreases in serum HDL, increases in serum Apo B, or the smaller, denser LDL particles that often accompany high triglyceride levels. Triglyceride concentrations greater than 500 mg/dl increase the risk of acute pancreatitis.

7. What is lipoprotein(a)?
Apoprotein(a) has approximately 85% sequence homology with plasminogen. When an apoprotein(a) binds to an apoprotein B-100 on the surface of an LDL particle, the new particle is referred to as lipoprotein(a). Lipoprotein(a) promotes atherosclerosis, possibly because it is easily oxidized and engulfed by macrophages and/or because it has antithrombolytic activity.

8. What are the primary dyslipidemias?
Primary dyslipidemias are lipid disorders that are totally or partially inherited. The major dyslipidemias are listed below.

Primary Dyslipidemia	Phenotype
Familial hypercholesterolemia	↑↑ Cholesterol
Familial combined hyperlipidemia	↑ Cholesterol and ↑ triglycerides
Familial dysbetalipoproteinemia	↑ Cholesterol and ↑ triglycerides
Polygenic hypercholesterolemia	↑ Cholesterol
Familial hypertriglyceridemia	↑↑ Triglycerides

9. What is familial hypercholesterolemia?
Familial hypercholesterolemia is caused by defective or absent peripheral LDL receptors. Homozygotes frequently have serum cholesterol levels of 800–1,200 mg/dl and die of coronary artery disease (CAD) before age 20 years. Heterozygotes have cholesterol levels of 300–600 mg/dl and often manifest CAD before age 50 years. Tendon xanthomas are characteristic of this disorder.

10. What is familial combined hyperlipidemia?
Familial combined hyperlipidemia is due, at least in part, to excessive hepatic synthesis of apoprotein B. Affected patients have elevations of both cholesterol and triglycerides and are susceptible to premature CAD.

11. What is familial dysbetalipoproteinemia?
Familial dysbetalipoproteinemia is caused by an abnormal apoprotein E (phenotype E2/E2), which binds poorly to hepatic receptors and thus impairs clearance of circulating VLDL remnants by the liver. Affected patients have elevations of both cholesterol and triglycerides as well as premature CAD. Planar xanthomas in the creases of the palms and soles are characteristic of this disorder.

12. What is polygenic hypercholesterolemia?
Polygenic hypercholesterolemia is due to one or more defects in lipoprotein metabolism similar to, but less severe than, those which cause the other primary dyslipidemias. Patients have mild to moderate cholesterol elevations and are at increased risk for premature CAD.

13. What is familial hypertriglyceridemia?
Familial hypertriglyceridemia is caused by excessive hepatic triglyceride synthesis. Affected patients have significantly elevated serum triglycerides but normal cholesterol and are not prone to develop CAD.

14. What are the secondary dyslipidemias?
Secondary dyslipidemias are lipid elevations due to other systemic diseases, such as diabetes mellitus, hypothyroidism, nephrotic syndrome, renal disease, obstructive liver disease, dysproteinemias, or drug toxicity. The dyslipidemia usually corrects when the primary disorder resolves or is treated appropriately.

15. When should lipid disorders be treated?
The guidelines of the National Cholesterol Education Program are based on risk factors and the serum LDL level. Recognized risk factors include male sex with age over 45 years, female sex

after menopause without estrogen replacement, family history of premature CAD, smoking, hypertension, diabetes mellitus, and HDL < 35 mg/dl. HDL ≥ 60 mg/dl warrants subtraction of one risk factor.

Treatment of Lipid Disorders

PATIENT RISK	GOAL	DIET, IF	DRUGS, IF
No CAD and < 2 risk factors	LDL < 160	LDL > 160	LDL > 190
No CAD and ≥ 2 risk factors	LDL < 130	LDL > 130	LDL > 160
Known CAD	LDL < 100	LDL > 100	LDL > 130

Triglyceride levels over 250 mg/dl should be treated with diet. Drugs should be added if the levels exceed 500 mg/dl after dietary intervention.

16. What dietary alterations lower cholesterol and triglycerides?

Serum cholesterol generally can be lowered approximately 5–10% by decreasing dietary intake of cholesterol and saturated fat. The American Heart Association step 1 or step 2 diet is recommended. Serum triglycerides often respond to the same measures coupled with reductions in the intake of refined carbohydrates and alcohol. Increasing dietary fiber also appears beneficial.

17. What medications most effectively lower serum cholesterol?

Medication	LDL Reduction
3-Hydroxy-3-methylglutaryl co-enzyme A (HMG CoA) reductase inhibitors	20–40%
Bile acid resins	15–30%
Niacin	15–30%
Gemfibrozil	10–15%

18. Which medications significantly lower triglycerides?

Medication	Triglyceride Reduction
Gemfibrozil	30–50%
Niacin	20–30%
HMG CoA reductase inhibitors	10–20%

19. Which medications most effectively raise serum HDL cholesterol?

Medication	HDL Increase
Niacin	10–25%
Gemfibrozil	10–25%
HMG CoA reductase inhibitors	5–10%

20. Can coronary artery disease be prevented by alterations in the lipid profile?

Primary prevention trials involving either diet or drugs have demonstrated that for every 1% reduction in the serum cholesterol level, the risk of developing clinically apparent CAD is reduced by approximately 2%. Studies suggest that raising HDL and lowering triglycerides also may be beneficial.

21. Can established coronary artery disease be reversed by alterations in the lipid profile?

Aggressive lipid-lowering programs have been reported to halt progression or induce regression of angiographically apparent coronary lesions in patients with known CAD or previous bypass surgery.

22. Is antioxidant therapy effective in preventing coronary artery disease?

Because LDL is oxidized before it is taken up by subendothelial macrophages, antioxidant therapy with vitamin C, vitamin E, or beta carotene has come under investigation. Evidence suggests that higher vitamin E intakes are associated with a lower risk of CAD in both men and women. Although there is, as yet, no definitive proof of their efficacy, antioxidants have been recommended as adjunctive therapy by some experts.

BIBLIOGRAPHY

1. Blankenhorn DH, Nessim SA, Johnson RL, et al: Beneficial effects of combined colestipol-niacin therapy on coronary atherosclerosis and coronary venous bypass grafts. JAMA 257:3233–3240, 1987.
2. Bradford RH, Downton M, Chremos, et al: Efficacy and tolerability of lovastatin in 3390 women with moderate hypercholesterolemia. Ann Intern Med 118:850–855, 1993.
3. Brown G, Albers JJ, Fisher LD, et al: Regression of coronary artery disease as a result of intensive lipid-lowering therapy in men with high levels of apolipoprotein B. N Engl J Med 323:1289–1298, 1990.
4. Criqui MH: Cholesterol, primary and secondary prevention, and all-cause mortality. Ann Intern Med 115:973–976, 1991.
5. Criqui MH, Heiss G, Cohn R, et al: Plasma triglyceride level and mortality from coronary heart disease. N Engl J Med 328:1220–1225, 1993.
6. East C, Bilheimer DW, Grundy SM: Combination drug therapy for familial combined hyperlipidemia. Ann Intern Med 109:25–32, 1988.
7. Expert Panel on Detection, Evaluation, and Treatment of High Blood Cholesterol in Adults: Summary of the Second Report of the National Cholesterol Education Program (NCEP) Expert Panel on Detection, Evaluation, and Treatment of High Blood Cholesterol in Adults (Adult treatment panel II). JAMA 269:3015–3023, 1993.
8. Frick MH, Elo O, Haapa K, et al: Helsinki heart study: Primary-prevention trial with gemfibrozil in middle-aged men with dyslipidemia; safety of treatment, changes in risk factors, and incidence of coronary heart disease. N Engl J Med 317:1237–1245, 1987.
9. Hunninghake DB, Stein EA, Dujovne CA, et al: The efficacy of intensive dietary therapy alone or combined with lovastatin in outpatients with hypercholesterolemia. N Engl J Med 328:1213–1219, 1993.
10. Lavie CJ, Gau GT, Squires RW, Kottke BA: Management of lipids in primary and second prevention of cardiovascular disease. Mayo Clin Proc 63:605–621, 1988.
11. Muldoon MF, Manuck SB, Matthews KA: Lowering cholesterol concentrations and mortality: A quantitative review of primary prevention trials. BMJ 301:309–314, 1990.
12. National Cholesterol Education Program Expert Panel on Detection, Evaluation, and Treatment of High Blood Cholesterol in Adults: Report of the National Cholesterol Education Program Expert Panel on Detection, Evaluation, and Treatment of High Blood Cholesterol in Adults. Arch Intern Med 148:36–69, 1988.
13. Rimm EB, Stampfer MJ, Ascherio A, et al: Vitamin E consumption and the risk of coronary heart disease in men. N Engl J Med 238:1450–1456, 1993.
14. Rossouw JE, Lewis B, Rifkind BM: The value of lowering cholesterol after myocardial infarction. N Engl J Med 323:1112–1119, 1990.
15. Scanu AM, moderator: Lipoprotein(a) and atherosclerosis. Ann Intern Med 115:209–218, 1991.
16. Silverman DI, Ginsburg GS, Pasternak RC: High-density lipoprotein subfractions. Am J Med 94:636–645, 1993.
17. Stampfer MJ, Hennekens, CH, Manson JE, et al: Vitamin E consumption and the risk of coronary disease in women. N Engl J Med 238:1444–1449, 1993.
18. Steinberg D, Parthasarathy S, Carew TE, et al: Beyond cholesterol: Modifications of low-density lipoprotein that increase its atherogenicity. N Engl J Med 320:915–924, 1989.
19. Wood PD, Stefanick ML, Dreon DM, et al: Changes in plasma lipids and lipoproteins in overweight men during weight loss through dieting as compared with exercise. N Engl J Med 319:1773–1779, 1988.
20. Wood PD, Stefanick ML, Williams PT, Haskell WL: The effects on plasma lipoproteins of a prudent weight-reducing diet, with or without exercise, in overweight men and women. N Engl J Med 325:461–466, 1991.

8. OBESITY

Daniel H. Bessesen, M.D.

1. How common is the problem of obesity in the United States?

Since 1960 the National Center for Health Statistics has conducted surveys of the prevalence of obesity every 10 years. These surveys, known as the NHANES studies, have shown a steady rise in the prevalence of obesity every 10 years. In 1980, 34 million Americans, almost 30% of all adults, were overweight. Of these, 12.4 million were severely overweight. The figures from 1990 reportedly show a continued rise. Obesity is more common among minorities. In black women between the ages of 45 and 54 years the prevalence of obesity exceeds 50%. A recent Health Technology Assessment Conference at the National Institutes of Health identified a paradox in the United States today. On the one hand, most of those who need to lose weight are not succeeding, whereas many people who do not need to lose weight are trying to do so. In a recent survey a surprising 44% of female and 15% of male high school students reported trying to lose weight. At a time when they should be growing, 14% of female and 4% of male high school students reported the use of self-induced vomiting as a weight loss strategy. The prevalence of obesity continues to increase despite an expenditure of over 30 billion dollars annually on commercial weight-loss products.

2. What is medically significant obesity?

Most Americans are concerned about their body weight for cosmetic rather than health reasons. Medically significant obesity is a degree of obesity associated with excessive morbidity or mortality.

3. What is the best way to determine if an individual has medically significant obesity?

Although visual inspection and total body weight may give an estimate of the degree of obesity, a simple measurement that correlates with more sophisticated measurements of fatness is the body mass index (BMI).

BMI is calculated as follows: BMI = weight (kg)/height^2 (meters)

The accompanying table uses the height (inches) and weight (lbs) of the patient to estimate BMI. An ideal BMI is less than 25. BMIs above this level appear to correlate with increases in morbidity and mortality.

Body Weights in Pounds According to Height and Body Mass Index[*]

HEIGHT	BODY MASS INDEX, kg/m^2													
	19	20	21	22	23	24	25	26	27	28	29	30	35	40
in	← ———————————————— BODY WEIGHT, lb ———————————————— →													
58	91	96	100	105	110	115	119	124	129	134	138	143	167	191
59	94	99	104	109	114	119	124	128	133	138	143	148	173	198
60	97	102	107	112	118	123	128	133	138	143	148	153	179	204
61	100	106	111	116	122	127	132	137	143	148	153	158	185	211
62	104	109	115	120	126	131	136	142	147	153	158	164	191	218
63	107	113	118	124	130	135	141	146	152	158	163	169	197	225
64	110	116	122	128	134	140	145	151	157	163	169	174	204	232
65	114	120	126	132	138	144	150	156	162	168	174	180	210	240
66	118	124	130	136	142	148	155	161	167	173	179	186	216	247
67	121	127	134	140	146	153	159	166	172	178	185	191	223	255
68	125	131	138	144	151	158	164	171	177	184	190	197	230	262
69	128	135	142	149	155	162	169	176	182	189	196	203	236	270
70	132	139	146	153	160	167	174	181	188	195	202	207	243	278

Table continued on following page.

49

Body Weights in Pounds According to Height and Body Mass Index* (Continued)

HEIGHT					BODY MASS INDEX, kg/m²								
	19	20	21	22	23	24	25	26	27	28	29	30	35	40
in	◄──────────────────────────── BODY WEIGHT, lb ────────────────────────────►													
71	136	143	150	157	165	172	179	186	193	200	208	215	250	286
72	140	147	154	162	169	177	184	191	199	206	213	221	258	294
73	144	151	159	166	174	182	189	197	204	212	219	227	265	302
74	148	155	163	171	179	186	194	202	210	218	225	233	272	311
75	152	160	168	176	184	192	200	208	216	224	232	240	279	319
76	156	164	172	180	189	197	205	213	221	230	238	246	287	328

*Each entry gives the body weight in pounds (lb) for a person of a given height and body mass index. Pounds have been rounded off. To use the table, find the appropriate height in the left-hand column. Move across the row to a given weight. The number at the top of the column is the body mass index for the height and weight. (From NIH Technology Assessment Conference Panel: Methods for voluntary weight loss and control. Ann Intern Med 116:942–949, 1992, with permission.)

4. What is meant by the term "regional adiposity"? What is its significance?

The health consequences of obesity are a function not only of body weight but also of the distribution of adipose tissue. Adipose tissue located around the hips and thighs, which is common in women (gynoid pattern), carries fewer health risks than excess adipose tissue located in the abdominal region, which is common in men (android pattern or abdominal obesity). Women who carry excess adipose tissue in the abdominal region have substantially increased risks for diabetes mellitus, hypertension, and hyperlipidemia. Because men are more likely to distribute adipose tissue in the abdominal region, obese men are generally at increased risk for such complications. Adipose tissue located within the abdominal cavity itself (intraabdominal fat) may be correlated most strongly with adverse health consequences. This correlation may be due to increased delivery of free fatty acids to the liver from the mesenteric fat beds drained by the portal vein. The distribution of adipose tissue may be estimated by the waist-to-hip ratio, which is calculated by measuring the minimal waist circumference and the maximal hip circumference with a tape measure. Central obesity is defined as a waist-to-hip ratio of more than 1.0 men and 0.8 for women. Thus, the BMI and the waist-to-hip ratio are the two most important indices of medically significant obesity.

5. What causes obesity?

Obesity arises when caloric intake exceeds energy expenditure. In addition to a positive caloric balance, obesity develops in the presence of a positive fat balance; that is, the individual consumes more fat calories than he or she burns. Several processes play important roles in the development of obesity: genetic factors, increased appetite and dietary factors, abnormalities in energy expenditure, and enhanced storage of ingested calories.

6. How important are genetic factors in the development of obesity?

Twin and adoption studies indicate that an individual's genotype is important in determining the rate of energy expenditure and fat distribution. The specific genes that cause obesity have not been identified yet but this is an area of active investigation. Genetic factors account for only 25–30% of the weight variation seen within a population.

7. What dietary factors predispose to obesity?

Perhaps the most important factor in the increasing incidence of obesity is the consumption of a high-fat diet. The prevalence of obesity in the United States has risen coincidentally with a rise in the average fat content of the diet. In a number of cultures, such as the Pima Indians of Arizona and the Nahru people of Polynesia, obesity was unheard of when people ate a native diet. With the introduction and subsequent easy access to high-fat foods, the prevalence of obesity among adults in both groups has reached 80–90%. This "western" or "modern" diet promotes a positive fat balance, in part because the body does not adjust with much accuracy the oxidation of fat in response to increased consumption. Recent data suggest that obese individuals have an increased preference for high-fat food and that with weight loss they may acquire a preference for foods with high caloric density. A high-fat diet also produces obesity in experimental animals.

Increased appetite also may play a role in the development of obesity, although this factor probably accounts for only part of the problem. The understanding of the neurobiology of appetite is a rapidly expanding area. A number of neurotransmitters, including norepinephrine, serotonin, and the peptides neuropeptide-Y and cholecystokinin, act within specific brain nuclei and play important roles in regulating not only total food intake but also preference for fat, carbohydrate, or protein. Neural pathways that regulate food intake are present in the hypothalamus, brain stem, and peripheral nervous system.

8. Do alterations in energy expenditure predispose to obesity?

Because weight gain occurs when caloric intake exceeds caloric expenditure, another important factor in the development of obesity is decreased energy expenditure. There are three components of energy expenditure: (1) basal metabolic rate (BMR) is the amount of energy required to keep the body warm, to keep Na^+ out of cells and K^- in cells, to breathe, and to keep the heart beating; (2) the thermic effect of food (TEF) is the amount of energy expended during digestion; and (3) the energy of activity is the amount of energy expended during physical activity or exercise. BMR is strongly related to lean body mass; almost no evidence suggests that obesity is caused by decreases in BMR. Whether TEF decreases in obese individuals is controversial. Increasing evidence, however, suggests that decreased physical activity may play an important role in the development and maintenance of obesity. When immigrants came to the United States, many changed from labor-intensive agricultural jobs to more sedentary office jobs. Obesity soon followed. Recent evidence using stable isotopes to measure total energy expenditure in free-living children suggests that decreased energy expenditure may be a highly important contributor to weight gain.

9. What are the economic consequences of obesity?

In 1980, 34 million Americans were obese. The overall costs of obesity in 1986 dollars was estimated to be $39.3 billion or 5.5% of national health costs for that year. Included were $22.2 billion for cardiovascular disease, $11.3 billion for diabetes, $1.5 billion for hypertension, and $1.9 billion for breast and colon cancer. This estimate does not include costs of musculoskeletal disorders, which may almost double the total figure. In addition, the loss in wages and productivity attributed to obesity approaches $20 billion per year.

10. What are the psychosocial consequences of obesity?

Situational depression and anxiety related to obesity are common. The obese person may suffer from discrimination that contributes further to difficulty with poor self-image and social relationships. In a recent study, obese adolescents were compared with adolescents who had other chronic health problems. Both groups were followed for 7 years. At the end of this period, the obese women were 20% less likely to be married, made $6,700/yr less in income, and had 10% more poverty than controls. This effect was independent of baseline aptitude test scores and socioeconomic status.

11. What diseases are more common in obese individuals?

Coronary artery disease (CAD)	Pulmonary emboli
Type II diabetes mellitus	Cholesterol stones
Hypertension	Osteoarthritis
Sleep apnea	

In the Nurses Health Study, which examined 115,886 women, participants with a BMI of 25–29 were 1.8 times more likely to have CAD compared with those with a BMI <21, the lowest risk group. Women with a BMI>29 were 3.3 times more likely to have CAD. Although a relative risk of 1.8 may not seem to be large, millions of women have this moderate level of obesity. The actual number of cases of CAD attributable to a moderate level of obesity (attributable risk = relative risk × population at risk) is therefore substantial. For this reason the largest public health impact of obesity lies not with the morbidly obese, but with the millions of moderately obese individuals seen by primary providers for other medical problems.

12. Is the presence of obesity associated with increased mortality rates?

Increased mortality is correlated with the severity of obesity as defined by BMI. The exact nature of this relationship, however, is complex. Early studies by life insurance companies established a relationship between weight and mortality. Such studies, which form the basis of the widely used "ideal body-weight tables," suggest that underweight individuals also have increased mortality. When these studies were reanalyzed however, the excess mortality in the lightest individuals was found to be due to cancer or complications of smoking (the average weight of smokers is significantly lower than that of nonsmokers). This finding suggests that the excess mortality in the lightest individuals was not due to reduced weight. Instead, both reduced weight and excessive mortality were due to a third factor, either preexisting cancer or cigarette smoking. In a recent study of Seventh Day Adventists, overall mortality decreased with lower body weight; the lowest overall mortality occurred in people with a BMI<21.

To establish firmly the role of obesity in overall mortality, a study needs to examine individuals over a long period of time and to control for confounding variables. Two studies have done so: the Framingham Study and the Harvard Growth Study. In the Framingham Study the relative risk of nonsmoking men 10–20% above ideal body weight was twice as high as that for men of ideal body weight. In the Harvard Growth Study, 500 lean or obese (BMI>25) adolescents were followed for 55 years. Mortality among obese men was 1.8 times higher than among lean controls. Obesity in adolescence predicted a broad range of adverse health effects. Again, the relative risk of moderate obesity may not be large, but given the millions of Americans who are moderately obese, the mortality attributable to moderate obesity is likely to be substantial.

13. Which malignancies are more common in obese individuals?

Obese women have an increased incidence of endometrial cancer, postmenopausal breast cancer, and gallbladder and biliary cancers. Obese men have a higher mortality rate from cancers of the prostate, rectum, and colon.

14. What are the common metabolic abnormalities found in obese patients?

Insulin resistance. Obesity is associated with a decrease in the ability of insulin to stimulate peripheral glucose disposal and to suppress hepatic output of glucose. The body then increases insulin secretion to compensate. This insulin resistance and hyperinsulinemia may be caused by increased delivery of free fatty acids to the liver from the adipose tissue located within the abdomen. This may be why abdominal obesity is associated with more metabolic complications.

Lipid abnormalities. Plasma triglycerides are frequently elevated in obese individuals. This leads to decreases in HDL cholesterol levels due to increases in HDL catabolism. Concentration of LDL cholesterol also may be increased.

Sex hormone abnormalities. Obese men show evidence of decreased testosterone and follicle-stimulating hormone (FSH). Obese women may have increased levels of estrogen after menopause, which may predispose to endometrial cancer. The increased level of androgens seen in women with upper-body obesity may lead to hirsutism, anovulatory menstrual cycles, and dysfunctional uterine bleeding. Increased levels of androgen appear to be causally related to the hyperinsulinemia seen in obese women.

15. What is the pickwickian syndrome?

The pickwickian syndrome, named for the fat boy Joe in Dickens' *Pickwick Papers,* is characterized by obesity, hypoventilation, somnolence, secondary polycythemia, right ventricular failure, and sleep apnea. Daytime hypertension may be the presenting complaint. Signs and symptoms improve markedly with weight loss; surprisingly, pulmonary problems may improve markedly with only a 20–30-lb weight loss.

16. When do organic causes of obesity need to be considered?
Rarely. Less than 1% of obese patients have underlying medical disorders as the primary cause of obesity. Cushing's syndrome, with excessive production of cortisol, results in central obesity and the associated risks of hypertension and diabetes. Hypothyroidism also may cause a gain of 10–15 lbs, and individuals with a recent onset of weight gain should be screened. Hypothyroidism and hypercortisolism virtually never cause massive obesity independently.

Although typically we think of weight loss as a sign of major depression, some individuals manifest depression as weight gain. Signs of depression should be carefully sought, because depression may result from and contribute to the weight-control difficulties of the obese patient.

17. How do you take a nutritional history from an obese individual?
As with any medical condition, the evaluation should begin with a complete history. To make a dietary intervention, one must first know what the patient is currently eating. Many physicians are not comfortable taking a nutritional history and defer this task to the dietitian. In fact, taking a nutritional history is no more difficult than taking any other kind of history, and having a physician discuss the details of the patient's diet reinforces the importance of the diet in overall health.

Dietitians often use two tools in taking a nutritional history: the diet recall and food frequency. A nutritionist asks the patient to record all foods eaten for 2–5 days. Whereas this approach is far more accurate than a 1–2 day oral recall history, it is also more time-consuming. It is easier for physicians to ask individuals what they ate the day before and the day of the clinic visit. Even from this limited information, one learns a great deal about how the person eats. Many obese individuals do not eat breakfast, eat lunch occasionally, then snack on high-fat foods through much of the late afternoon and early evening. They may eat while doing other things; thus they find it difficult to assess what they are actually eating. Having this information allows you to begin to make simple nutritional suggestions. To take a food frequency history, the nutritionist may use a questionnaire to find out how often certain foods are eaten. A simpler approach for the physician is to ask about the frequently eaten meals. Many people have a limited repertoire of meals that are eaten repetitively. Many individuals eat the same breakfast and lunch 3–5 times/week. If one can help individuals to modify frequently consumed meals, one has substantially modified their diet.

History taking tools are combined with dietary advice. Such steps do not replace good nutritional counseling, but they are a powerful adjunct to the work of a registered dietitian. They demonstrate that the patient's physician is committed to dietary therapy and interested in working in this important area.

18. What is an appropriate goal for a weight-loss program?
A number of important issues should be remembered when helping obese individuals to control their weight:

1. **What is the goal?** The patient may want to lose 40 lbs in 40 days. This approach is guaranteed to fail in the long term. A better goal is mild, sustained weight loss. A more realistic goal may be prevention of further weight gain. Perhaps the best goal is to improve habits of eating and activity. Such habits are the only factors that most individuals can influence in the long term. To take the focus off weight and to place it on personal habits allows individuals to succeed today if they change their habits and to fail next month if habits revert, even if the weight target has been achieved.

2. **Habits change slowly and gradually.** It is not realistic to expect anyone to go from a 50% fat diet to a vegetarian diet overnight. It is neither reasonable nor appropriate to expect an obese individual to become an aerobic athlete in 2 weeks. Patience on the part of both the provider and the patient is a cornerstone of success.

3. **Any meaningful change in behavior must be lifelong.** Because of the biologic basis for obesity, as soon as the individual stops the weight-loss strategy, weight tends to return to its

previous level. Thus the changes have to be simple and to fit into the patient's lifestyle. More extensive, radical, and labor-intensive techniques are not likely not be sustained and the weight predictably returns.

19. What kind of nutritional counseling should the average obese patient receive?

The usual problem with the eating habits of obese individuals is not that they do not know what to eat; instead, they pay no attention to what they eat. A major goal of diet therapy for novice dieters is to pay more attention to what they eat. The physician should encourage the individual (1) to eat 3 meals per day; (2) to eat only at mealtimes; and (3) to eat only one serving at each meal. Following these three steps requires active decisions about food choices. The physician then works with the dietitian to prescribe a flexible and balanced diet of intake restricted to approximately 1,200 calories, which will result in consistent and appropriate weight loss. The diet should minimize fat intake. One must remember that habits change slowly and need to be changed for the long term. Anyone who has switched from whole milk to 1–2% milk has experienced how a gradual, incremental change is far more tolerable than a radical one. If the patient eats at fast-food restaurants 5 times/week perhaps he or she can initially change to 4 times/week, eating something lower in fat once a week. Over time the patient can replace more and more of the "usual meals" with new meals. Another approach is not to eliminate foods, but simply to reduce portion size or frequency of consumption.

20. Is exercise an important part of a weight-loss program?

Exercise plays an important role in a successful weight-loss program. Studies of the effect of exercise in addition to diet show that exercise does not produce a great deal of added weight loss; most often, however, individuals who succeed in long-term weight reduction exercise regularly. Studies of body composition show that diet alone reduces total body weight, fat mass, and lean body mass. Diet plus exercise, on the other hand, may produce a similar decrease in total weight but a much greater decrease in fat mass, because lean body mass actually increases. An increase in lean body mass may allow the individual to liberalize an otherwise unacceptably restricted diet. Many patients who are too focused on total weight loss and who engage in a vigorous exercise program are frustrated, because they do not lose enough weight. For such individuals, it may help to measure body composition by underwater weighing to demonstrate that they have lost substantial fat mass and gained lean body mass. Although most experts advocate aerobic training, recent evidence suggests that a balanced program of strength training and aerobic exercise may be better than either alone.

21. What medicines should be prescribed to aid in weight loss?

Various medications have been used to induce weight loss. In the past, amphetamines, thyroid hormone, and diuretics were used for this purpose, but they have far too many side effects to be acceptable. Phenylpropanolamine (PPA) (Dexatrim, Acutrim) is an over-the-counter aid for weight loss. Controlled data suggest that PPA has a statistically significant but quantitatively small effect on body weight. In a recent survey by *Consumer Reports,* less than 5% of people who used PPA were satisfied with the effects. Half were dissatisfied, and many experienced troubling side effects. Various drugs that affect serotonin metabolism have been used in clinical trials. Fenfluramine, perhaps the best studied, has been shown to afford a greater degree of weight loss than diet alone. This weight loss is maintained as long as the drug is continued; the added weight lost returns when the drug is discontinued.

A number of new medications—including pancreatic lipase inhibitors, which inhibit the absorption of dietary fat; atypical beta-agonists, which increase thermogenesis; and neurotransmitter reuptake blockers, which reduce appetite—are in clinical trials. Each shows promise, although none is without side effects. The central problem with drug therapy for obesity is that it must be lifelong; to date, the long-term risk-benefit ratio of such compounds has not been established. At this time, therefore, drug therapy for obesity cannot be advocated.

22. What role do education and psychosocial support play in the treatment of obesity?
The patient should be encouraged to become educated specifically about nutrient content of foods, individual caloric intake, and trigger patterns that lead to increased eating. Often the failure of a dietary program occurs during periods of high stress. Eating is a pleasurable experience for most people, and when life is difficult, they may use it for comfort. One of the most important components of a weight-loss program is follow-up by a physician, health care team, or weight-loss group. Groups such as Weight Watchers and TOPS have worked well for many individuals. The article in *Consumer Reports* is well written for lay persons and reviews the efficacy, cost, and advantages and disadvantages of several proprietary and nonproprietary weight-loss programs.[5]

23. Should liposuction be advocated for obese patients?
In the only controlled trial, weight lost by liposuction was regained. Sometimes the adipose tissue reaccumulated in the same site, other times it reaccumulated elsewhere. Liposuction cannot be advocated as a weight-loss strategy for patients with medically significant obesity.

24. What is morbid obesity?
Morbid obesity has been variably defined as weight that is 100% or 100 lbs above ideal. Another definition is obesity that has resulted in a substantial compromise in health. Most morbidly obese people have sleep apnea and hypoventilation with or without right-heart failure. Their relative risk of sudden death is 15–30 times higher than in lean controls. Affected individuals have a significant medical problem with a high risk of dying in the short term. Although the issue is controversial, many experts advocate aggressive weight-loss therapy in morbidly obese individuals, including the use of very-low-calorie diets and surgical treatment.

25. What is a very-low-calorie diet (VLCD)? When should its use be considered?
A VLCD is a diet of 800 kcal/day, which produces rapid weight loss. Most patients lose 1.5–2.5 kg/wk on a VLCD. Such diets should be administered by an experienced team in a supervised manner; in this setting, serious complications are unusual. The most common of the complications is cholelithiasis. General physicians probably should not be involved in the administration of VLCD, unless they are prepared to work with someone with more experience or to engage in such therapy regularly. The long-term results with VLCDs are no better than with other diet programs. For this reason VLCDs have limited usefulness and should be used only in individuals with a BMI > 30.

26. What mechanical methods are available for consideration in the treatment of morbidly obese individuals?
For patients who are morbidly obese and suffer severe medical complications from obesity, gastric operations that result in a small gastric pouch (gastroplasty) or gastric bypass (to bypass absorption of food) may be undertaken.

For patients with a BMI > 40, surgical therapy may offer the best long-term chance for reduced body weight. Surgery should be considered only after more traditional approaches have failed and after the patient has been evaluated by a multidisciplinary team with experience in this area. The surgeon must have extensive and ongoing experience with such procedures for the patient to have the best chance at a good outcome. Placing the patient on a VLCD preoperatively may improve surgical outcome by reducing hepatic volume and thereby improving visualization of the stomach, as well as by reducing perioperative pulmonary complications.

CONTROVERSY

27. Does weight loss reduce the morbidity and mortality associated with obesity?
Although increased body weight is associated with adverse health consequences, it is not clear that weight loss is accompanied by a concurrent decrease in such consequences. Successful

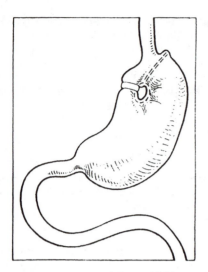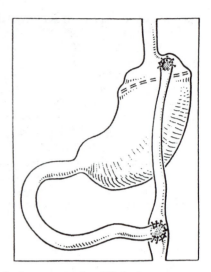

Gastroplasty (left) and gastric bypass (right) operations for the treatment of morbid obesity.

weight loss clearly lowers blood pressure, improves insulin action and blood glucose control, puts less stress on joints, and improves the lipid profile. However, the effects on overall mortality and morbidity are less clear. Numerous large, population-based studies, including NHANES, MRFIT, and the Framingham Study, have shown that weight loss is associated with a higher mortality rate than weight stability, perhaps because weight loss is usually associated with weight regain. The real culprit may be weight cycling (yo-yo dieting). It is unfortunate that, despite billions of dollars spent on weight-loss products, we still do not have a single prospective, randomized trial designed to look at the long-term health effects of weight loss. Until such a trial is done, a reasonable approach is to encourage patients to develop good eating habits and to engage in regular exercise; to discourage inappropriate weight-loss strategies; and to focus less on the cosmetics of obesity and more on a healthy lifestyle.

BIBLIOGRAPHY

1. Bray GA: Drug treatment of obesity. Am J Clin Nutr 55:538S–544S, 1992.
2. Gortmaker SL, Must A, Perrin JM, et al: Social and economic consequences of overweight in adolescence and young adulthood. N Engl J Med 329:1008–1012, 1993.
3. Grundy SM: Gastrointestinal surgery for severe obesity. Ann Intern Med 115:956–961, 1991.
4. Kuczmarski RJ: Prevalence of overweight and weight gain in the United States. Am J Clin Nutr 55:495S–502S, 1992.
5. Losing weight: What works, what doesn't. Consumer Reports June:347–357, 1993.
6. Manson JE, Colditz GA, Stampfer MJ, et al: A prospective study of obesity and risk of coronary heart disease in women. N Engl J Med 322:882–889, 1990.
7. Must A, Jacques PF, Dallai GE, et al: Long-term morbidity and mortality of overweight adolescents. N Engl J Med 327:1350–1355, 1992.
8. National Institutes of Health Consensus Development Panel on the Health Implications of Obesity: Health implications of obesity. Ann Intern Med 103:147, 1985.
9. National Task Force on the Prevention and Treatment of Obesity: Very low-calorie diets. JAMA 270:967–974, 1993.
10. Technology Assessment Conference Panel: Methods for voluntary weight loss and control: Technology Assessment Conference statement. Ann Intern Med 116:942–949, 1992; 119(7 Pt2):641–764, 1993.
11. Wadden TA, Van Itallie TB, Blackburn GL: Responsible and irresponsible use of very-low-calorie diets in the treatment of obesity. JAMA 263:83, 1990.
12. Wing RR: Behavioral treatment of severe obesity. Am J Clin Nutr 55:545S–551S, 1992.

II.   Bone and Mineral Disorders

9. OSTEOPOROSIS

Michael T. McDermott, M.D.

1. What is osteoporosis?
Osteoporosis is a predisposition to skeletal fractures resulting primarily from a reduction in total or regional bone mass.

2. What fractures are most commonly associated with osteoporosis?
Fractures of the vertebrae, the hips, and the distal radius (Colles' fractures) are characteristic, but any fracture may occur.

3. What are the complications of osteoporotic fractures?
Pain and disability result from fractures of any type. Vertebral fractures also cause loss of height and anterior spinal kyphosis. Hip fractures are associated with increased mortality due primarily to thromboembolic disease.

4. What are the risk factors for low bone mass?

Family history	Cigarette smoking
Slender build	Excessive alcohol consumption
Fair skin	Excessive caffeine consumption
Early menopause	Medications (corticosteroids, levothyroxine,
Sedentary lifestyle	anticonvulsants, heparin)
Low calcium intake	

5. How is bone mass currently measured?
Standard roentgenography is inadequate for accurate bone mass assessment. Single-photon absorptiometry, dual-photon absorptiometry, CT scan, and dual-energy x-ray absorptiometry are more recently developed techniques that offer far greater accuracy and reproducibility and may be used to evaluate multiple skeletal sites.

6. What are the accepted indications for bone mass measurement?
    1. Decision making regarding the initiation or continuation of estrogen replacement therapy.
    2. Evaluation of osteopenia or vertebral deformities discovered on routine radiographs.
    3. The presence of modifiable conditions, such as steroid therapy and hyperparathyroidism, that may cause osteopenia.

7. What other disorders must be considered as a cause of low bone mass?

Osteomalacia	Multiple myeloma
Osteogenesis imperfecta	Rheumatoid arthritis
Hyperparathyroidism	Renal failure
Hyperthyroidism	Idiopathic hypercalciuria
Cushing's syndrome	

8. What is the function of bone remodeling?
Remodeling is an adaptation to mechanical stresses. Osteoclasts continually resorb existing bone. Osteoblasts form new bone by secreting osteoid, a protein matrix that is subsequently mineralized by calcium and phosphate from the extracellular fluid. Remodeling maintains skeletal strength and integrity.

9. What modalities are available for the prevention and treatment of osteoporosis?
The prevention and treatment of osteoporosis involve interventions that inhibit bone resorption or stimulate bone formation. Antiresorptive agents include calcium, estrogen, calcitonin, and bisphosphonates. Formation-stimulating agents include fluoride, parathyroid hormone, androgens, and growth hormone. Exercise favorably effects both resorption and formation.

10. What are the best sources of dietary calcium?
The major sources of bioavailable calcium are dairy products and calcium fortified citrus juices.

Source	Approximate Calcium Content
Milk	300 mg/cup
Cheese	200 mg/oz
Yogurt	350 mg/cup
Citrus juice with calcium	300 mg/cup

Patients should be asked about their use of these foods. If dietary calcium consumption is inadequate, calcium supplements should be added to achieve the desired intake.

11. What are the current recommendations for oral calcium intake?
Young women and men should consume 1,000 mg of calcium daily. Postmenopausal women and patients with osteoporosis should receive 1,500 mg daily.

12. What is the role of estrogen replacement therapy in osteoporosis?
Estrogens inhibit bone resorption, moderately increase bone mass, and reduce the risk of spine, hip and wrist fractures. Estrogens are the most effective means of preventing postmenopausal osteoporosis, and recent studies indicate that they are also useful in treating established osteoporosis.

13. How effective is calcitonin in the management of osteoporosis?
Calcitonin directly inhibits osteoclasts. Treated patients show a slight gain in bone mass similar to that seen with estrogens. Skeletal fractures also appear to be reduced. In addition, calcitonin reduces pain significantly in 80% of patients with fractures. The mechanism appears to be release of a central nervous system opioid.

14. Are bisphosphonates effective agents for osteoporosis?
Cyclic bisphosphonates, with or without phosphate, have also been shown to increase bone mass modestly and to reduce the incidence of fractures over a 2-year treatment course. Concern about longer-term effects exists, but results thus far appear promising.

15. What is the status of fluoride therapy?
Sodium fluoride stimulates bone formation, resulting in significant and progressive increases in bone mass. The bone is structurally abnormal, however, and studies have failed to show a reduction in skeletal fractures. Many experts feel that fluoride should be avoided until such issues are resolved by ongoing research.

16. What is the role of exercise?
Exercise stimulates bone formation and inhibits resorption. It also may reduce the incidence and severity of falls by improving muscular strength and coordination. Both aerobic and weight training are beneficial.

17. How can falls be prevented?

The major risk factors for falls include the use of sedatives, sensorium-altering drugs and antihypertensive medications, visual impairment, proprioceptive loss, and lower-extremity disability. Minimizing modifiable risk factors and removing obstacles to ambulation in the home are inexpensive and effective measures for reducing fractures due to falls.

18. How do steroids cause osteoporosis?

Corticosteroids in supraphysiologic doses directly inhibit bone formation and indirectly increase bone resorption through antagonism of intestinal calcium absorption and promotion of renal calcium excretion. Because of these dual effects significant osteoporosis may develop within 6 months of initiating corticosteroid therapy.

19. How can steroid-induced osteoporosis be prevented and treated?

Patients on steroid therapy should receive calcium (1,500 mg) and vitamin D (400 U) each day. If urinary calcium excretion exceeds 300 mg/day, a thiazide diuretic may be added. Both calcitonin and bisphosphonates have been reported to reduce or prevent bone loss. As an alternative, bone-sparing steroids such as deflazacort are currently under investigation.

BIBLIOGRAPHY

1. Civitelli R, Gonnelli S, Zacchel F, et al: Bone turnover in postmenopausal osteoporosis. Effect of calcitonin treatment. J Clin Invest 82:1268–1274, 1988.
2. Consensus Development Conference: Diagnosis, prophylaxis, and treatment of osteoporosis. Am J Med 94:646–650, 1993.
3. Grisso JA, Kelsey JL, Strom BL, et al: Risk factors for falls as a cause of hip fracture in women. N Engl J Med 324:1326–1331, 1991.
4. Heaney RP, Baylink DJ, Johnston CC Jr, et al: Fluoride therapy for the vertebral crush fracture syndrome: A status report. Ann Intern Med 111:678–680, 1989.
5. Johnston CC Jr, Slemenda CW, Melton LJ: Clinical use of bone densitometry. N Engl J Med 324:1105–1108, 1991.
6. Johnston CC Jr, Miller JZ, Slemenda CW, et al: Calcium supplementation and increases in bone mineral density in children. N Engl J Med 327:82–87, 1992.
7. Lufkin EG, Wahner HW, O'Fallon WM, et al: Treatment of postmenopausal osteoporosis with transdermal estrogen. Ann Intern Med 117:1–9, 1992.
8. Lukert BP, Raisz LG: Glucocorticoid-induced osteoporosis: pathogenesis and management. Ann Intern Med 112:352–364, 1990.
9. Marx CW, Dailey GE III, Cheney C, et al: Do estrogens improve bone mineral density in osteoporotic women over age 65? J Bone Miner Res 7:1275–1279, 1992.
10. Overgaard K, Hansen MA, Jensen SB, Christiansen C: Effect of salcatonin given intranasally on bone mass and fracture rates in established osteoporosis: A dose-response study. BMJ 305:556–561, 1992.
11. Prince RL, Smith M, Dick IM, et al: Prevention of postmenopausal osteoporosis: A comparative study of exercise, calcium supplementation, and hormone-replacement therapy. N Engl J Med 325:1189–1195, 1991.
12. Raisz LG: Local and systemic factors in the pathogenesis of osteoporosis. N Engl J Med 318:818–828, 1988.
13. Reid IR, Ames RW, Evans MC, et al: Effect of calcium supplementation on bone loss in postmenopausal women. N Engl J Med 328:460–464, 1993.
14. Riggs BL, Hodgson SF, O'Fallon WM, et al: Effect of fluoride treatment on the fracture rate in postmenopausal women with osteoporosis. N Engl J Med 322:802–809, 1990.
15. Riggs BL, Melton LJ III: The prevention and treatment of osteoporosis. N Engl J Med 327:620–627, 1992.
16. Sambrook P, Birmingham J, Kelly P, et al: Prevention of corticosteroid osteoporosis: A comparison of calcium, calcitriol, and calcitonin. N Engl J Med 328:1747–1752, 1993.
17. Storm T, Thamsborg G, Steiniche T, et al: Effect of intermittent cyclical etidronate therapy on bone mass fracure rate in women with postmenopausal osteoporosis. N Engl J Med 322:1265–1271, 1990.
18. Tinetti ME, Speechley M, Ginter SF: Risk factors for falls among elderly persons living in the community. N Engl J Med 319:1701–1707, 1988.

10. OSTEOMALACIA AND RICKETS

William E. Duncan, M.D., Ph.D., COL, MC

1. What are osteomalacia and rickets?

Osteomalacia and rickets are terms that describe the clinical, histologic, and radiologic abnormalities of bone that are associated with more than 50 different diseases and conditions. Osteomalacia is a disorder of mature bone in which mineralization of newly formed osteoid (the bone protein matrix) is inadequate or delayed. Rickets is a disease of children in which defective mineralization occurs both in the bones and in the cartilage of the epiphyseal growth plates. Thus, rickets is associated with growth retardation and a variety of skeletal deformities not typically seen in osteomalacia. Osteomalacia is the predominant histologic lesion in rachitic bones. Although rickets and osteomalacia were initially described separately and thought of as distinct clinical entities, it is now realized that the same pathologic processes may result in either disorder, depending upon whether a growing or nongrowing skeleton is involved.

2. Why is it important to know about these bone diseases?

In the United States at the beginning of the 20th century, rickets caused by a deficiency of vitamin D was common in urban areas. In the 1920s, an appreciation of the antirachitic properties of sunlight and cod liver oil (which contains vitamin D) virtually eliminated this bone disease. With the development of effective treatments for previously fatal diseases (such as chronic renal failure) and with an improved understanding of both vitamin D and mineral metabolism, many additional syndromes with osteomalacia or rickets as a feature have subsequently been recognized. In addition, in a significant number of adult women with osteoporosis, osteomalacia may be an unsuspected component of their bone disease.

3. List the causes of osteomalacia and rickets.

The primary abnormality in osteomalacia and rickets is defective mineralization of the bone matrix. The primary bone mineral is hydroxyapatite ($Ca_{10} (PO_4)_6 (OH)_2$). Thus, any disease that limits the availability of calcium or phosphorus may result in osteomalacia or rickets. The causes of osteomalacia and rickets fall into three categories: (1) those associated with abnormalities of vitamin D metabolism or action; (2) those associated with abnormalities of phosphorus metabolism; and (3) a small group of disorders with normal vitamin D and mineral metabolism.

4. What disease processes interfere with the metabolism of vitamin D?

The disease processes associated with abnormal vitamin D metabolism or action (see table) are best understood with a knowledge of the normal metabolism of vitamin D (see figure).

Because vitamin D is produced in the skin, except when exposure to sunlight or the intake of vitamin D–fortified milk and dairy products is limited, nutritional deficiency of vitamin D is rarely found in the United States. The elderly are particularly at risk for vitamin D deficiency because of: (1) an age-related decrease in the dermal synthesis of vitamin D; (2) impaired hepatic and renal hydroxylation of vitamin D; and (3) a diminished intestinal responsiveness to 1,25-dihydroxyvitamin D.

Also at risk for vitamin D deficiency are persons with intestinal malabsorption associated with diseases of the small intestine, hepatobiliary tree, and pancreas. Celiac disease or sprue, regional enteritis, intestinal bypass surgery, partial gastrectomy, chronic liver disease, primary biliary cirrhosis, and pancreatic insufficiency have been associated with the development of osteomalacia.

Two extremely rare syndromes are also associated with rickets. Vitamin D–dependent rickets (VDDR) type I is associated with an almost complete absence of renal 25-hydroxyvitamin

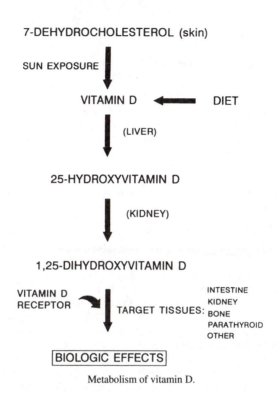

7-DEHYDROCHOLESTEROL (skin)

SUN EXPOSURE

VITAMIN D ⬅ DIET

(LIVER)

25-HYDROXYVITAMIN D

(KIDNEY)

1,25-DIHYDROXYVITAMIN D

VITAMIN D RECEPTOR

TARGET TISSUES: INTESTINE KIDNEY BONE PARATHYROID OTHER

BIOLOGIC EFFECTS

Metabolism of vitamin D.

D-1α-hydroxylase activity. VDDR type II is caused by a defective vitamin D receptor resulting in end-organ resistance to 1,25-dihydroxyvitamin D. Anticonvulsant drugs (e.g., phenytoin, phenobarbital) may interfere with the action of 1,25-dihydroxyvitamin D in the peripheral tissues and accelerate the hepatic metabolism of this steroid hormone.

Conditions Associated with Osteomalacia and Rickets

CONDITION	MECHANISM*
Abnormal Vitamin D Metabolism or Action	
Nutritional deficiency	Vitamin D deficiency
Malabsorption	Vitamin D deficiency
Primary biliary cirrhosis	Malabsorption of vitamin D
Chronic renal disease	Impaired 1-hydroxylation
Chronic liver disease	Defective 25 hydroxylation
VDDR type I	1-Hydroxylase deficiency
VDDR type II	Abnormal vitamin D receptor
Drugs (phenytoin, barbiturates, cholestyramine)	Increased catabolism and/or excretion
Phosphate Deficiency or Renal Phosphate Wasting	
Diminished phosphate intake	Phosphate deficiency
Excess aluminum hydroxide intake	Increased binding of intestinal phosphate
X-linked hypophosphatemic rickets	Renal phosphate transport defect
Tumor-induced osteomalacia	Renal phosphate transport defect
Miscellaneous renal tubular defects	Renal phosphate transport defect
(renal tubular acidosis, Fanconi syndrome)	

Table continued on following page.

Conditions Associated with Osteomalacia and Rickets (Continued)

CONDITIONS	MECHANISM*
Normal Vitamin D and Phosphate Metabolism	
Hypophosphatasia	Alkaline phosphatase deficiency
Drugs (bisphosphonates, fluoride, aluminum)	Inhibition of mineralization or stimulation of matrix synthesis
Osteogenesis imperfecta	Abnormal bone collagen
Fibrogenesis imperfecta ossium	Defective bone matrix

*Although only one mechanism for osteomalacia and rickets is given for each condition, other mechanisms may also contribute to the bone disease.
VDDR = vitamin D–dependent rickets.

5. What conditions associated with abnormalities of phosphate metabolism result in osteomalacia or rickets?

The second category of disorders associated with osteomalacia and rickets is a heterogenous group of diseases resulting from a deficiency of phosphate or an abnormality of renal phosphate handling. Nutritional phosphate deficiency, decreased intestinal absorption of phosphate due to binding by ingested phosphate binders such as aluminum hydroxide, or renal phosphate wasting due to renal tubular acidosis may result in osteomalacia or rickets.

Hypophosphatemic rickets (also called vitamin D–resistant rickets) is the most common inherited form of rickets in man and is transmitted as an X-linked dominant trait. The abnormal gene for this disorder has been localized to the short arm of the X chromosome. The main abnormality is renal phosphate wasting and decreased renal synthesis of 1,25-dihydroxyvitamin D. Tumor-induced osteomalacia is an uncommon syndrome in which usually benign neoplasms (frequently of a mesenchymal nature) are found in association with nonfamilial acquired osteomalacia. These tumors appear to elaborate an as yet unidentified humoral factor that is responsible for renal phosphate wasting and impaired renal production of 1,25-dihydroxyvitamin D. The tumors usually responsible for this disease include sarcomas, hemangiomas, and giant cell tumors of bone and, rarely, carcinoma of the breast and prostate.

6. How does chronic renal failure cause osteomalacia and rickets?

Chronic renal failure is associated with three kinds of bone disease: osteomalacia or rickets, osteitis fibrosa cystica (due to long-standing secondary hyperparathyroidism), and a combination of these two bone diseases (also termed mixed renal osteodystrophy). Rickets and osteomalacia are usually late findings in the course of the kidney disease and are rarely seen before patients begin dialysis. Rickets and osteomalacia are caused by aluminum intoxication from aluminum-containing antacids used as phosphate binders or from use of an aluminum-contaminated dialysate, low circulating 1,25-dihydroxyvitamin D concentrations, and possibly the chronic metabolic acidosis associated with the renal failure.

7. What are the clinical findings associated with osteomalacia and rickets?

In adults, osteomalacia may be asymptomatic. When symptomatic, osteomalacia may present with diffuse skeletal pain, proximal muscle weakness, and sometimes even muscle wasting. The muscle weakness often involves the proximal muscles of the lower extremities and may result in a waddling gait. The bone pain is described as dull and aching and is usually located in the back, hips, knees, legs and at sites of fractures. The pain is increased by physical activity or by palpation. Fractures may result from only minor trauma.

In children with rickets, because of the impaired calcification of cartilage at the growth plates, additional clinical manifestations are often observed. Especially prominent are widening of the metaphyses (the growth zone between the epiphysis and the diaphysis), slowed growth, and various skeletal deformities. The effects of rickets are greatest where the growth of bone is most rapid. Since the rate of growth of the skeleton varies with age, the manifestations of rickets likewise vary with age. One of the earliest signs of rickets in the infant is craniotabes (abnormal softness of the skull). In older infants and young children, thickening of the forearm at the wrist and of the costochondral junctions (also known as the rachitic rosary) may be manifestations of rickets. Harrison's groove, a lateral indentation of the chest wall at the site of attachment of the diaphragm may also be present. In older children, bowing of the tibia and fibula may be observed. At any age, if the affected individual is hypocalcemic, paresthesias, tetany, and seizures may also be present.

8. Describe the biochemical findings associated with osteomalacia and rickets.

The laboratory abnormalities associated with osteomalacia or rickets depend on the underlying defect or process causing the bone disease. For example, the biochemical abnormalities observed in conditions associated with the abnormal metabolism of vitamin D are predicted by understanding the body's response to hypocalcemia and a knowledge of the vitamin D metabolic pathway. Thus in patients with nutritional vitamin D deficiency or malabsorption, the low vitamin D concentrations result in a low to low-normal serum calcium concentration, which serves as a stimulus for increased secretion of parathyroid hormone (secondary hyperparathyroidism). This hyperparathyroid state in turn causes an increased renal excretion of phosphate, a low serum phosphate, an elevated alkaline phosphatase, and a reduced urinary calcium excretion.

Depending on the abnormality of vitamin D metabolism, different vitamin D metabolite patterns will be observed. In nutritional vitamin D deficiency, 25-hydroxyvitamin D concentrations are low. In VDDR type I, where there is a deficiency of the renal 25-hydroxyvitamin D-1α-hydroxylase enzyme, normal or increased serum 25-hydroxyvitamin D and low or undetectable serum 1,25-dihydroxyvitamin D concentrations are observed. On the other hand, in VDDR type II, which is caused by a mutation of the vitamin D receptor resulting in resistance of target organs to 1,25-dihydroxyvitamin D, concentrations of both 25-hydroxyvitamin D and 1,25-dihydroxyvitamin D are elevated.

The hallmarks of the hypophosphatemic and osteomalacia syndromes are fasting hypophosphatemia and renal phosphate wasting (as assessed by a decrease in the maximum renal tubular reabsorption of phosphate/glomerular filtration rate [TmP/GFR]). Serum calcium and parathyroid hormone concentrations are usually normal. Inexplicably, serum 1,25-dihydroxyvitamin D concentrations are inappropriately low for the degree of hypophosphatemia (which is normally a stimulus for increased renal 1α-hydroxylation of 25-hydroxyvitamin D).

In the third group of disorders causing osteomalacia and rickets (those with normal vitamin D and phosphate metabolism), there are few associated biochemical abnormalities. In patients with hypophosphatasia, an abnormally low alkaline phosphatase concentration is usually observed. Serum calcium, 25-hydroxyvitamin D, 1,25-dihydroxyvitamin D, and parathyroid hormone concentrations in patients with this disorder are normal. About half of these subjects are hyperphosphatemic due to an increased TmP/GFR. Serum concentrations of calcium and phosphate in fibrogenesis imperfecta ossium are normal but the serum alkaline phosphatase activity is usually increased.

9. What are the radiographic findings associated with osteomalacia and rickets?

The histologic and biochemical abnormalities associated with rickets and osteomalacia are usually found before radiographic abnormalities are observed. The most common radiographic change seen in patients with osteomalacia is a reduction in skeletal density (generalized osteopenia). Pseudofractures (also called Looser zones or Milkman fractures) or complete fractures may also be observed. Pseudofractures are straight transverse radiolucent bands ranging from a few millimeters to several centimeters in length, usually perpendicular to the surface of the bones. They are most often bilateral and are particularly common in the femur, pelvis, and small bones of the hands and feet.

Abnormalities, including fraying of the metaphyses of the long bones, widening of the unmineralized epiphyseal growth plates, and bowing of the legs, are observed in children with rickets. Skeletal deformities in patients with rickets may persist into adulthood.

Patients with osteomalacia may have additional radiographic findings due to the associated secondary hyperparathyroidism. Such findings may include subperiosteal resorption of the phalanges, loss of the lamina dura of the teeth, widening of the spaces at the symphysis pubis and sacroiliac joints, and the presence of brown tumors or bone cysts.

10. List the histologic features of osteomalacia.

The two diagnostic bone biopsy features of osteomalacia are the presence of wide osteoid seams and an increased mineralization lag time (the time necessary for newly deposited matrix to mineralize). The mineralization lag time is assessed clinically by administration of two short courses of oral tetracycline given several weeks apart. Because the tetracycline is deposited at the mineralization front, the lag time may be determined by measuring the distance between the two fluorescent tetracycline bands in the biopsied bone. Depending on the cause of the osteomalacia, hyperparathyroid bone changes may occur. Because of the varied clinical signs and symptoms, radiographic findings, and biochemical abnormalities associated with osteomalacia and rickets, none of these tests or findings is pathognomonic for these bone diseases. The bone biopsy remains the ''gold standard'' in establishing the diagnosis of rickets and osteomalacia. The evaluation of the bone biopsy must be performed by experienced personnel.

11. Describe the therapy for osteomalacia and rickets.

In patients with osteomalacia and rickets caused by an abnormality of vitamin D metabolism, the goal of therapy is to correct the hypocalcemia and the deficiency of active vitamin D metabolites by administration of calcium salts and vitamin D preparations. In the United States, vitamin D_2 (ergocalciferol), vitamin D_3 (cholecalciferol), 25-hydroxyvitamin D (calcifediol), 1,25-dihydroxyvitamin D (calcitriol), and dihydrotachysterol are available. Each of these preparations has a different half-life and potency. The choice of vitamin D preparation and dose is determined by the underlying pathologic defect of vitamin D metabolism. For example, in patients with vitamin D deficiency, 5,000–10,000 IU of ergocalciferol (along with 1 gram of elemental calcium) per day is often sufficient to heal the osteomalacia. In contrast, in the treatment of the osteomalacia associated with VDDR type II, where there is a profound resistance to the effects of vitamin D, administration of the most potent vitamin D metabolite, 1,25-dihydroxyvitamin D, in doses up to 60 µg/day (an extraordinarily high dose) along with large doses of oral calcium is necessary. In severe cases, high-dose intravenous calcium infusions are required to heal the rickets in patients with VDDR type II.

In the treatment of hypophosphatemic rickets, both phosphate supplements and calcitriol are effective in healing the bone disease. Tumor removal or irradiation is required to treat tumor-induced osteomalacia.

In chronic renal failure with aluminum-induced osteomalacia, aluminum is removed from the affected bone by treatment with the chelating agent desferoxamine. The osteomalacia can then be treated by calcium together with either 25-hydroxyvitamin D or 1,25-dihydroxyvitamin D. Osteomalacia associated with renal tubular acidosis is treated with vitamin D and with bicarbonate to correct the acidosis.

12. What are the complications of treatment with vitamin D or vitamin D metabolites?

When using high doses of vitamin D or one of the potent vitamin D metabolites, it is important to monitor carefully for the development of hypercalcemia. Mild hypercalcemia may be asymptomatic. However, severely hypercalcemic patients may complain of anorexia, nausea, vomiting, weight loss, headache, constipation, polyuria, polydipsia, and altered mental status. Impaired renal function, nephrocalcinosis, nephrolithiasis, and even death may eventually ensue. Should vitamin D intoxication occur, all calcium supplements and vitamin D preparations should be immediately discontinued and therapy for the hypercalcemia instituted.

BIBLIOGRAPHY

1. Bardin CW (ed): Current Therapy in Endocrinology and Metabolism, 5th ed. St Louis, Mosby-Year Book, Inc., 1994.
2. Bingham CT, Fitzpatrick LA: Noninvasive testing in the diagnosis of osteomalacia. Am J Med 95:519, 1993.

3. Bliziotes M, Yergey AL, Nanes MS, et al: Absent intestinal response to calciferols in hereditary resistance to 1,25-dihydroxyvitamin D: Documentation and effective therapy with high-dose intravenous calcium infusions. J Clin Endocrinol Metab 66:294, 1988.

4. Drezner MK: Vitamin D–resistant rickets/osteomalacia. Endocrinologist 3:392, 1991.

5. Favus MJ (ed): Primer on the Metabolic Bone Diseases and Disorders of Mineral Metabolism, 2nd ed. New York, Raven Press, 1993.

6. Harvey JN, Gray C, Belchetz PE: Oncogenous osteomalacia and malignancy. Clin Endocrinol 37:379, 1992.

7. Hutchison FN, Bell NH: Osteomalacia and rickets. Semin Nephrol 2:127, 1992.

8. Parfitt AM: Osteomalcia and related disorders. In Avioli LV, Krane SM (eds): Metabolic Bone Diseases and Clinically Related Disorders, 2nd ed. Philadelphia, W.B. Saunders, 1990, p 329.

9. Pitt MJ: Rickets and osteomalacia are still around. Radiol Clin North Am 29:97, 1991.

10. Reichel H, Koeffler HP, Norman AW: The role of the vitamin D endocrine system in health and disease. N Engl J Med 320:980, 1989.

11. PAGET'S DISEASE OF BONE

William E. Duncan, M.D., Ph.D., COL, MC

1. What is Paget's disease of bone?

Paget's disease is characterized by an abnormality of bone architecture resulting from an imbalance between osteoblastic bone formation and osteoclastic bone resorption. Sir James Paget first described the disease in 1877. Although he used the term osteitis deformans, we now know that Paget's disease of bone is not an inflammation of bone (osteitis) and only rarely results in deformity.

2. How do you diagnose Paget's disease?

The diagnosis is generally based on the presence of a combination of clinical manifestations, radiographic signs, and characteristic biochemical changes. Although histologic examination of pagetic bone is diagnostic for the disease, bone biopsy is unnecessary and too invasive for routine use, unless the diagnosis of Paget's disease is unclear or osteogenic sarcoma or metastatic carcinoma has to be excluded.

3. What are the signs and symptoms of Paget's disease?

The majority of patients with Paget's disease are asymptomatic, and the diagnosis is suspected from radiographs done for other reasons or from an unexpected elevation of the serum alkaline phosphatase concentration. The most common symptom of Paget's disease, however, is bone or joint pain. Headache, bony deformity, skull enlargement, fracture, change in skin temperature over an involved bone, high-output congestive heart failure, and entrapment neuropathies that cause loss of hearing or other neurologic deficits are much less common. Neurologic deficits arise from bony impingement on the brain and cranial nerves exiting from the skull, spinal nerve entrapment, and direct pressure of pagetic vertebrae on the spinal cord. Deformity is usually seen in patients with longstanding Paget's disease. Most commonly the skull, clavicles, and long bones are deformed and exhibit both an increase in size and an abnormal contour. There is speculation that Ludwig van Beethoven's hearing loss, headaches, and progressive hyperostosis frontalis were the result of longstanding Paget's disease of bone.

Complications Associated with Paget's Disease of Bone

Bone pain
Bone deformity
Secondary arthritis adjacent to pagetic bone
Neurologic abnormalities
Spinal stenosis
Hearing loss and other cranial nerve palsies
Radiculopathy
Obstructive hydrocephalus
Cardiovascular complications
Increased blood flow to involved bone
Increased cardiac output
Vascular and aortic valve calcifications
Fracture
Malignant transformation
Immobilization hypercalcemia

4. Describe the radiographic abnormalities seen with Paget's disease.

Paget's disease of bone appears to progress through several distinct phases: the early osteolytic phase, in which osteoclastic bone resorption predominates; a phase of mixed osteoclastic and osteoblastic overactivity; and subsequently a less active period of bone remodeling and marked sclerosis. The radiographic appearance of involved bone differs with each phase. About 1–2% of patients exhibit a purely lytic phase of the disorder. The characteristic findings of this phase are an advancing wedge-shaped resorption front at either end of the long tubular bones and large circumscribed osteolytic lesions (termed osteoporosis circumscripta) in the skull. During the mixed phase of the disease, both osteoclastic bone resorption and osteoblastic bone formation may be appreciated on radiographs. Evolution of osteolytic lesions into the osteoblastic phase may require years or even decades, during which the affected bone may become sclerotic and enlarged or demonstrate bowing deformities, incomplete transverse fractures (pseudofractures), or complete pathologic fractures. The osteoblastic phase in the skull is characterized by thickening of the calvarium and a patchy increase in bone density that gives the skull a "cotton wool" appearance. Sometimes the sclerotic bone changes are so extensive that they may be confused with metastatic disease. Both metastatic cancer (e.g., prostate cancer) and Paget's disease are common in the elderly and may coexist in the same patient.

The metabolic activity of osteoblastic pagetic bone lesions is most easily assessed by radionuclide scanning. The active pagetic bone lesions avidly take up technetium-labeled bisphosphonate. CT and MRI scans add little in the work-up of patients with uncomplicated Paget's disease.

5. Give the laboratory abnormalities associated with Paget's disease.

The laboratory values that are abnormal in Paget's disease reflect either increased bone formation or increased bone resorption. Unless a patient with widespread Paget's disease is immobilized, the serum calcium and phosphate concentrations are normal. The tests that reflect increased osteoblastic function are the concentrations of serum alkaline phosphatase and osteocalcin, whereas those reflecting increased bone resorption are the urinary levels of hydroxyproline and pyridinium-collagen crosslinks. To determine accurately the urinary excretion of hydroxyproline, patients should be placed on a meat-free diet; a 24-hour urine collection is required.

When disease is primarily lytic, the alkaline phosphatase concentration may be normal. Otherwise the activity of serum alkaline phosphatase generally parallels the indices of bone resorption. For these reasons, the concentration of serum alkaline phosphatase is the simplest and least expensive laboratory test with which to follow the course of Paget's disease and its response to treatment. Of interest, a markedly elevated concentration of alkaline phosphatase (e.g., 10 times the upper limit of normal) is usually associated with Paget's disease involving the skull, whereas widespread disease in the rest of the skeleton may be associated with a more modest elevation. In patients with increased concentrations of alkaline phosphatase, liver disease should be excluded since this enzyme is abundant in both liver and bone. If liver-specific tests, such as 5'-nucleotidase or gamma-glutamyl transferase, are normal, however, it is most likely that the elevated alkaline phosphatase originates from bone.

6. What are the histologic findings in bone affected by Paget's disease?

The early lesions of Paget's disease are characterized by increased numbers of large, multinucleated osteoclasts, some containing up to 100 nuclei. In the mixed osteolytic-osteoblastic phase, large numbers of active osteoblasts form bone at sites of prior osteoclastic resorption. The intense osteoblastic reaction seen in this phase is characterized by the deposition of structurally weakened bone in a chaotic fashion (the so-called mosaic pattern) rather than in the orderly lamellar pattern of uninvolved bone.

7. Which patients are most likely to have Paget's disease?

The incidence of Paget's disease varies with age, gender, and geographic location. Although Paget's disease may present in younger individuals, it is most common in patients over 50 years of age. Men are more commonly affected than women (male-to-female ratio of about 3:2).

Although there is no definite hereditary pattern, a significant number of patients with the disorder (12% in one large study) report affected family members. Paget's disease is more common in the populations of eastern and northern Europe and in areas where Europeans have immigrated (such as the United States, Australia, New Zealand, and South Africa). This condition is uncommon in Scandinavia, Asia, and Africa and in black Americans.

8. Which bones are involved in Paget's disease?

Paget's disease may be monostotic, involving only one skeletal site (in about 20% of patients), or polyostotic, involving several different areas of the skeleton. Common sites of pagetic involvement include the pelvis, hip, spine, skull, tibia, and humerus. Less common sites of involvement (in less than 20% of the cases) include the forearm, clavicles, scapulae, and ribs.

9. What is the current thinking about the cause of Paget's disease?

Although the cause of Paget's disease is unknown, the primary defect in Paget's disease appears to be an abnormality of the osteoclast. Reports of viruslike inclusions within the osteoclasts in pagetic bones are suggestive of a viral etiology. These nuclear inclusions resemble paramyxovirus nucleocapsids. The measles virus, respiratory syncytial virus, and canine distemper virus have been implicated as etiologic agents. The finding of viruslike inclusions, however, may simply reflect the fact that pagetic bone is perhaps more susceptible to infection by such viruses.

10. What medications are available to treat Paget's disease?

There is no cure for Paget's disease, but several medications are used to decrease the accelerated rate of osteoclastic bone resorption. Currently in the United States, the medications used for the treatment of Paget's disease include calcitonin, etidronate, and plicamycin. Salmon calcitonin (Calcimar, Miacalcin) and human calcitonin (Cibacalcin) are parenteral preparations that require intramuscular or subcutaneous injection. A nasal calcitonin spray is currently available in Europe and should become available in the United States in the future. Etidronate disodium (Didronel) is an oral preparation usually administered for 3–6 months and then followed by a 3–6 month drug-free interval. Etidronate is a member of a class of agents termed bisphosphonates. Several recently developed bisphosphonates (such as pamidronate) have been found to be highly effective in the treatment of Paget's disease refractory to conventional therapies. Although not approved for the treatment of Paget's disease, plicamycin (Mithracin) has been used occasionally. Gallium nitrate (Ganite), which is used to threat hypercalcemia, is also under investigation for the treatment of Paget's disease.

After treatment with etidronate disodium, suppression of disease activity is usually prolonged, sometimes lasting for several years, whereas the response to calcitonin or plicamycin is generally short-lived after treatment is discontinued. Thus, for uncomplicated Paget's disease, oral etidronate is usually the treatment of choice. Calcitonin should be reserved for patients with primarily lytic disease, for patients who are resistant to bisphosphonates, for patients in whom a particularly rapid response is required (e.g., patients with high-output cardiac failure or symptomatic disease of the spine), or before elective surgery on pagetic bone. Treatment of symptomatic patients also should include other therapeutic modalities, such as analgesics, nonsteroidal anti-inflammatory drugs, canes, shoe lifts, hearing aids, and surgery.

11. Give the indications for treatment of Paget's disease.

The primary indication for treatment is the presence of symptoms. However, not all symptoms respond to treatment. Bone pain usually responds, as do certain neurologic compression syndromes. However, hearing loss, bony deformities, and mechanically dysfunctional joints are not likely to improve with therapy. Additional indications for treatment of Paget's disease are the prevention of local progression and complications (see below), planned surgery at a pagetic site, and widespread pagetic involvement in patients in whom prolonged immobilization is anticipated (immobilization increases the risk for hypercalcemia).

Indications for Treatment of Paget's Disease of Bone

Symptoms (bone pain, headache, neurologic abnormalities)
Osteolytic bone disease
Active asymptomatic disease in:
  Weight-bearing bones
  Areas adjacent to major joints
  Vertebral bodies
  Skull
Young patients
Before elective surgery on pagetic bone
Immobilization hypercalcemia

Treatment of asymptomatic Paget's disease is controversial. However, untreated Paget's disease appears to be progressive with time, and not all asymptomatic patients will remain so. Thus, many physicians treat patients with primarily osteolytic disease or asymptomatic patients with active disease involving weight-bearing bones, vertebral bodies, the skull, and areas adjacent to major joints.

12. In asymptomatic patients, at what concentration of alkaline phosphatase concentration should treatment begin?

This is another area of controversy. The level of alkaline phosphatase should be viewed in the context of the radiographic picture. A concentration of alkaline phosphatase only 2–3 times the upper limit of normal in the context of polyostotic changes on radiographs may simply represent the late "burned-out" phase of the disease. Little benefit results from treating such an individual. However, the same test result in a patient with monostotic Paget's disease in a weight-bearing bone or in an area adjacent to a major joint would lead most physicians to consider treatment. Because lytic lesions are often associated with normal or near-normal alkaline phosphatase values, most physicians would treat patients with such lesions.

13. When should malignant degeneration be suspected?

One of the most serious complications of Paget's disease is the development of malignant sarcomas in pagetic bone. Such tumors are usually isolated, but 20% may be multicentric. Fortunately this complication of Paget's disease is rare, occurring in less than 1% of patients with clinically apparent disease. The tumors are extremely aggressive and generally result in death within 3 years of diagnosis. The pelvis and the long bones (humerus, femur, and tibia) are the most common sites for malignant transformation. Malignant transformation is heralded by the onset of new or worsening bone pain and/or soft-tissue swelling. Usually progressive destruction of pagetic bone is found on radiographs. Less commonly, increasing sclerosis or masses of dense amorphous deposits in bone are also suggestive of malignant change. The concentration of serum alkaline phosphatase may rise rapidly in an otherwise previously stable patient. The tumors are usually osteogenic sarcomas, but fibrosarcomas and chondrosarcomas have been reported in bone affected by Paget's disease. It is not known whether treatment of Paget's disease lessens the incidence of this complication.

Technetium bone scans and gallium scans may be useful to differentiate tumor from Paget's disease. Although technetium bone scans show intense uptake throughout pagetic bone, the uptake is less intense in osteogenic sarcomas. On the other hand, the gallium scan generally localizes in areas of tumor involvement but not in pagetic bone. A biopsy of the involved bone is usually diagnostic.

Other bone neoplasms are also associated with Paget's disease, such as benign giant cell tumors. These tumors do not carry the grave prognosis associated with malignant degeneration.

BIBLIOGRAPHY

1. Altman RD: Long-term follow-up of therapy with intermittent etidronate disodium in Paget's disease of bone. Am J Med 79:583, 1985.
2. Bone HG, Kleerekoper M: Paget's disease of bone. J Clin Endocrinol Metab 75:1179, 1992.
3. Cantrill JA, Anderson DC: Treatment of Paget's disease of bone. Clin Endocrinol 32:507, 1990.
4. Fogelman I, Collier BD, Brown ML: Bone scintigraphy. Part 3: Bone scanning in metabolic bone disease. J Nucl Med 34:2247, 1993.
5. Hadjipavlou A, Lander P, Srolovitz H, Enker IP: Malignant transformation in Paget disease of bone. Cancer 70:2802, 1992.
6. McClung M: Treating Paget's disease of bone. Endocrinologist 2:22, 1992.
7. Merkow RL, Lane JM: Paget's disease of bone. Endocrinol Metab Clin North Am 19:177, 1990.
8. Sellars SL: Beethoven's deafness. S Afr Med J 48:1585, 1974.
9. Singer FR, Wallach S (eds): Paget's Disease of Bone: Clinical Assessment, Present and Future Therapy. New York, Elsevier, 1991.
10. Singer FR: Clinical efficacy of salmon calcitonin in Paget's disease of bone. Calcif Tissue Int 49(Suppl 2):S7, 1991.
11. Siris ES, Ottman R, Flaster E, Kelsey JL: Familial aggregation of Paget's disease of bone. J Bone Miner Res 6:495, 1991.
12. Siris ES: Paget's Disease of Bone. In Farus MJ (ed): Primer on the Metabolic Bone Diseases and Disorders of Mineral Metabolism, 2nd ed. New York, Raven Press, 1993, p 375.
13. Wimalawansa SJ, Gunasekera RD: Pamidronate is effective for Paget's disease of bone refractory to conventional therapy. Calcif Tissue Int 53:237, 1993.

12. HYPERCALCEMIA

Leonard R. Sanders, M.D.

1. What is hypercalcemia? How does protein binding affect the calcium level?

Hypercalcemia is a total serum calcium value above the normal range (8.5–10.5 mg/dl) in the presence of normal serum proteins. Calcium is 50% free (ionized), 40% protein-bound, and 10% complexed to phosphate, citrate, bicarbonate, and lactate. Only elevations in the free calcium are associated with symptoms and signs. Of the protein-bound calcium, about 80% is bound to albumin and 20% to globulins. A 1 g/dl decrease or increase in serum albumin from 4 g/dl decreases or increases the serum calcium by 0.8 mg/dl. An increase or decrease in serum globulin by 1 g/dl increases or decreases serum calcium by 0.16 mg/dl. Such protein changes do not affect free calcium and do not cause calcium-related symptoms.

2. How frequent are hypercalcemia and its main associated conditions?

Hypercalcemia affects 0.5–1% of the general population. The incidence may increase to 3% among postmenopausal women. Primary hyperparathyroidism causes 70% of outpatient and 20% of inpatient hypercalcemia. Cancer-associated hypercalcemia causes 50% of inpatient hypercalcemia, and 10% of patients with malignancy develop hypercalcemia. Combined, hyperparathyroidism and cancer cause 90% of all hypercalcemia. About 5–10% of patients with hyperparathyroidism develop nephrolithiasis.

3. How are mild, moderate, and severe hypercalcemia classified?

First, consider the patient's general health and hypercalcemic symptoms. For example, a patient with renal failure and a serum phosphorus of 8.5 mg/dl may have metastatic calcification with a serum calcium of 10.5 mg/dl. Then correct the serum calcium for the albumin concentration. $Ca_{corrected} = Ca_{observed} + [4.0 - albumin] \times 0.8$. With this in mind, a serum calcium between 1.5 and 3 mg/dl above the upper normal limit defines moderate hypercalcemia. Mild hypercalcemia occurs below this range and severe hypercalcemia above. Thus, if the upper normal limit for calcium is 10.5 mg/dl, a serum calcium between 12.0 and 13.5 mg/dl defines moderate hypercalcemia. A serum calcium < 12.0 mg/dl is mild and > 13.5 mg/dl is severe hypercalcemia.

4. What are the symptoms and signs of hypercalcemia?

No symptoms are usually present with mild hypercalcemia (<12 mg/dl). Moderate or severe hypercalcemia and rapidly developing mild hypercalcemia cause more frequent symptoms and signs. Common symptoms and signs involve the central nervous system (lethargy, stupor, coma, mental changes, psychosis); the gastrointestinal tract (anorexia, nausea, constipation, acid peptic disease); the kidneys (polyuria, nephrolithiasis); the musculoskeletal system (arthralgias, myalgias, weakness); and the vascular system (hypertension). The classic EKG change associated with hypercalcemia is a short Q-T interval. Occasionally severe hypercalcemia also causes dysrhythmias, ST segment depression, sinus arrest, and disturbances in atrioventricular (A-V) conduction.

5. What are the sources of serum calcium?

Bone contains 99% of body calcium. Of the remaining 1%, most is intracellular; a small amount is extracellular. Bone calcium approximates 1 kg in young people and 0.5 kg in the elderly. One percent of the skeletal calcium is freely exchangeable with the extracellular fluid. Normal serum calcium is maintained by integrated regulation of calcium absorption, resorption, and reabsorption. These processes occur respectively in the gut, bone, and kidney. The gut absorbs about 30% of dietary calcium; absorption varies from 15–70%, depending on dietary calcium and age. Calcium absorption decreases with age. The kidney reabsorbs 98% of the filtered calcium. A normal dietary calcium intake is 1,000 mg/day. Of this amount, the gut absorbs 300 mg, excretes

700 mg, and secretes 100 mg. The net intestinal excretion is 800 mg/day. The bone exchanges 500 mg/day with serum, and the kidney excretes 200 mg/day for normal calcium balance.

6. What are the major anatomic and physiologic determinants of serum calcium?

Bone, gut, kidney, liver, skin, parathyroid, and thyroid are the main organs affecting serum calcium. They control the serum calcium by regulating serum levels of parathyroid hormone (PTH), 1,25-dihydroxyvitamin D (1,25-D), calcitonin, phosphate, and calcium itself. The parathyroid glands secrete PTH and the thyroid gland makes calcitonin. Diet, skin, liver, and kidney control the synthesis and secretion of 1,25-D. Vitamin D2 is ingested in the diet, and vitamin D3 is synthesized in the skin. In the liver, 25-hydroxylase hydroxylates both vitamins to form 25-hydroxyvitamin D2 and D3 (25-OHD). Both forms of the vitamin (hormone) circulate, and their biologic activities are the same. In the mitochondria of the proximal renal tubule, 1-alpha-hydroxylase converts 25-OHD to 1,25-D. All three forms of the vitamin affect calcium metabolism. However, only 1,25-D is sufficiently potent to have a noticeable effect at physiologic levels.

7. How do hormones affect the level of serum calcium?

PTH and 1,25-D provide the main control of serum calcium. Calcitonin may play a role, but its significance is not well defined in humans. PTH and calcitonin affect bone and kidney but have no direct effects on the intestine. 1,25-D has effects on bone, kidney, and intestine. A major effect of 1,25-D is to increase intestinal absorption of calcium. Both PTH and 1,25-D increase bone resorption by increasing osteoclast activity. Because osteoclasts have no known receptors for either hormone, PTH and 1,25-D stimulate osteoclast activity indirectly. PTH enhances activity of osteoblasts that secrete factors that stimulate osteoclastic bone resorption. 1,25-D promotes osteoclast differentiation from promonocytes to monocytes to macrophages to osteoclasts. 1,25-D also increases calcium transport from bone to blood. Both hormones promote normal bone formation by actions on osteoblasts, and 1,25-D maintains a favorable calcium-phosphate product necessary for normal bone mineralization. Calcitonin inhibits osteoclastic bone resorption, decreases renal tubular reabsorption of calcium, and may also enhance osteoblast activity. Other actions and interactions of these hormones on bone, kidney, and gut are described below. Estrogen receptors have been identified in osteoblasts and osteoclasts. Estrogens inhibit bone resorption, increase bone growth, and modestly lower serum calcium.

8. Outline the interactions of calcium and phosphate with the main calcium regulating hormones.

Interaction of Factors Controlling Serum Calcium

	PTH	1,25-D	CALCITONIN	CALCIUM	PO₄
PTH		↑+	+	↑ +	↓ ↑ +
1,25-D	↓ −	↓ −	+	↑	↑
Calcitonin	+	+		↓	↓
Calcium	↓	↓	↑		↓
PO₄	+	↓	−	↓	

The above table summarizes the main factors controlling the serum calcium. The arrows show direct and the symbols (+/−) indirect actions of factors in the left column on factors in the top row. As a rule, the direct effects predominate as the net effect. Recall that absorption, resorption, and reabsorption are the respective effects of gut, bone, and kidney. PTH directly stimulates kidney production of 1,25-D and indirectly increases renal synthesis of 1,25-D by its phosphaturic and net hypophosphatemic effect. PTH increases calcium by stimulating bone resorption and distal renal tubular reabsorption. The increased calcium increases calcitonin secretion, and the increased bone resorption also increases serum phosphate. Increased 1,25-D increases absorption of calcium and phosphate (PO₄). 1,25-D directly inhibits PTH secretion and renal synthesis of 1,25-D. However, 1,25-D stimulates absorption, resorption, and probably reabsorption of both calcium and phosphate. The result is a net increase in serum calcium and phosphate. The increased calcium inhibits synthesis of PTH and 1,25-D and stimulates secretion of calcitonin. The increased phosphate also inhibits synthesis of 1,25-D. Calcitonin inhibits resorption and reabsorption of calcium and phosphate. This decreases serum calcium and phosphate which in turn increases 1,25-D. The decreased calcium also increases PTH. Calcium decreases secretion of PTH and renal production of 1,25-D. In addition, calcium stimulates thyroid secretion of calcitonin. By complexing with phosphate, calcium decreases serum phosphate. Phosphate inhibits renal synthesis of 1,25-D and complexes with calcium, causing a fall in serum calcium that stimulates PTH and inhibits release of calcitonin.

9. What are the main causes of hypercalcemia?
The mnemonic **VITAMINS TRAP** includes most causes of hypercalcemia:[18]

V	=	Vitamins
I	=	Immobilization
T	=	Thyrotoxicosis
A	=	Addison's disease
M	=	Milk-alkali syndrome
I	=	Inflammatory disorders
N	=	Neoplastic-related disease
S	=	Sarcoidosis
T	=	Thiazide diuretics and other drugs (lithium)
R	=	Rhabdomyolysis
A	=	AIDS
P	=	Paget's disease, Parenteral nutrition, Pheochromocytoma, and Parathyroid disease

10. How do various causes of hypercalcemia increase the serum calcium?
True hypercalcemia results from altered bone resorption, renal tubular reabsorption, and gut absorption of calcium. From the discussions above, one appreciates that mechanisms of hypercalcemia are usually multifactorial. However, most hypercalcemic syndromes have a primary effect as follows:

Increased bone resorption: hyperparathyroidism, neoplastic diseases, thyrotoxicosis, pheochromocytoma, excessive vitamin A (>50,000 u/day), and immobilization. Malignant tumors cause hypercalcemia primarily by producing humoral or local substances that increase osteoclastic bone resorption. Direct osteolysis by the tumor is now believed to be an unusual cause of hypercalcemia. Immobilization may cause hypercalcemia when associated with hyperparathyroidism, malignancy, young age, Paget's disease, or renal failure. Lithium carbonate alters the set point for PTH secretion, causing secretion at higher levels of calcium.

Increased renal reabsorption or decreased excretion: milk-alkali syndrome, rhabdomyolysis, thiazide diuretics, familial hypocalciuric hypercalcemia (FHH). Hypercalcemia may cause diuresis. The resulting dehydration decreases the glomerular filtration rate (GFR) and this increases renal reabsorption of calcium and bicarbonate. In milk-alkali syndrome, alkalosis increases renal reabsorption of calcium, and hypercalcemia increases reabsorption of bicarbonate. Associated renal insufficiency from nephrocalcinosis decreases excretion of calcium. In rhabdomyolysis, the injured muscles release calcium and myoglobin. The myoglobin causes renal failure that further increases calcium retention. Thiazides decrease intravascular volume. This decreases GFR, increases proximal tubular reabsorption of calcium, and concentrates the plasma. These factors increase plasma calcium. Thiazides also directly increase renal distal tubular reabsorption of calcium and may potentiate PTH action on bone. Patients with FHH have a genetically determined defect in renal excretion of calcium.

Increased gut absorption: excessive vitamin D, sarcoidosis, other inflammatory disorders, AIDS, and lymphomas increase 1,25-D. Excessive dietary vitamin D (usually > 50,000 units/week) may be associated with hypercalcemia. Inflammatory and granulomatous disorders include sarcoidosis, tuberculosis, coccidioidomycosis, histoplasmosis, candidiasis, eosinophilic granuloma, berylliosis, and silicone implants. Certain lymphomas also produce excessive 1,25-D. In all, hypercalcemia is related to excessive production of 1,25-D and associated increase in gut absorption of calcium. However, 1,25-D acts to increase bone resorption and probably renal reabsorption as well. Milk-alkali syndrome is also associated with increased absorption of calcium and nephrocalcinosis.

Unknown: vasoactive intestinal polypeptide-secreting tumor (VIPoma), Addison's disease, parenteral nutrition, theophylline.

11. What is humoral hypercalcemia of malignancy (HHM)?
HHM is a hypercalcemic syndrome that results when a malignant tumor produces a humoral substance (PTH-related peptide [PTHrP]) that usually increases bone resorption and causes hypercalcemia. HHM is the most common cause of tumor-related hypercalcemia.

12. In HHM, is the malignancy always obvious before hypercalcemia?
The usual teaching is that advanced malignancy is nearly always present before cancer-associated hypercalcemia. However, up to 20% of patients with cancer-associated hypercalcemia may present with hypercalcemia before malignancy is diagnosed.

13. What malignancies and humoral mediators cause hypercalcemia?
The most common malignancies causing hypercalcemia, in order of descending frequency, are lung (squamous and adenocarcinoma), breast, myeloma, lymphoma, and renal cell carcinoma. Less commonly carcinomas of the colon, thyroid, and stomach cause hypercalcemia from humoral or local metastases. Rarely, small cell lung cancer and ovarian carcinomas cause hypercalcemia by making native PTH. However, PTHrP is the most common humoral mediator of hypercalcemia, accounting for 80% of malignancy-associated hypercalcemia. Sources of excessive production of PTHrP include squamous malignancies of the lung, esophagus, cervix, vulva, skin, head and neck; breast carcinoma; and renal cell carcinoma. Lymphomas due to human T-cell leukemia virus-I also make excessive PTHrP. However, most lymphomas and myeloma do not make excessive PTHrP. Certain lymphomas produce 1,25-D. Myeloma may produce excess lymphotoxin and interleukin-1 (IL-1). Lymphomas and other malignancies metastatic to bone produce osteoclastic activating factors (OAFs) that stimulate osteoclastic bone resorption and cause hypercalcemia. OAFs include transforming growth factors (TGF-α and TGF-β), prostaglandins (PGE$_2$), tumor necrosis factor-alpha (TNF-α), lymphotoxin (LT), interleukins (IL-1 and IL-6), and PTHrP. TGF-α and TGF-β may stimulate bone metastases to make excessive local amounts of PTHrP. Although breast and other cancers metastatic to bone make proteases that may cause direct osteolysis, local tumoral production of OAFs is probably the usual mechanism of hypercalcemia associated with metastases to bone.

14. How is HHM distinguished from primary hyperparathyroidism?

Hypercalcemia, Primary Hyperparathyroidism, and Malignancy

	INTACT PTH	PTHrP	1,25-D	CALCIUM
Primary hyperparathyroidism	↑	↓	↑	↑
PTHrP malignancy	↓	↑	↓	↑
Non-PTHrP malignancy	↓	↓	↓	↑

The main distinguishing features are the levels of intact PTH, PTHrP, and 1,25-D. The classic and most common patterns of these hormones are shown in the table above. Primary hyperparathyroidism (HPT) usually has elevated levels of intact PTH. Malignancy-associated hypercalcemia usually has low levels of intact PTH. Of hypercalcemic patients with HHM, 80% have increased levels of PTHrP, and 20% have both low intact PTH and PTHrP. Patients with HPT have low levels of PTHrP. Thus, measuring the two hormones distinguishes all three disorders. At times the levels overlap. HPT has been reported with low-normal to high-normal intact PTH. PTHrP is a protein with 141 amino acids, whereas PTH has 84 amino acids. The region of homology to PTH is primarily within the first 13 N-terminal amino acids. PTHrP simulates the same receptors as PTH and has the same biologic effects. However, the two hormones have different effects on levels of 1,25-D. PTHrP stimulates receptors that activate renal 1-alpha hydroxylase. However, continuous secretion of PTHrP by malignant tumors may downregulate the receptors. This inhibits 1-alpha-hydroxylase activity and decreases 1,25-D. Continuous infusion of PTH causes similar decreases in 1,25-D. Secretion of PTH in HPT is intermittent. Intermittent secretion avoids downregulation and results in increased 1,25-D. In addition, serum calcium levels are higher in HHM than in HPT. The higher calcium levels decrease production of 1,25-D. Traditional associations of primary HPT include mild renal tubular acidosis, hypophosphatemia, hyperchloremia, and an increased ratio of chloride to phosphate. Unfortunately, such associations are nonspecific and too insensitive to predict diagnosis.

15. How are the three types of hyperparathyroidism (HPT) distinguished?

PTH and Calcium in Hyperparathyroidism

	PTH	CALCIUM
Primary	Normal ↑	↑
Secondary	↑	↓ Normal
Tertiary	↑↑	↑

Primary HPT is idiopathic and results from excessive secretion of PTH in patients with a single adenoma (85%), multiple adenomas (5%), parathyroid hyperplasia (10%), and parathyroid carcinoma (< 1%). The calcium is high, and PTH is normal or high. **Secondary HPT** results from normal compensation of the parathyroid glands to hypocalcemia. The most common cause of secondary HPT is chronic renal failure (CRF), which results in hyperphosphatemia that causes hypocalcemia. Other causes of hypocalcemia are renal calcium leak, dietary calcium malabsorption, and vitamin D deficiency. Hypocalcemia causes parathyroid hyperplasia. Attempting to return the calcium to normal, the enlarged glands secrete excessive PTH. Prolonged hypocalcemia may cause autonomous parathyroid function and hypercalcemia. Spontaneous change from low or normal calcium levels to hypercalcemia marks the transition from secondary to **tertiary HPT.** In tertiary HPT, PTH levels are usually >10–20 times normal.

Occasionally, patients with secondary HPT have hypercalcemia. This usually occurs when hypocalcemic patients with CRF receive a kidney transplant. The new kidney returns the phosphate levels to normal, causing the calcium levels to rise. Because the parathyroid glands are hyperplastic, basal PTH secretion continues, despite normal-to-high calcium levels. If the transplant patient has secondary HPT, the parathyroid glands involute, and the serum calcium returns to normal. This process may take months and occasionally years. If the increased calcium and PTH fail to correct spontaneously or with calcitriol therapy, the patient has tertiary HPT. Tertiary HPT usually requires resection of at least 3.5 parathyroid glands to correct the hypercalcemia.

16. What PTH assay is most useful in the work-up of hypercalcemia?
Parathyroid hormone (PTH) has 84 amino acids. The first 34 amino acids of the N-terminus contain the full biologic activity of the hormone. However, intact PTH (1–84) causes final biologic activity in vivo. The preferred assays for measurement are the immunochemiluminometric (ICMA) and immunoradiometric (IRMA) assays for intact PTH. Both are highly sensitive and specific. Because of availability, the IRMA assay is more commonly used. Neither assay is affected by renal failure. The parathyroid gland secretes intact PTH and carboxy terminal fragments. The liver metabolizes intact PTH to its amino terminal and carboxy terminal fragments. In renal failure, carboxy terminal fragments accumulate. Because the liver and

peripheral tissues quickly metabolize intact PTH and N-terminal fragments, they do not accumulate in renal failure.

17. What methods best localize the parathyroid tumor in hyperparathyroidism?

The normal parathyroid gland is < 5 mm and < 40 mg. Parathyroid adenomas are > 5 mm and usually > 500 mg. Ninety percent of the time, a skilled parathyroid surgeon can localize and remove a parathyroid adenoma without preoperative localization. Thus, usually no preoperative localization is used. Because 5–10% of parathyroid adenomas are in aberrant locations, however, preoperative localization helps when accurate noninvasive techniques are readily available; the surgeon requests preoperative localization; or the parathyroid tumor was not found during an initial operation. Noninvasive localization techniques include high frequency (7.5–10 MHz) ultrasound, ^{99m}technetium pertechnetate or 123-iodine (^{123}I) with thallium (^{201}T1) subtraction scanning, ^{99m}technetium-Sestamibi scanning, cervical CT or MRI scanning, and intravenous digital subtraction angiography (IVDSA). These techniques average 75% sensitivity with false-positive rates of 10–30%. Invasive techniques include arteriography and selective venous sampling; sensitivity rates are 90% with few false-positive results.

18. What are the multiple endocrine neoplasia (MEN) syndromes?

MEN is associated with three familial syndromes, two of which present with hypercalcemia due to hyperparathyroidism. MEN 1 or Wermer's syndrome includes the 3 Ps: pituitary, parathyroid, and pancreatic tumors. MEN 2 has two variants, both of which have medullary carcinoma of the thyroid (MCT) and pheochromocytoma. Patients with MEN 2a or Sipple's syndrome have MCT, pheochromocytoma, and hyperparathyroidism. Patients with MEN 2b have MCT, pheochromocytoma, multiple mucosal neuromas, and marfanoid habitus. The importance of MEN syndromes with hypercalcemia is that parathyroid tumors are more often bilateral, hyperplastic, and malignant. Moreover, anesthesia and surgery can stimulate a pheochromocytoma to cause a hypertensive crisis. Thus, patients with suspected MEN 2 need screening for pheochromocytoma before parathyroid surgery. MCT may cause other endocrine syndromes by secreting excessive adrenocorticotropic hormone (ACTH), antidiuretic hormone (ADH), vasoactive intestinal polypeptide (VIP), prostaglandins, somatostatin, serotonin, and other hormones.

19. What is familial hypocalciuric hypercalcemia (FHH)? How is it diagnosed?

FHH, also called benign familial hypercalcemia, results from an autosomal dominant defect mapped to the long arm of chromosome 3 or the short arm of chromosome 19. FHH has decreased renal clearance of calcium, normal-to-high serum levels of PTH, mild relative hypermagnesemia, normal or low serum phosphorus, and a fractional excretion of calcium (FE_{Ca}) < 1%. In FHH, PTH is inappropriately high for the level of serum calcium. Therefore, FHH can mimic primary hyperparathyroidism. However, patients with FHH are usually asymptomatic, have no associated complications, and require no therapy. In unusual cases, neonates with FHH may have severe symptomatic hypercalcemia. The clinical importance of FHH is to distinguish it from primary hyperparathyroidism so that invasive procedures such as parathyroidectomy are not done needlessly. Near-total parathyroidectomy does not usually correct the hypercalcemia in FHH. However, total parathyroidectomy causes hypoparathyroidism and hypocalcemia. The most important diagnostic feature of FHH is the combination of a family history of benign hypercalcemia and a FE_{Ca} < 1%. Patients with primary hyperparathyroidism usually have an FE_{Ca} > 2%.

20. What is the likely diagnosis in the following hypercalcemic patient?

An 18-year-old man had a normal screening history and physical exam for college. His physician referred him to an endocrinologist because his screening lab showed a calcium of 11.3 mg/dl. He is asymptomatic and still has a normal exam. Repeat serum calcium is 11.5 mg/dl. Family history reveals that his mother and brother also have asymptomatic hypercalcemia. Review of his old records shows calcium levels of 10.5–11.8 for at least 2 years. Additional lab tests showed the following values: intact PTH = 70 pg/ml (nl < 60); serum creatinine (Cr) = 1 mg/dl; spot urine calcium = 5 mg/dl; and urine Cr = 90 mg/dl. The FE_{Ca} is calculated in the same manner as a fractional excretion of Na (FE_{Na}), but Ca is substituted for Na as follows:

$$FE_{Ca} = [U_{Ca}/P_{Ca}] / [U_{Cr}/P_{Cr}] = [U_{Ca}/P_{Ca}] \times [P_{Cr}/U_{Cr}]$$

$$FE_{Ca} = [5 \text{ mg/dl} / 11.5 \text{ mg/dl}] \times [1 \text{ mg/dl} / 90 \text{ mg/dl}] \times 100\% = 0.5\%$$

A more accurate FE_{Ca} calculation uses a calcium value of 6.9 mg/dl (0.6 × 11.5), because circulating proteins bind 40% of the calcium and the kidney filters only 60%. The FE_{Ca} value for the patient is still < 1% (0.8%), indicating renal reabsorption of > 99% of the filtered calcium. In the presence of hypercalcemia, this value is clearly abnormal. The FE_{Ca} < 1% supports the diagnosis of FHH. This, plus a family history of hypercalcemia and absence of symptoms, signs, or complications, makes the diagnosis of FHH. No further work-up is needed. A random (spot) urine sample is sufficient for a FE_{Ca} as it is for a FE_{Na}.

21. What drug therapy is useful in hypercalcemia?

Drug Therapy of Hypercalcemia

THERAPY	DOSE	ROUTE	MONITOR / COMMENT
Saline	250–1,000 ml/hr	IV	Cardiopulmonary function with exam, CVP/PCWP, and CXR
Furosemide	20–80 mg q 2–4 hr or 40 mg/hr CI	IV	Serum and urine electrolytes. Replace K, Mg, and PO_4 based on serum levels and urinary losses.
Salmon calcitonin	4–8 IU/kg q 6–12 hr	IM/SC	Allergic reaction. Give a skin test of 1 IU intradermally before treatment.
Prednisone/ methylprednisolone	20 mg bid-tid	PO/IV	Possible adjunct to calcitonin. Effective in 1,25-D–associated hypercalcemia.
Pamidronate	30–90 mg q wk	IV	Infuse over 4–24 hr. Give ¹/₂ dose and maximum infusion time in severe renal failure.
Etidronate	7.5 mg/kg/day	IV	Infuse over 4 hr. prn qd × 5 days. Give ¹/₂ dose in renal failure.
Plicamycin	25 µg/kg/day	IV	Infuse over 4 hr. prn q 2–3 days. Avoid in hepatic dysfunction and thrombocytopenia. Monitor CBC, platelets, PT/PTT, and liver enzymes.
Gallium nitrate	200 mg/m² BSA/day	IV	Infuse over 24 hr. prn qd × 5 days. Avoid in renal failure. Monitor serum Cr, PO_4, and CBC.
Neutral sodium phosphate	500–1,000 mg tid	PO	Adjunct to other therapy. Avoid if serum PO_4 > 3.5 mg/dl.
Dialysis	Low or no calcium dialysate	HD/PD CAVHD	Hypercalcemic crisis or refractory hypercalcemia. Useful in renal failure. Nephrology consultation.
Na or K Phosphate (1 mmol phosphate = 31 mg elemental phosphorus)	1–3 mmol phosphate per hr × 12 hr	IV	Hypercalcemic crisis. Renal and cardiac toxicity and sudden death. Avoid in renal failure and serum PO_4 > 3 mg/dl.
Edetate disodium (EDTA)	50 mg/kg/day	IV	Hypercalcemic crisis. Infuse over 3–4 hr. Max. dose < 3 g/24 hr. prn qd × 5 days. Avoid in renal failure.

CI = continuous infusion; BSA = body surface area; IV = intravenously; IM = intramuscularly; SC = subcutaneously; PO = orally; HD = hemodialysis; PD = peritoneal dialysis; CAVHD = continuous arteriovenous hemodialysis; CVP = central venous pressure; PCWP = pulmonary capillary wedge pressure; CXR = chest radiograph; Na = sodium; K = potassium; Mg = magnesium; PO_4 = phosphate; PRN = as required; CBC = complete blood count; PT = prothrombin time; PTT = partial thromboplastin time; Cr = creatinine.

The preceding table summarizes the current guidelines for drug therapies for hypercalcemia. Most patients with severe hypercalcemia require combined treatment with multiple drugs. The lowest amount and least frequent dose that will achieve and maintain acceptable levels of serum calcium should be given. All patients with hypercalcemia are dehydrated and require rehydration with normal saline as initial therapy. This is frequently followed by furosemide. Both therapies increase urinary excretion of sodium and calcium but normalize the serum calcium in < 10% of patients. Furosemide prevents volume overload. Saline and diuretic therapy require meticulous monitoring of the patient's blood and urine for volume and electrolyte problems. Calcitonin, diphosphonates, plicamycin, and gallium nitrate inhibit bone resorption. Calcitonin effectively normalizes serum calcium in 20% of patients within 2–4 hrs and lasts 2–3 days. Combined use with glucocorticoids arguably prolongs the modest (1–2 mg/dl) hypocalcemic effect for about a week. Glucocorticoids inhibit synthesis and action of 1,25-D. A single infusion of pamidronate is 90% effective within 48 hours, lasts 2–8 weeks, and is the drug of choice for HHM. Etidronate normalizes the calcium in 40% of patients and requires repeated infusions. Plicamycin is 60% effective, works within 24 hrs, and lasts up to a week. Repeated infusions cause bone marrow and hepatic toxicity that limit its long-term use. Gallium nitrate is 75% effective, requires multiple 24-hour infusions, and is nephrotoxic. Oral phosphate is adjunctive therapy in patients with a serum phosphate < 3.5 mg/dl. Hypercalcemic crisis causes severe cardiac dysrhythmias and neurologic dysfunction. For extreme emergencies, sodium EDTA or IV phosphate immediately lowers the calcium by chelation and complexation. Both drugs, however, are dangerous. EDTA may cause severe acute renal failure. Intravenous phosphate may cause metastatic calcification, acute renal failure, cardiac dysrhythmias, and death from cardiac arrest. Dialysis against a low or no calcium bath can effect immediate lowering of the calcium while other medications take effect. It is of particular benefit in patients with hypercalcemic renal failure and removes chelated calcium EDTA. Dialysis is emergency therapy but probably should be used before IV EDTA or IV phosphate. Mobilization decreases bone resorption. Limiting oral and IV calcium supplements decreases calcium input.

22. What is the mechanism of action and appropriate dose of diphosphonate therapy?
Diphosphonates bind to hydroxyapatite crystals, making them toxic and less accessible to osteoclasts. The current diphosphonate preparations, etidronate (EHDP) and pamidronate (APD), are poorly absorbed and effective only intravenously as therapy for hypercalcemia. Pamidronate is the most effective antiresorptive drug available. Doses for pamidronate and etidronate are outlined in question 21. The usual intravenous dose of pamidronate is 30, 60, or 90 mg for mild, moderate, and severe hypercalcemia, respectively. Because diphosphonates are renally excreted, half the recommended dose should be infused over 24 hours for patients with significant renal failure (estimated GFR < 20 ml/min). Side effects of pamidronate are unusual, but mild, transient fever may occur.

23. A 65-year-old woman on thiazide diuretics presents with altered mentation, nausea, and vomiting. Lab tests show a calcium of 18 mg/dl and a creatinine of 4.5 mg/dl. Urine output was marginal. How should her hypercalcemia be managed initially?
Most patients presenting with hypercalcemia of this severity have an underlying malignancy. They are frequently debilitated and have compromised cardiovascular function. All are dehydrated. Admit her to the ICU. Order an EKG and CXR. Repeat STAT SMA-11 (Na, K, Cl, CO_2, BUN, Cr, glucose, Ca, PO_4, Mg, albumin). Place a central line to assess volume status (CVP or PCWP). Give normal saline at 500–1000 ml/hr, depending on volume status. Give salmon calcitonin, 1 IU intradermally, and check the site after 15–20 minutes. If no wheal or significant erythema develops, give 8 IU/kg salmon calcitonin IM (effective within 2–4 hrs). Repeat the IM calcitonin injection every 6 hours. Begin a 60-mg infusion of pamidronate and continue over a 24-hour period (maximal dose reduced for renal failure). Once volume is replete, give 20–100 mg IV furosemide every 2–4 hours to maintain urine output at 4–5 liters/day. If urine output is not adequate, give 200 mg furosemide IV over 30 minutes and start 40 mg/hr as a continuous

infusion. Replace the urine output with IV normal saline, or alternate with half normal saline, depending on volume and electrolyte status. Obtain SMA-11 every 6 hours and spot urine sample for Na, K, Cl, Cr once a day to estimate losses. Replace potassium and magnesium losses as required. If hypercalcemia worsens, CNS function deteriorates, or urine output declines, get nephrology consultation for dialysis. Consider plicamycin if above measures remain ineffective. Then consider gallium nitrate. Obtain a noncontrast CT scan of the head. If possible, because of nephrotoxicity, avoid intravenous iodinated contrast. Reserve intravenous EDTA and phosphate for life-threatening, hypercalcemia-induced dysrhythmias. Stop the thiazide diuretic.

CONTROVERSY

24. Do all hypercalcemic patients with hyperparathyroidism require surgical treatment?
No. Most clinicians recommend parathyroidectomy for patients with symptoms and signs of hypercalcemia (see question 4) and asymptomatic patients < 50 years old with serium calcium > 12 mg/dl. The experienced parathyroid surgeon performs a parathyroidectomy with > 90% success rate, < 5% complication rate, rare mortality, and brief hospitalization. Symptomatic patients usually improve after parathyroidectomy. However, not all patients have access to an experienced parathyroid surgeon, and operative morbidity increases to > 15% if the surgeon is not experienced. Most patients with mild hyperparathyroidism are asymptomatic, remain asymptomatic, and are older than 50 years; many have increased risks for surgical complications. In addition, no controlled data suggest that asymptomatic mild hyperparathyroidism causes clinically symptomatic osteoporosis, renal failure, or other major complications. Conversely, recent data suggest that mild increases in PTH may increase bone formation. Thus, asymptomatic patients with serum calcium < 11.5–12 mg/dl do not need surgery. They benefit from careful follow-up, increased activity and hydration, a normal calcium intake, and estrogen replacement (in postmenopausal women). Selected patients may benefit from oral phosphate and diphosphonate therapy.

BIBLIOGRAPHY

1. Bilezikian JP: Hypercalcemia. In Bardin CW: Current Therapy in Endocrinology and Metabolism, 5th ed. St. Louis, C.V. Mosby, 1994, pp 511–514.
2. Bilezikian JP: Clinical review 51: Management of hypercalcemia. J Clin Endocrinol Metab 77:1445–1449, 1993.
3. Burtis WJ, Stewart AF: Nonparathyroid hypercalcemia. In Becker KL, Bilezikian JP, Bremner WJ, et al (eds): Principles and Practice of Endocrinology and Metabolism. Philadelphia, J.B. Lippincott, 1990, pp 437–447.
4. Deftos LJ, Parthemore JG, Stabile BE: Management of primary hyperparathyroidism. Annu Rev Med 44:19–26, 1993.
5. Delmez JA, Slatopolsky E: Clinical review 20: Recent advances in the pathogenesis and therapy of uremic secondary hyperparathyroidism. J Clin Endocrinol Metab 72:735–739, 1991.
6. Eisenberg H, Pallotta J, Sacks B, et al: Parathryroid localization, three-dimensional modeling, and percutaneous ablation techniques. Endocrinol Metab Clin North Am 18:659–700, 1989.
7. Fujino T, Watanabe T, Yamaguchi K, et al: The development of hypercalcemia in a patient with an ovarian tumor producing parathyroid hormone-related protein. Cancer 70:2845–2850, 1992.
8. Hall TG, Schaiff RA: Update on the medical treatment of hypercalcemia of malignancy. Clin Pharmacol 12:117–125, 1993.
9. Heath H: Primary hyperparathyroidism: Recent advances in pathogenesis, diagnosis, and management. Adv Intern Med 37:275–293, 1992.
10. Kahky MP, Weber RS: Complications of surgery of the thyroid and parathyroid glands. Surg Clin North Am 73:307–321, 1993.
11. Mallette LE: Regulation of blood calcium in humans. Endocrinol Metab Clin North Am 18:601–610, 1989.
12. Marcus R: Estrogens and progestins in the management of primary hyperparathyroidism. J Bone Miner Res 6 (Suppl 2):S125–S129, S151–S152, 1991.
13. Melton LJ: Epidemiology of primary hyperparathyroidism. J Bone Miner Res 6 (Suppl 2)S25–S30, S31–S32, 1991.

14. Mosekilde L, Eriksen EF, Charles P: Hypercalcemia of malignancy: Pathophysiology, diagnosis and treatment. Crit Rev Oncol Hematol 11:1–27, 1991.
15. Mundy GR: Hypercalcemia in hematologic malignancies and in solid tumors associated with extensive localized bone destruction. In Murray MJ, Christakos S, Kleerekoper M, et al (eds): Primer on the Metabolic Bone Diseases and Disorders of Mineral Metabolism. New York, Raven Press, 1993, pp 173–176.
16. National Institutes of Health: Diagnosis and management of asymptomatic primary hyperparathyroidism: consensus development conference statement. Ann Intern Med 114:593–597, 1991.
17. Nussbaum SR: Pathophysiology and management of severe hypercalcemia. Endocrinol Metab Clin North Am 22:343–362, 1993.
18. Pont A: Unusual causes of hypercalcemia. Endocrinol Metab Clin North Am 18:753–764, 1989.
19. Ratcliffe WA, Hutchesson AC, Bundred NJ, et al: Role of assays for parathyroid-hormone-related protein in investigation of hypercalcaemia [see comments]. Lancet 339:164–167, 1992.
20. Tonner DR, Schlechte JA: Neurologic complications of thyroid and parathyroid disease. Med Clin North Am 77:251–263, 1993.

13. HYPOCALCEMIA

Reed S. Christensen, M.D.

1. Define hypocalcemia.
Hypocalcemia is the state in which the serum calcium level drops below the normal range of 8.5–10.5 mg/dl (2.1–2.5 mmol) despite correction for serum albumin, to which calcium is bound. Calcium levels are corrected for hypoalbuminemia by adding 0.8 mg/dl to the serum calcium level for every 1.0 g/dl that the albumin level is below 4.0 g/dl. The adjusted level of serum calcium correlates with the level of ionized calcium, which is the physiologically active form of serum calcium.

2. What is the normal level of serum ionized calcium?
Approximately 50% of serum calcium is bound to albumin, other plasma proteins, and related anions, such as citrate, lactate, and sulfate. Of this, 40% is bound to protein and 10–13% is attached to anions. The remaining 50% is unbound, giving a normal ionized calcium level of 1.00–1.15 mmol/L.

3. What factors, other than albumin, influence the levels of serum ionized calcium?
Serum pH influences levels of ionized calcium by causing decreased binding of calcium to albumin in acidosis and increased binding in alkalosis. As an example, respiratory alkalosis, which is seen in hyperventilation, causes a drop in the level of serum ionized calcium. A shift of 0.1 pH unit is associated with an ionized calcium change of 0.04–0.05 mmol/L. Increased levels of chelators, such as citrate, also may lower the levels of ionized calcium, as does heparin.

4. How is calcium regulated?
Three hormones maintain calcium homeostasis: parathyroid hormone (PTH), vitamin D, and calcitonin. PTH acts in three ways to raise serum calcium levels: (1) it stimulates osteoclastic activity in bone; (2) it increases conversion of 25-hydroxyvitamin D to 1,25-dihydroxyvitamin D (calcitriol) and thereby increases intestinal absorption of calcium; and (3) it increases renal reabsorption of calcium. Calcitriol is produced by a pathway that includes formation of vitamin D (cholecalciferol) in the skin in the presence of ultraviolet light, conversion of cholecalciferol to 25-hydroxyvitamin D in the liver, and finally hydroxylation to the most active form, 1,25-dihydroxyvitamin D in the kidney. Calcitonin, which is produced by the C-cells of the thyroid, decreases the level of serum calcium by suppressing osteoclast activity in bone. The interplay of hormones maintains calcium levels within a very narrow range in a normal individual.

5. What are the major causes of hypocalcemia?
The etiology of hypocalcemia must be considered in relation to the level of serum albumin, the secretion of PTH, and the presence or absence of hyperphosphatemia. The potential for multiple causes of hypocalcemia is due to the multiple organ and hormonal regulatory systems involved in calcium homeostasis. Initially hypocalcemia may be approached by looking for failure in one or more of these systems. The systems primarily involved are the parathyroid glands, bone, kidney, and liver.

Clinical Entity	Mechanism
Hypoparathyroidism	Decreased PTH production
Hypomagnesemia	Decreased PTH release
Pseudohypoparathyroidism	PTH ineffective at target organ
Liver disease	Decreased albumin production
	Decreased 25-hydroxyvitamin D production
	Drugs that stimulate 25-hydroxyvitamin D metabolism

Clinical Entity	Mechanism
Renal disease	Renal calcium leak
	Decreased 1,25-dihydroxyvitamin D production
	Elevated serum PO_4 level from decreased PO_4 clearance
	Drugs that increase renal clearance of calcium
Bone disease	Drugs suppressing bone resorption
	"Hungry bone syndrome"—recovery from hyper-parathyroidism or hyperthyroidism
Phosphate load	Endogenous: tumor lysis syndrome, hemolysis, rhabdomyolysis
	Exogenous: phosphate-containing enemas and lax-atives, phosphorus burns
Other illness	
Pancreatitis	Sequestration of calcium to pancreas
Toxic shock syndrome	
Other critical illness	Decreased PTH production

6. What laboratory tests are clinically useful in distinguishing among the causes of hypocalcemia?

In the evaluation of an individual patient, many causes can be excluded on the basis of history and physical examination. The following table summarizes the laboratory findings in conditions for which these values define the diagnosis.

Differential Diagnosis of Laboratory Evaluation of Hypocalcemia

	CA.	PHOS.	PTH	25-VIT. D	1,25-VIT.D
Hypoparathyroidism	↓	↑	↓	Normal	↓
Pseudohypoparathyroidism	↓	↑	↑	Normal	↓ or Normal
Liver disease	↓	↓	↑	↓	↓ or Normal
Renal disease	↓	↑	↑	Normal	↓ or Normal

7. What are the neurologic and psychologic symptoms of hypocalcemia?

Hypocalcemia may present with numbness, tingling, muscle cramps, and fasciculations. Psychiatric symptoms of irritability, paranoia, depression, psychosis, and organic brain syndrome may also develop. Subnormal intelligence also has been reported with hypocalcemia. Individuals may be unaware of symptoms because of the gradual onset and may realize an abnormality only when their sense of well-being improves with treatment.

Neurologic symptoms may progress to tetany and seizures. Seizures occur because of a lowered threshold that reveals underlying epilepsy or as "cerebral tetany" (see below), which is not a true seizure.

Chvostek's and Trousseau's signs are useful in detecting hypocalcemia. Chvostek's sign is a facial twitch elicited by tapping over the zygomatic arch. Trousseau's sign is forearm spasm induced by inflation of an upper-arm blood-pressure cuff for up to 3 minutes. It is important to note that 4–25% of normal individuals have a positive response.

Calcifications of basal ganglia may occur in the small blood vessels in the region. These occasionally may cause extrapyramidal signs but usually are asymptomatic. Of note, 0.7% of routine computed tomographic (CT) scans of the brain show calcification of basal ganglia.

8. In hypocalcemia, how does cerebral tetany differ from a true seizure?

Cerebral tetany results in generalized tetany without loss of consciousness, tongue biting, incontinence, or postictal confusion. Anticonvulsants may relieve the symptoms, but as noted above, they also may worsen the hypocalcemia.

9. How does hypocalcemia affect cardiac function?

Calcium is involved in cardiac automaticity and required for muscle contraction. Hypocalcemia then results in arrhythmias and decreased contractile strength. This decrease in force of contraction may be refractory to pressor agents, especially those that involve calcium in the mechanism of action. Beta blockers and calcium channel blockers, which decrease calcium availability to intracellular processes, may exacerbate cardiac failure. The Q-T interval is prolonged with low serum calcium and, although the relationship is variable, the calcium level best correlates with the interval from the Q-wave to the peak of the T-wave.

10. What are the potential ophthalmologic findings in hypocalcemia?

Papilledema may occur with subacute and chronic hypocalcemia. Patients are most often asymptomatic. With normalization of calcium levels the papilledema usually resolves. If symptoms develop or if papilledema does not resolve when the patient is normocalcemic, cerebral tumor and benign intracranial hypertension must be excluded. Optic neuritis with unilateral loss of vision occasionally develops. Lenticular cataracts also may occur with longstanding hypocalcemia but usually do not increase in size once hypocalcemia is corrected.

11. With what autoimmune disorders is hypocalcemia sometimes associated?

Hypoparathyroidism may result from autoimmune destruction of the parathyroid glands. Hypoparathyroidism has been associated with adrenal, gonadal, and thyroid failure as well as with alopecia areata, vitiligo, and chronic mucocutaneous candidiasis. Because specific antibodies have been associated with the above organs, adrenal, gonadal, and thyroid failure is classified as autoimmune polyglandular syndrome, type I.

12. Hypocalcemia is frequently encountered in intensive care settings. What are the potential causes?

Total serum calcium levels, which are low in 70–90% of intensive care patients, result from multiple causes. Hypoalbuminemia is one major cause. In addition, administration of anionic loads (i.e. citrate, lactate, oxalate, bicarbonate, phosphate, ethylenediamine tetraacetic acid [EDTA], and radiographic contrast) may lower ionized calcium levels by chelation, as noted above. Parathyroid failure and decreased vitamin D synthesis are also believed to play a role. Underlying disease states and malnutrition also frequently contribute. Furthermore, rapid blood transfusion with citrate ion as a preservative and anticoagulant therapy may transiently decrease ionized calcium by 14–40%.

13. Hypercalcemia is not unusual in patients with cancer. What conditions may lead to hypocalcemia in this patient group?

Tumor lysis syndrome with hyperphosphatemia is associated with hypocalcemia because of the formation of intravascular and tissue calcium-phosphate complexes. Multiple chemotherapeutic agents, such as vincristine/prednisone-16 (VP-16), and antibiotics, such as amphotericin B and the aminoglycosides, may induce hypomagnesemia, which leads to hypocalcemia. Hypomagnesemia impairs calcium homeostasis by reducing secretion of PTH and causing resistance to PTH in skeletal tissue. Thyroid surgery and neck irradiation may cause hypoparathyroidism transiently or permanently. Medullary carcinoma of the thyroid and pheochromocytoma may secrete calcitonin and on rare occasions cause hypocalcemia.

14. What drugs may cause hypocalcemia?

Phenobarbital, diphenhydramine, and glutethimide increase hepatic metabolism of 25-hydroxyvitamin D and may cause hypocalcemia. Aminoglycosides, diuretics (Furosemide), chemotherapeutic agents that induce renal magnesium wasting, and laxatives or enemas that create a large phosphate load also may be associated with hypocalcemia.

15. Which vitamin D metabolite is best for assessing total body vitamin D stores, 25-hydroxyvitamin D, or 1,25-dihydroxyvitamin D?

The serum level of-25 hydroxyvitamin D best reflects total body stores of vitamin D, because conversion to 1,25-dihydroxyvitamin D is tightly controlled. The level of serum 1,25-dihydroxyvitamin D is maintained despite significant vitamin D depletion.

16. How is hypocalcemia treated?

Hypocalcemia, when asymptomatic, requires supplementation with oral calcium and vitamin D derivatives to maintain the serum calcium level in the range of 7.5–8.5 mg/dl. When the serum calcium level falls acutely to a level at which the patient is symptomatic, intravenous supplementation is recommended. The dose of calcium depends on the amount of elemental calcium delivered in a given preparation. Approximately 90 mg of elemental calcium is given intravenously as a bolus for a hypocalcemic emergency, followed by an infusion of 0.5–2.0 mg/kg/hr.

Elemental Calcium Contents of Commonly Used Preparations

PREPARATION	ORAL DOSE	ELEMENTAL CALCIUM
Calcium citrate	950 mg	200 mg
Citracal		
Calcium acetate	667 mg	169 mg
PhosLo		
Calcium carbonate		
Tums	500 mg	200 mg
Tums Ex	750 mg	300 mg
Tums 500	1,250 mg	500 mg
OsCal	625 mg	250 mg
	1,250 mg	500 mg
Calcium 600	1,500 mg	600 mg
Titralac (suspension)	1,000 mg/5 ml	400 mg

INTRAVENOUS AGENT	VOLUME	ELEMENTAL CALCIUM
Calcium chloride	2.5 ml of 10% solution	90 mg
Calcium gluconate	10 ml of 10% solution	90 mg
Calcium gluceptate	5 ml of 22% solution	90 mg

17. How does the treatment of hypoparathyroidism differ from the treatment of other causes of hypocalcemia?

Decreased levels of PTH result in reduced conversion of 25-hydroxyvitamin D to 1,25-dihydroxyvitamin D and thereby reduce intestinal absorption of calcium. To overcome this defect, the patient must be given either very large doses of vitamin D or physiologic doses of 1,25-hydroxyvitamin D (calcitriol).

BIBLIOGRAPHY

1. Lebowitz MR, Moses AM: Hypocalcemia. Semin Nephrol 12:146–158, 1992.
2. McEvoy G (ed): Calcium salts. In AHFS Drug Information. Bethesda, MD, American Society of Hospital Pharmacists, 1992, pp 1498–1501.
3. Olinger ML: Disorders of calcium and magnesium metabolism. Emerg Med Clin North Am 7:795–822, 1989.
4. Potts JT: Hypocalcemia. In Wilson JD (ed): Principles of Internal Medicine, 12th ed. New York, McGraw-Hill, 1991, pp 1920–1921.
5. Shane E: Hypocalcemia: Pathogenesis, differential diagnosis and management. In Fauus MJ (ed): Primer on the Metabolic Bone Diseases and Disorders of Mineral Metabolism, 2nd ed. New York, Raven Press, 1993, pp 188–190.
6. Zaloga GP: Hypocalcemia in critically ill patients. Crit Care Med 20:251–262, 1992.

14. NEPHROLITHIASIS

Leonard R. Sanders, M.D.

1. Define hypercalciuria, nephrolithiasis, renal stones, and nephrocalcinosis.
Hypercalciuria is urinary excretion of > 300 mg/day of calcium in men and > 250 mg/day in women. A more accurate definition is urinary calcium excretion > 4 mg/kg ideal body weight per day in either sex. Nephrolithiasis, urolithiasis, and renal lithiasis are synonymous terms that define the clinical syndrome of formation and movement of stones in the urinary collecting system. Renal stones or calculi are abnormally hard, insoluble, substances that form in the renal collecting system. Nephrocalcinosis is deposition of calcium salts in the renal parenchyma.

2. Who is at risk to develop kidney stones?
Two to 4 percent of the United States population is at risk to develop one stone, and 50–60% have recurrence within 5–10 years. Stones occur most commonly between ages 18 and 45 and 2 to 3 times more commonly in men than women. However, the gap between men and women has narrowed in recent years. The cause of the increase in renal stones in women is not clear. It may represent changes in diet (increased calcium and protein intake), exercise (dehydration), or other causes. Anyone with a family history of renal calculi is also at high risk as are people with autosomal dominant polycystic kidney disease and medullary cystic disease. Others at risk have urine volume < 2 L/day, dietary sodium > 2 g/day, hypercalciuria, hyperoxaluria, hyperuricosuria, hypocitraturia, hypomagnesiuria, low calcium intake, and high protein intake.

3. What are the composition and approximate frequency of most kidney stones?
There are six major types of renal stones: mixed calcium oxalate and phosphate (41%), calcium oxalate (27%), calcium phosphate (7%), struvite (magnesium ammonium phosphate) (15%), uric acid (7%), and cystine (2%). On rare occasions, kidney stones may form from xanthine. Triamterene may serve as a nidus for stone formation.

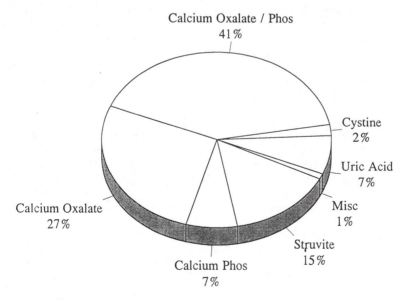

Frequency of renal stones.

4. What are the main causes of nephrolithiasis?

The most common causes of nephrolithiasis are associated with idiopathic hypercalciuria. These include absorptive hypercalciuria type I, type II, and type III (renal phosphate leak), and renal hypercalciuria. Other causes include primary hyperparathyroidism, hyperoxaluric calcium nephrolithiasis, hyperuricosuric calcium nephrolithiasis, hypocitraturic calcium nephrolithiasis, hypomagnesiuric calcium nephrolithiasis, infection stones, gouty diathesis, and cystinuria. Patients with idiopathic nephrolithiasis make up 10–20% of stone formers and have no identifiable cause after routine work-up.

5. What conditions are associated with both renal stone disease and hypercalciuria?

Calcium stones account for 70–80% of all kidney stones. About 40–50% of calcium stone formers have hypercalciuria. Most of these patients (40%) have idiopathic hypercalciuria. About 5% have primary hyperparathyroidism, and 3% have renal tubular acidosis. Other causes of hypercalciuria include excessive dietary vitamin D, excessive calcium and alkali intake, sarcoidosis, Cushing's syndrome, hyperthyroidism, Paget's disease of bone, and immobilization.

6. What are the most important causes of normocalciuric calcium nephrolithiasis?

The most important and most common causes of normocalciuric calcium nephrolithiasis are hypocitraturia (50%), hyperuricosuria (25%), hyperoxaluria (10%), and urinary stasis (5%).

7. Describe the process of renal stone formation.

Initially, urinary crystallization or precipitation of sparingly soluble salts and acids occurs. Nucleation follows as the initial crystals and urinary matrix ions form a stable framework for crystal enlargement through growth and aggregation. Once sufficiently large, the crystals are trapped in a narrow portion of the urinary collecting system. The trapped particles then serve as a nidus or focus for further growth and development of the stone. Usually stones originate in the renal papilla. Once formed, the stone may detach, move distally, and cause obstruction. Common sites for obstruction are the ureteropelvic junction, the mid ureter, and the ureterovesical junction.

8. What pathophysiologic factors influence formation of renal stones?

Renal stones do not form without quantitative or qualitative imbalances of stone precursors, inhibitors, or promoters. Hereditary or acquired defects may cause such imbalances. Other factors that increase stone formation include urinary stasis (medullary sponge kidney), decreased flow (obstruction), increased urine ammonium (infection), dehydration (concentrated urine), and level of urinary acidity (renal tubular acidosis). Renal tubular acidosis combines problems of hypercalciuria, hypocitraturia, and alkaline urine.

9. What are the main chemical precursors of renal stones?

Relatively high concentrations of salt and acid solutes are the main determinants of crystalluria and stone formation. Calcium oxalate is most common and is supersaturated in normal urine to 4–5 times its solubility. Other precursors are calcium phosphate (hydroxyapatite) and calcium phosphate monohydrate (brushite). Uric acid, cystine, struvite (magnesium ammonium phosphate), and mucoprotein are undersaturated stone precursors. Drugs, such as ascorbic acid (conversion to oxalate) and triamterene (nidus for stone formation), also may promote renal stone formation.

10. List the main inhibitors of renal stone formation. Describe how they work.

Inhibitors include urinary citrate, pyrophosphate, nephrocalcin, magnesium, glycosaminoglycans, Tamm-Horsfall protein, and uropontin. Most inhibitors bind crystal precursors, thus improving solubility, and impair precipitation, nucleation, crystal growth, or aggregation.

11. What is nephrocalcin? What role does it play in formation of renal stones?

Nephrocalcin is an anionic protein produced by the proximal renal tubule and the loop of Henle. It normally inhibits the nucleation, crystal growth, and aggregation phases of stone formation.

However, nephrocalcin isolated from many stone formers has defective structure and function and is found in the matrix of many calcium stones. Thus, nephrocalcin may have a dual role in stone formation. When normal, it acts as an inhibitor of stone formation. When abnormal, it may act as a promoter by binding calcium and forming a nidus for crystallization.

12. What are promoters of renal stone formation?

Promoters of renal stone formation are poorly characterized but are believed to be primarily urinary mucoproteins and glycosaminoglycans. Under certain conditions, promoters enhance the formation of renal stones.

13. Summarize the basic determinants of serum calcium.

In the serum, calcium is 40% protein bound, 10% complexed and 50% ionized. The three sources of serum calcium are intestinal absorption, bone resorption, and renal reabsorption. Intestinal calcium absorption is a variable proportion of the intake (15–70%); renal calcium reabsorption is a variable portion of the filtered load (95–99.5%). The net flux of calcium from bone varies, depending on changes in the intestines and kidney. Under normal physiologic conditions flux of calcium into and out of bone is the same. Parathyroid hormone (PTH) and vitamin D control the normal bone, gastrointestinal, and renal handling of calcium.

14. How does the kidney handle calcium?

The ionized and complex portions of the serum calcium are filterable. Thus, about 60% of the serum calcium is filtered by the glomerulus. The kidney reabsorbs 97–98% of the filtered calcium. Calcium reabsorption is passive throughout the nephron. The proximal convoluted tubule (PCT) reabsorbs 60%; the loop of Henle, 30%; and the distal nephron, about 10%. In the PCT, calcium is passively reabsorbed with water and other solutes. In the loop of Henle and the distal nephron, passive calcium reabsorption depends on favorable electrochemical gradients linked to active transport of sodium (Na), potassium (K), and chloride. In the loop of Henle, Na-K-2CL transport generates a positive potential difference that enhances calcium transport. Therefore, inhibition of Na-K-2CL transport by furosemide depresses calcium transport and increases urinary calcium. On the other hand, inhibition of Na transport by thiazides in the distal convoluted tubule makes the interior of the cell more electronegative and enhances calcium entry (reabsorption). PTH also may impair sodium entry in the distal nephron and increase calcium absorption by enhancing calcium channel activity.

15. Calculate the normal filtered and excreted load of calcium per day.

The serum calcium is normally 10 mg/dl. The kidney filters the complexed and free calcium that make up 60% of the total or 6 mg/dl. The normal glomerular filtration rate (GFR) = 120 ml/min. Thus, the filtered load of calcium of 6 mg/100 ml $\times$ 120 ml/min $\times$ 1440 min/day = 10,368 mg/day. Because the kidney reabsorbs 98% of the filtered calcium, only 2% is excreted. Thus, normally the kidney excretes about 200 mg of calcium/day. The calculation is 10,368 mg/day $\times$ 0.02 = 207 mg/day. If the excreted calcium increased to 5%, the urinary calcium increases to 500 mg/day.

16. How does hypercalciuria occur?

Normal mechanisms of calcium homeostasis prevent hypercalcemia by increasing urinary calcium. Thus, any nonrenal elevation in serum calcium causes increased filtered calcium and increased urinary calcium. Increased sodium delivery to the loop of Henle and the distal tubule also increases urinary calcium. For each 100 mEq/day increase in Na^+ excretion, the urinary calcium excretion increases by 40–50 mEq/day. Impairment of any calcium reabsorbing site in the nephron also increases urine calcium.

17. What is the pathophysiology of idiopathic hypercalciuria?

Idiopathic hypercalciuria (IH) is a heterogeneous disorder associated with elevated urinary calcium from intestinal hyperabsorption (absorptive hypercalciuria) or decreased renal tubular reabsorption (renal leak) of calcium. Absorptive hypercalciuria may result from a primary gut abnormality causing hyperabsorption, from increased gut responsiveness to calcitriol, or from increased levels of calcitriol. Increased levels of calcitriol may be caused by a renal phosphate leak that sequentially causes urinary loss of phosphate, decreased serum phosphate, increased calcitriol production, increased gut absorption of calcium, increased serum calcium, and hypercalciuria. A primary renal calcium leak impairs tubular reabsorption of calcium and also may cause hypercalciuria. IH may be hereditary and occurs in 30–50% of calcium stone formers. Question 28 distinguishes the various forms of idiopathic hypercalciuria.

18. What causes hyperoxaluria? Why is it important in nephrolithiasis?
Normally, 14% of urinary oxalate comes from dietary absorption. The remainder comes in equal amounts from metabolism of glyoxylate and ascorbic acid. Hereditary hyperoxaluria is a rare autosomal recessive defect caused by increased oxidation of glyoxylate to oxalate. However, enteric hyperoxaluria is clinically more important. Free calcium in the gut normally binds oxalate and prevents its absorption. Small intestinal disease may cause fat malabsorption. Excessive fat in the gut binds calcium; thus it is no longer free to bind oxalate. The oxalate is then absorbed by the colon. The recent association of low calcium diets and recurrent calcium stones is based on presumed increases in oxalate absorption. Excessive dietary oxalate also leads to hyperoxaluria. Although ethylene glycol ingestion and methoxyflurane anesthesia increase urinary excretion of oxalate crystals, there are no documented associations with calcium oxalate stones. Ascorbic acid in doses > 2 g/day may promote calcium oxalate stones. Because hyperoxaluria causes calcium oxalate supersaturation more potently than calcium, it is a powerful stimulus of calcium oxalate stone formation.

19. How does hyperuricosuria contribute to renal stones?
About 25% of calcium stone formers have hyperuricosuria, and about 25% of patients with symptomatic tophaceous gout develop uric acid stones. Excessive urinary uric acid supersaturates the urine, crystallizes, and forms uric acid stones. In addition, uric acid crystals may form a nidus for calcium phosphate and calcium oxalate deposition, resulting in increased calcium stone formation. However, most formers of uric acid stones do not have gout, hyperuricemia, or hyperuricosuria. All formers of uric acid stones have acid urine.

20. How does acid urine predispose to uric acid renal stones?
Because uric acid has a pKa of 5.75, acid urine shifts the equilibrium so that concentrations of uric acid are greater than concentrations of sodium urate. Moreover, because uric acid is 100 times less soluble than urate, stones are more likely to form in acid urine. This equilibrium is so important that uric acid stones virtually never occur without acid urine.

21. What conditions cause low levels of urinary citrate?
Idiopathic hypocitraturia is a primary but uncommon cause of hypocitraturia. Secondary causes of low citrate are more common including metabolic acidosis, hypokalemia, thiazide diuretics, carbonic anhydrase inhibitors, magnesium depletion, renal tubular acidosis, and diarrhea. Citrate is freely filtered by the glomerulus, and 75% is reabsorbed by the proximal convoluted tubule. Little citrate is secreted. Most secondary causes of hypocitraturia decrease urinary citrate by increasing proximal renal tubular reabsorption. Diarrhea also causes direct gastrointestinal loss of citrate and magnesium.

22. What is the role of diet in the formation of kidney stones?
The high protein intake of the average American diet (1–1.5 gm/kg/day) may increase both sulfate and uric acid in the urine. High levels of sulfate and uric acid may act as cofactors in the formation of calcium oxalate stones. Sulfate provides an acid load, and acidosis decreases urinary citrate. High calcium intake, recommended for prevention or treatment of osteoporosis, may lead to hypercalciuria or at least higher urinary concentrations of calcium. High dietary oxalate increases calcium oxalate crystalluria. Common foods rich in oxalate include carrots, green beans, spinach,

tomatoes, sweet potatoes, rhubarb, strawberries, grapefruit, oranges, wheat germ, cocoa, cranberry juice, raspberry juice, tea, and roasted coffee.

23. What are the presenting symptoms and signs of renal stones?

Renal stones may be asymptomatic and found as incidental radiologic findings. They also may present as a dull ache in the posterior flank. However, the classic symptom of renal stones is excruciating and intermittent pain. The pain starts in the posterior lumbar area and then radiates anteroinferiorly into the abdomen, groin, genital region, and medial thigh. Symptoms of nausea, vomiting, sweating, and general prostration may occur. Intense pain may last several hours and be followed by dull flank pain. The patient with renal colic appears acutely ill and restless and moves from side to side attempting to relieve the pain. Fever, chills, and hematuria may be present. Physical examination shows tenderness and guarding of the respective lumbar area. Deep palpation worsens the patient's discomfort, but rebound tenderness is absent. Urinary tract infection may be present. Obstruction, if present, is usually unilateral. Clinical evidence of renal failure is usually absent.

24. Outline the general diagnostic approaches to the patient with kidney stones.

Present, past, and family histories provide the clues to diagnosis. Drug history should include triamterene and vitamins A, C, and D. Dietary history should include sources of excessive calcium, salt, oxalate, uric acid, and protein. Urinalysis should focus on pH, hematuria, pyuria, bacteriuria, and crystalluria. Acid urine suggests cystine or uric acid stones. Recurrent infections and alkaline urine suggest struvite stones. Radiographs of the kidney, ureter, and bladder (KUB) should be obtained for all stone formers. An intravenous pyelogram (IVP) should be obtained for all symptomatic patients who have not passed the stone and for patients who have passed the stone but continue to have symptoms, hematuria, or multiple stones on KUB. The IVP localizes the stone in the urinary tract. Before ordering an IVP, make sure that the patient has normal serum creatinine and no allergy to radiocontrast media. Ultrasonography is usually not helpful, because it does not detail the anatomic location of the stones. The only means of definitive diagnosis is crystallographic analysis of the stone. The patient should strain all urine and save the stone if passed. If the patient has no pain and the stone is < 5 mm, careful follow-up for several months is acceptable. Ninety percent of stones < 5 mm will pass spontaneously. If the patient has symptoms, if the stone is > 1 cm, or if obvious obstruction is present, a urologist should be consulted. A 1-cm stone is not likely to pass spontaneously. Besides an IVP, patients with microscopic and macroscopic hematuria need urology consultation and cystoscopy. Questions below cover specific issues about additional laboratory and radiographic work-up.

25. What is the clinical significance of urinalysis in patients with renal stones?

Most stone formers have macroscopic or microscopic hematuria. The remainder of the urinalysis is usually normal. Crystals are normally absent in freshly voided urine. Many crystals seen on microscopic examination of warm, freshly voided urine suggest the diagnosis. However, most urine specimens cool before examination, and crystals may form in normal urine with time and cooling. Therefore, most crystalluria has little clinical significance. An exception is the presence of cystine crystals, which are diagnostic of cystinuria. Persistently acidic urine (pH below 5.5–5.0) suggests uric acid or cystine stones. Uric acid renal stones never form, unless the urine pH is acid. Persistently alkaline urine (pH above 7.5–8) and recurrent urinary tract infection strongly suggests struvite stones. Struvite stones never form, unless the urine pH is alkaline. The patient may use nitrazine paper to help follow the response to therapy. However, accurate measurement of urine pH with a pH meter is important for diagnosis. For accurate pH measurement, the patient should collect the urine in a chilled container, seal it, and keep it on ice. The urinary pH should be measured with a pH meter within 24 hours. Collection under oil is not necessary.

26. What are the characteristics of urinary crystals seen in renal-stone patients?

Calcium oxalate monohydrate crystals are oval-shaped and resemble red blood cells. Calcium oxalate dihydrate crystals are pyramid-shaped and have an envelope appearance. Calcium phosphate crystals are too small for standard light microscopic resolution and look like amorphous debris. Uric acid crystals also usually resemble amorphous debris. However, uric acid crystals have a characteristic yellow-brown color. The less common uric acid dihydrate crystals may be rhomboid-shaped or resemble the six-sided diamonds on a deck of cards. Any of these crystals may be found in normal urine; their presence is not diagnostic of disease. However, the presence of cystine crystals always means cystinuria. Cystine crystals are flat, hexagonal plates resembling benzene rings. Unlike benzene rings, however, the rings of cystine crystals may have equal or unequal sides. Struvite (magnesium ammonium phosphate) crystals are rectangular prisms that resemble coffin lids.

27. What radiographic tests are useful for evaluating patients with renal stones?
The KUB shows calcium stones but does not differentiate the type. KUB with tomograms or a digitally enhanced KUB better localizes and identifies renal stones. Calcium oxalate stones are usually small, dense, and circumscribed. Cystine stones are faint, soft, and waxy. Struvite stones are irregular and dense. Uric acid stones are radiolucent and not seen on KUB. An IVP will localize stones in the urinary tract and show the degree of obstruction and renal function. If needed during pregnancy, a limited IVP (KUB + 10-min postcontrast film) may be appropriate. A radiolucent obstruction on IVP suggests a uric acid stone. However, a noncontrast CT scan may be required to rule out uroepithelial malignancy. Ultrasonography is not helpful in evaluating renal stones, unless there are contraindications to the IVP. Ultrasound may identify obstruction and give the size and location of larger stones.

28. Distinguish among the various forms of idiopathic hypercalciuria.
Idiopathic hypercalciuria involves four primary syndromes: absorptive hypercalciuria (AH) types I, II, and III and renal hypercalciuria (RH). They have the following features.

Idiopathic Hypercalciuria

LAB VALUE	AH-I	AH-II	AH-III	RH
Serum calcium	Normal	Normal	Normal	Normal
Serum phosphorus	Normal	Normal	↓	Normal
Serum intact PTH	Normal	Normal	Normal	↑
24-hr urinary calcium (1-gm calcium diet)	↑	↑	↑	↑
Urine calcium/creatinine (1-gm calcium load)	↑	↑	↑	↑
24-hr urinary calcium (400-mg calcium diet)	↑	Normal	↑	↑
Fasting urinary calcium (mg/dl GFR)	Normal	Normal	↑	↑

Serum phosphorus is low in AH-III because of a primary renal phosphate leak. Intact PTH is high in renal hypercalciuria, because the primary defect is decreased calcium reabsorption, which causes relative hypocalcemia and stimulates PTH. All patients by definition have high 24-hour urinary calcium on a 1-gram calcium diet and a high urine calcium/creatinine (Ca/Cr) ratio after a 1-gram calcium load. AH-II normalizes 24-hr urine calcium on a restricted calcium diet (400 mg/day) because the absorptive excess is not as severe. However, the 24-hour urine calcium during calcium restriction remains high in AH-I, AH-III, and RH. It remains high in AH-I because of marked hyperabsorption of calcium, in AH-III, because hypophosphatemia decreases renal tubular reabsorption of calcium, and in RH, because decreased renal tubular reabsorption is the primary defect. Low serum phosphorus is < 2.5 mg/dl on an 800-mg/day phosphorus diet. High 24-hour urinary calcium is > 4 mg/kg ideal body weight. Normal 24-hour urinary calcium on a 400-mg/day calcium restriction is < 200 mg/day. Normal fasting urine calcium is < 0.11 mg per 100 ml GFR. Normal urine Ca/Cr is < 0.20 after a 1-gram oral load of calcium. Occasionally, the above work-up varies in the same patient, overlaps in different categories, and may not change initial therapy. For these reasons most clinicians do not differentiate the various forms of idiopathic hypercalciuria. However, complicated stone disease probably requires the above thorough evaluation.

29. **Match the drugs with the stone-forming condition that they are useful for treating.**

Drug Therapy for Renal Stones

DISORDER	DRUG	DOSAGE
Absorptive type I	Hydrochlorothiazide	25–50 mg bid
	Potassium citrate	10–30 mg tid
	Cellulose sodium phosphate	5 g qd–tid with meals
	Magnesium gluconate	10 mEq bid
Absorptive type II	Hydrochlorothiazide	25–50 mg bid
Renal phosphate leak	Neutral sodium phosphate	500 mg tid
Renal hypercalciuria	Hydrochlorothiazide	25–50 mg bid
Hypocitraturia	Potassium citrate	10–40 mg tid
Hyperuricosuria	Potassium citrate	10–30 mg tid
	Allopurinol	200–600 mg qd
Enteric hyperoxaluria	Potassium citrate	10–30 mg tid
	Magnesium gluconate	10 mEq bid
	Calcium citrate	950 mg qid
	Calcium carbonate	250–500 mg qid
	Cholestyramine	4 g tid
	Pyridoxine	100 mg qd
Cystinuria	Potassium citrate	10–30 mg tid
	α-Mercaptopropionylglycine	250–500 mg qid
	D-Penicillamine	250–500 mg qid
	Pyridoxine	50 mg qd
Struvite stones	Acetohydroxamic acid	250 mg bid–qid

30. **What therapy is appropriate in all stone formers?**
Fluid intake should be increased to increase urine output to 2–3 L/day, and dietary sodium should be restricted to 2 g/day. Dietary protein shall be restricted to 0.8–1 g/kg ideal body weight/day. The patient should avoid excesses of foods high in oxalate. Think twice before starting drug therapy. Do not start drug therapy unless there is certainty or a strong suspicion that the drug will improve or correct the underlying disease mechanism. Know the mechanism of action and side effects of the drugs used. When indicated, use the drugs listed above alone or in combination. Tailor the dose to the patient's metabolic disturbance.

CONTROVERSIES

31. **What patients with calcium renal stones need a thorough metabolic evaluation?**
There is little controversy that patients with cystine or uric acid stones need evaluation. However, patients with calcium stones usually respond to thiazide therapy. If hypokalemia develops, potassium citrate improves the hypokalemia and the thiazide-induced hypocitraturia. Thus, some experts suggest treating any calcium stone former who requires drug therapy with one or both drugs. However, therapy for renal stone disease is life-long. Thiazides can cause hyponatremia, hypokalemia, hypocitraturia, dehydration, hyperuricemia, gout, hyperglycemia, hypersensitivity reactions, and other problems. Furthermore, patients may have combined defects that will be missed without at least a limited metabolic work-up. An alternate approach is to get a basic work-up on all stone formers before starting life-long therapy. The work-up may improve selection of therapy by revealing several defects that promote stone formation.

32. **What is the best initial work-up for renal stone formers?**
Initially the approach summarized in question 24 should be followed. The initial approach to testing varies from no evaluation to several tests. For the symptomatic patient or the patient who

requires drug therapy, the following work-up is rational. Order an SMA-12 that includes Na, K, Cl, CO_2, BUN, creatinine, glucose, calcium, phosphorus, albumin, magnesium, and uric acid. These plus a 24-hour urine test for creatinine, Na, K, Cl, calcium, phosphorus, magnesium, oxalate, and citrate will screen for most causes of nephrolithiasis. These tests may document baseline abnormalities pathogenic for renal stones, and therapy may change such values. Some laboratories require acidification of the urine for oxalate and citrate measurement. Thus, the patient should collect a 24-hour urine sample at least twice. Some experts obtain only one urine collection; others obtain three. Some do not acidify the urine. Because diet and other factors may cause the results to change, most experts suggest 2–3 urine collections before starting life-long therapy.

33. How should patients with complicated renal calculi be further evaluated?

With any given patient, some experts in renal stone disease do all the following tests initially; some do some of the tests; some do none. Further testing depends on the severity of the stone disease and the response to initial therapy. Specialized testing should be done when the patient has serious recurrent stone disease that has failed initial medical therapy. Such tests include repeating the baseline tests and obtaining values of serum intact PTH, 1,25-dihydroxyvitamin D, and 24-hour urine sulfate and urea. If the diagnosis remains in question, specialized urine testing is appropriate. After an overnight fast with nothing by mouth but distilled water, tests should be done to determine values for serum calcium and creatinine and 2-hr urine calcium and creatinine. This should be followed by a 4-hour urine sample for calcium and creatinine after giving 1-gram of elemental calcium orally. From these measurements, the fasting urinary calcium can be calculated in mg/dL GFR (normal < 0.11) and the absorption of calcium can be estimated by calculating the urinary Ca/Cr ratio (mg/mg) (normal < 0.20). These measurements may identify the cause of hypercalciuria.

34. What are some pitfalls in the therapy of renal stone formers?

Alkalinization of the urine is recommended for treatment of uric acid and cystine stones to increase solute solubility. However, use of sodium bicarbonate increases excretion of sodium and thus of calcium. The increased calcium and alkali may increase calcium stone formation. Potassium citrate is the better alkalizing agent because it increases the citrate inhibitor without increasing the urinary sodium and calcium load. Cellulose sodium phosphate (CSP) binds calcium in the gut of patients with AH-I and decreases both calcium and magnesium absorption. Patients with AH-I often have osteopenia. CSP may predispose them to further osteopenia and a hypomagnesemic tendency to renal stones. Therefore, thiazides and potassium citrate should be tried first; CSP should be reserved for refractory stone disease, and magnesium should be replaced, as required. Calcium restriction may decrease hypercalciuria; however, it also may decrease gut binding of oxalate, increase oxalate absorption, promote hyperoxaluria, and increase calcium oxalate stones. Thiazide diuretics decrease hypercalciuria but may cause hypokalemia and hypocitraturia. Potassium should be replaced with potassium citrate, and urine values should be measured after 2 months of therapy to assess effects.

35. What is the best thiazide diuretic to use in renal stone formers?

Any thiazide diuretic decreases urinary excretion of calcium. Options include hydrochlorothiazide, 25–50 mg bid; trichlormethiazide, 2–4 mg qd; indapamide, 2.5–5 mg qd; and chlorthalidone, 25–50 mg qd. All may have problems with potassium wasting. Because hypokalemia may cause hypocitraturia, potassium citrate is reasonable replacement therapy. Triamterene should be avoided because of its possible role in stone formation. However, amiloride, 5 mg qd, is reasonable. Various experts may choose any of the above.

36. What is the treatment for an asymptomatic patient with a 1–2-cm stone?

Most experts treat a symptomatic patient with a 1–2-cm calcium stone in the renal pelvis or a significant proximally obstructing stone (0.6–2 cm) with extracorporeal shock-wave lithotripsy (ESWL). The asymptomatic patient is a toss-up. Each expert has an opinion based on the experience of the local medical community. Nephrology and urology consultations are appropriate. Other forms of lithotripsy include percutaneous ultrasonic lithotripsy (PUL) and endoscopic ultrasonic lithotripsy (EUL). All these therapies are expensive and can easily cost more than $5,000–10,000 per treatment.

BIBLIOGRAPHY

1. Bush WH: Radiology and treatment of urinary tract stone disease. Curr Opin Radiol 4:32–38, 1992.
2. Favus MJ, Coe FL: Nephrolithiasis. In Becker KL, Bilezikian JP, Bremner WJ, et al (eds): Principles and Practice of Endocrinology and Metabolism. Philadelphia, J.B. Lippincott, 1990, pp 536–544.
3. Goldfarb S: The role of diet in the pathogenesis and therapy of nephrolithiasis. Endocrinol Metab Clin North Am 19:805–820, 1990.
4. Khatchadourian J, Pak CYC: Nephrolithiasis. In Bardin CW (ed): Current Therapy in Endocrinology and Metabolism, 5th ed. St. Louis, C.V. Mosby, 1994, pp 528–532.
5. Kohrmann KU, Rassweiler J, Alken P: The recurrence rate of stones following ESWL. World J Urol 11:26–30, 1993.
6. Laufer J, Boichis H: Urolithiasis in children: Current medical management. Pediatr Nephrol 3:317–331, 1989.
7. Lemann J Jr, Worcester EM, Gray RW: Hypercalciuria and stones. Am J Kidney Dis 17:386–391, 1991.
8. Massey LK, Roman-Smith H, Sutton RA: Effect of dietary oxalate and calcium on urinary oxalate and risk of formation of calcium oxalate kidney stones. J Am Diet Assoc 93:901–906, 1993.
9. Menon M, Koul H: Clinical review 32: Calcium oxalate nephrolithiasis. J Clin Endocrinol Metab 74:703–707, 1992.
10. Pak CY: Etiology and treatment of urolithiasis. Am J Kidney Dis 18:624–637, 1991.
11. Pak CY: Calcium metabolism. J Am Coll Nutr 8 (Suppl):46S–53S, 1989.
12. Pak CY: Urolithiasis. In Schrier RW, Gottschalk CW (eds): Diseases of the Kidney, 5th ed. Boston, Little, Brown, 1993, pp 729–741.
13. Preminger GM: Renal calculi: Pathogenesis, diagnosis, and medical therapy. Semin Nephrol 12:200–216, 1992.
14. Riese RJ, Sakhaee K: Uric acid nephrolithiasis: pathogenesis and treatment. J Urol 148:765–771, 1992.
15. Segura JW: Current surgical approaches to nephrolithiasis. Endocrinol Metab Clin North Am 19:919–935, 1990.
16. Stewart C: Nephrolithiasis. Emerg Med Clin North Am 6:617–630, 1988.
17. Torres VE, Wilson DM, Hattery RR, et al: Renal stone disease in autosomal dominant polycystic kidney disease. Am J Kidney Dis 22:513–519, 1993.
18. Uribarri J, Oh MS, Carroll HJ:J The first kidney stone. Ann Intern Med 111:1006–1009, 1989.
19. Van Arsdalen KN, Banner MP, Pollack HM: Radiographic imaging and urologic decision making in the management of renal and ureteral calculi. Urol Clin North Am 17:171–190, 1990.
20. Wickham JE: Treatment of urinary tract stones. BMJ 307:1414–1417, 1993.

III. Pituitary and Hypothalamic Disorders

15. PITUITARY INSUFFICIENCY

William J. Georgitis, M.D., COL, MC

CAUSES

1. What causes pituitary insufficiency?

Pituitary insufficiency results from pituitary, hypothalamic, or parasellar diseases that disrupt the normal function of the hypothalamic-pituitary unit by displacement, infiltration, or destruction.

2. What happens to anterior pituitary hormones after stalk section?

All of the anterior pituitary hormones regulated by hypothalamic releasing hormones decline, including thyrotropin (TSH), luteinizing hormone (LH), follicle-stimulating hormone (FSH), growth hormone (GH), and corticotropin (ACTH). Prolactin rises. This response, which is unique among adenohypophysial hormones, results from the loss of the inhibitory effect of hypothalamic dopamine on the lactotroph.

3. What is a craniopharyngioma?

In childhood, craniopharyngioma is the most common tumor in the region of the hypothalamus and pituitary. It is a squamous cell tumor that arises from Rathke's pouch remnants. Two-thirds are suprasellar, and one-third extend into or are within the sella. Most are cystic, but some are mixed cystic-solid structures. Cyst fluid is typically viscous and yellow-brown in color, resembling motor oil. Calcification of the rim of the tumor is a useful radiographic sign, demonstrated best by computerized tomography. Calcifications are present in 75% of children but only 35% of adults. Surgery is indicated both for treatment and pathologic confirmation.

4. What disorders adjacent to the pituitary or hypothalamus cause pituitary dysfunction?

Extrasellar diseases include meningiomas, chordomas, craniopharyngiomas, optic nerve gliomas, carotid aneurysms, sphenoid sinus mucoceles, and nasopharyngeal carcinomas.

5. If a young adult complains of polyuria and is also found to be hypogonadal, what diagnosis should be considered?

Pineal dysgerminoma. This tumor can grow to involve the hypothalamus and disrupt both posterior and anterior pituitary function.

PITUITARY APOPLEXY

6. What is pituitary apoplexy?

Apoplexy in general terminology means loss of consciousness followed by paralysis. Classic pituitary apoplexy is an acute life-threatening event characterized by severe headache and collapse caused by intrapituitary hemorrhage. The resultant expanding hemorrhagic mass may compress parasellar structures, including cranial nerves coursing through the adjacent cavernous sinuses. Ocular paralysis and ptosis from involvement of the third, fourth, and sixth cranial nerves as well as facial nerve involvement provide the element of paralysis necessary to meet the general definition of apoplexy. Anterior pituitary insufficiency is common, whereas the functions of the posterior pituitary are almost always preserved. Most patients recover spontaneously. Subacute forms of pituitary necrosis occur in patients with diabetes mellitus and sickle-cell disease. Radiologic evidence of pituitary infarction is an indication for a comprehensive functional evaluation.

EMPTY SELLA SYNDROME

7. Is primary empty sella syndrome frequently associated with symptomatic pituitary dysfunction?

No. Primary implies that the "empty" sella is totally or partially filled with cerebrospinal fluid and is not the end result of infarction, surgical removal, or irradiation of a tumor. Some believe that this disorder is an anatomical variant of normal or perhaps results from a congenital defect in the diaphragm covering the sella. The prevalence of evident hypopituitarism in primary empty sella is less than 10%.

8. What is Sheehan's syndrome? How common is it?

Sheehan's syndrome is an acquired form of empty sella syndrome associated with a difficult obstetrical delivery. Thirty percent of women suffering postpartum hemorrhage and vascular collapse may demonstrate some anterior pituitary insufficiency from ischemic pituitary necrosis.

DIAGNOSIS

9. Do hypopituitary features differ between children and adults?

In childhood the presence of hypopituitarism is usually signified by growth failure. In adolescents arrest or failure of sexual maturation indicates pituitary malfunction. In adults, signs of hypogonadism dominate the clinical picture. Hypogonadism may easily be overlooked in postmenopausal women or elderly men, who often fail to report declining sexual function or desire.

10. Is there an easy way to tell if the sella turcica is enlarged?

If a dime (diameter = 16 mm) fits within the sella, it is too big. The most common cause for sellar enlargement is pituitary adenoma. Carcinoma of the pituitary is extremely rare. Fortunately, metastases to this region within the cranium are also rare and more often involve the highly vascular hypothalamus, causing secondary hypopituitarism and diabetes insipidus.

11. What tests should be considered for hypopituitary patients?

The evaluation should include assessment of anterior pituitary hormones, radiographic imaging by computerized tomography or magnetic resonance imaging to assess anatomy, and formal visual fields with lesions near the optic chiasm or optic nerves. The tests for anterior pituitary hormones often include serum hormone levels measured with or without trophic factor stimulation. Nocturia, polyuria, or polydipsia suggest the need to test for adequacy of vasopressin secretion.

12. What characteristics of adrenal insufficiency are present in ACTH-deficient patients?

Nonspecific symptoms, such as fatigue and weight loss, are often displayed with ACTH deficiency. In women, axillary and pubic hair may diminish or disappear. Features of glucocorticoid deficiency are usually not as severe as those of primary adrenal failure.

13. What serum level of cortisol is consistent with adrenal insufficiency?

Morning values of cortisol less than 10 mcg/dl or ACTH-stimulated values less than 20 µg/dl may be indicative of secondary adrenal insufficiency.

14. Is secondary adrenal insufficiency as common as gonadotropin deficiency in patients with pituitary tumor?

No. The frequency of dysfunction among the anterior pituitary hormones at the time of diagnosis of a pituitary tumor presents a spectrum of prevalence with growth hormone > gonadotropins >

thyrotropin > corticotropin. Prolactin deficiency rarely is recognized clinically. Posterior pituitary dysfunction with diabetes insipidus is so infrequent that its presence should suggest diseases primarily of hypothalamic or pineal origin. Most patients with adenoma have surprisingly intact anterior pituitary function before treatment and usually acquire hypopituitarism after surgical or radiation treatment. For this reason the search for medical therapies as alternatives to ablative treatments for pituitary tumors continues.

15. What is the difference between secondary and primary hypothyroidism?
Hypothyroidism is primary when the thyroid itself fails. In secondary hypothyroidism, thyroid hormone deficiency is secondary to loss of the trophic hormones secreted by the pituitary or hypothalamus.

Elevation of TSH is the most sensitive and specific test for the diagnosis of primary hypothyroidism. As the thyroid's secretion of thyroxine declines, levels of TSH rise.

In secondary hypothyroidism, symptoms and signs are similar to those in primary hypothyroidism but milder. Even patients with massive pituitary tumors may not have obvious hypothyroidism. Laboratory tests, like the symptoms and signs, are less helpful than in primary hypothyroidism. Levels of TSH are usually in the normal range but may be low or slightly elevated. Levels of thyroxine (T_4) may be normal or low, but levels of triiodothyronine (T_3) are often normal. The low levels of T_4 despite normal immunoassayable TSH is evidence of diminished TSH bioactivity.

16. What is the Houssay phenomenon?
You can stump most attendings with this question. Houssay, an Argentinian Nobel laureate, showed that the diabetes of pancreatectomized dogs can be ameliorated by hypophysectomy. Later, he and other investigators demonstrated the diabetogenic actions of pituitary extracts. The clinical correlate of this phenomenon has been reported rarely. A diminishing requirement for insulin may serve as a sign that a diabetic patient has acquired hypopituitarism with deficiencies of insulin counterregulatory factors, such as growth hormone and cortisol. As a corollary, the diabetes secondary to growth hormone excess in acromegaly may improve or resolve after pituitary surgery or octreotide therapy.

TREATMENT

17. What is the most important hormone deficiency to identify and treat in patients with anterior pituitary disease?
Inadequate cortisol secretion is the most important to identify and treat.

18. Why is aldosterone deficiency not a concern in the patient with hypopituitarism?
Secretion of aldosterone is regulated primarily by the renin-angiotensin axis and is only secondarily modulated by potassium and ACTH.

19. Is anterior pituitary hormone deficiency always a commitment to life-long replacement?
In most cases, yes, but there are important exceptions. Primary hypothyroidism may present as amenorrhea-galactorrhea in a woman or as impotence and impaired libido in a man. Dramatic regression of pituitary hyperplasia and resolution of hypogonadism may occur with thyroid replacement. Hypopituitarism from hemochromatosis, an inherited disorder of iron storage, has improved with therapy directed at the underlying disorder. Another example is certain patients with pituitary macroadenomas. Mild elevations in prolactin sometimes resolve immediately after surgical excision of the tumor. Improvement in deficient hormones, especially ACTH, may also occur.

20. When one hormone deficiency in hypopituitarism is diagnosed, why is it important to define whether other hormone deficiencies are present?
Replacement with thyroid hormone alone in a patient with coexistent adrenal deficiency may

precipitate acute adrenal insufficiency. Furthermore, vasopressin deficiency may be masked by adrenal insufficiency. After glucocorticoid replacement, central diabetes insipidus may appear and require specific treatment with a vasopressin analogue.

21. Who should receive growth hormone treatment?

Treatment is indicated for children with short stature, open epiphyses, and documented growth hormone deficiency.

22. Should growth hormone deficiency be treated in adults?

In adults, growth hormone deficiency usually goes unrecognized but may contribute to asthenia, weakness, and poor wound healing. The role of biosynthetic growth hormone as replacement therapy or even as an interventional therapy targeted to improve skeletal mass, body composition, and muscle strength is presently an active area of investigation. Its clinical use for such purposes should be regarded as experimental until the risks and benefits have been clearly defined.

BIBLIOGRAPHY

1. Abboud CF: Hypopituitarism. In Conn RB (ed): Current Diagnosis, 8th ed. Philadelphia, W.B. Saunders, 1991, pp 811–819.
2. Arafah B: Reversible hypopituitarism in patients with large nonfunctioning pituitary adenomas. J Clin Endocrinol Metab 62:1173–1179, 1986.
3. Molitch ME: Hypopituitarism. In Rakel RE (ed): Conn's Current Therapy. Philadelphia, W.B. Saunders, 1993, pp 623–626.
4. Reichlin S, Thorner MO, Vance ML, et al: Hypothalamus and pituitary. In Wilson JD, Foster DW (eds): Williams' Textbook of Endocrinology, 8th ed. Philadelphia, W.B. Saunders, 1992, pp 135–356.

16. NONFUNCTIONING PITUITARY TUMORS

Michael T. McDermott, M.D.

1. What is a nonfunctioning pituitary tumor?

A nonfunctioning pituitary tumor arises from cells of the pituitary gland but does not secrete clinically detectable amounts of a pituitary hormone. These tumors are usually benign adenomas.

2. What other lesions can resemble nonfunctioning pituitary tumors?

Tumors not of pituitary origin also may occur within the sella turcica, including metastatic carcinomas, craniopharyngiomas, meningiomas, and tumors derived from neural tissues. In addition, nonneoplastic lesions such as Rathke's pouch cysts, arterial aneurysms, and granulomatous disease may be seen in the same area.

3. Differentiate between microadenoma and macroadenoma.

A pituitary microadenoma is less than 10 mm in its largest dimension, whereas a macroadenoma is 10 mm or larger. A macroadenoma may be contained entirely within the sella turcica or may have extrasellar extension.

4. Which structures may be damaged by growth of a pituitary tumor outside the sella turcica?

Pituitary tumors that grow superiorly may compress the optic chiasm and pituitary stalk. Tumors that grow inferiorly may erode into the sphenoid sinus. Laterally they may invade the cavernous sinuses and compress cranial nerves III, IV, and VI or the internal carotid artery. Anterior and posterior growth may erode the bones of the tuberculum sellae and dorsum sellae, respectively.

5. What are the clinical features of nonfunctioning pituitary tumors?

Nonfunctioning pituitary tumors usually present as space-occupying masses that compress nearby neurologic and/or vascular structures. Common clinical manifestations include headaches, visual field defects, visual loss, and extraocular nerve palsies. Pituitary insufficiency also may result from destruction of the remaining normal pituitary tissue.

6. What anatomic evaluation is necessary for a pituitary tumor?

Computed tomography (CT) or magnetic resonance imaging (MRI) of the pituitary gland and parasellar regions often allows a precise diagnosis and determines the presence and extent of extrasellar invasion. Visual field testing helps to assess function of the optic chiasm and tracts. Angiography may be needed in some cases to rule out the presence of an aneurysm.

7. What evaluation is necessary to determine that a pituitary tumor is nonfunctioning?

A thorough history and physical examination must be performed to detect any signs or symptoms of overproduction of pituitary hormones. Hormone testing should include determination of at least serum prolactin, growth hormone, thyroid-stimulating hormone (TSH), thyroxine (T_4), luteinizing hormone (LH), and follice-stimulating hormone (FSH), testosterone (men) and free cortisol in 24-hour urine sampling. Serum alpha subunit, when available, is also helpful.

8. Does an elevated level of serum prolactin mean that a tumor is functioning?

No. Secretion of prolactin is negatively regulated by hypothalamic inhibitory factors, such as dopamine, which reach the anterior pituitary through the pituitary stalk. Stalk compression may interfere, thus increasing release of prolactin. The serum prolactin rarely exceeds 100 ng/ml in such cases, whereas it is usually much higher with prolactin-secreting tumors.

9. What is the primary treatment for a nonfunctioning pituitary tumor?

The treatment of choice is transsphenoidal surgery, in which access to the pituitary gland is gained through the sphenoid sinus. Radiation therapy may be used if surgery is contraindicated or not desired. Medications such as bromocriptine are rarely helpful with these tumors.

10. Is postoperative radiation therapy recommended for incompletely resected tumors?

Older literature, mostly from uncontrolled studies, suggests that postoperative radiation therapy is beneficial. Currently, however, many experts advise radiation only for large tumor remnants that compress vascular or neural structures. Residual disease of lesser severity may be monitored with imaging studies and treated if growth occurs.

11. What endocrine complications occur in the immediate postoperative period?

Transient diabetes insipidus (vasopressin deficiency) is common and may be followed by transient water intoxication (vasopressin excess), both due to trauma or edema of the neurohypophysis. Fluid balance and serum electrolytes must therefore be closely monitored. Secondary adrenal insufficiency is of little immediate concern, because high-dose dexamethasone is generally given to reduce postoperative cerebral edema, but the insufficiency may become apparent after dexamethasone is stopped. Deficiencies of other pituitary hormones do not tend to be a problem if they were normal preoperatively.

12. What is the management of postoperative diabetes insipidus and water intoxication?

Mild postoperative diabetes insipidus may be managed with isovolumetric, isotonic fluid replacement. More severe cases should be treated with aqueous vasopressin, 5 units subcutaneously every 4–6 hours, until urine volumes become normal. If hyponatremia develops, vasopressin must be reduced or stopped and fluid intake restricted. If diabetes insipidus persists beyond 1 week, patients may be switched to desmopressin (DDAVP), 0.1 ml intranasally once or twice daily.

13. What endocrine problems may occur during long-term follow-up?

Deficiency of one or more pituitary hormones may develop weeks, months, or years after treatment, especially if radiation was given. The major concern in the first month is adrenal insufficiency. Once dexamethasone is discontinued, an adrenocorticotropin (ACTH) stimulation test, metyrapone test, or insulin tolerance test should be performed to assess the pituitary-adrenal axis. If the response is inadequate, treatment with hydrocortisone should be started, and the patient should be retested in 1–3 months. At that time serum T_4 and testosterone (men) also should be checked. Depending on the circumstances, the tests may need to be repeated at 6 months, 1 year, and then annually thereafter for up to 10 years.

14. What is the long-term management of pituitary insufficiency?

Deficiency	Replacement Regimen
Adrenal insufficiency	Hydrocortisone, 20 mg AM, 10 mg PM
Hypothyroidism	Levothyroxine, 0.1–0.125 mg every day
Hypogonadism, men	Depo-testosterone, 300 mg intramuscularly every 3 wk
Hypogonadism, women	Conjugated estrogens, 0.625–1.25 mg on days 1–25 of each month
	Medroxyprogesterone acetate, 5–10 mg on days 13–25 of each month
Diabetes insipidus	Desmopressin, 0.1 ml intranasally 1–2 ×/day

15. What are the clinical features of pituitary carcinomas?

Pituitary carcinomas, which are extremely rare, expand rapidly and cause mass effects. Some secrete hormones causing endocrine syndromes similar to those seen with adenomas. Metastatic disease to the central nervous system, cervical lymph nodes, liver, and bone are commonly associated.

16. What is the treatment for pituitary carcinomas?
Transsphenoidal surgery is the primary therapy, followed by postoperative radiation. No significant use of chemotherapy has been reported for pituitary carcinomas.

17. What is the prognosis for pituitary carcinoma?
The mean survival is approximately 4 years.

18. Which cancers metastasize to the pituitary gland?
Metastatic disease to the pituitary gland occurs in approximately 3–5% of patients with widely disseminated carcinoma. The most commonly reported primary tumors are breast, lung, kidney, prostate, liver, pancreas, nasopharynx, plasmacytoma, and sarcoma and adenocarcinoma of unknown primary site.

BIBLIOGRAPHY

1. Branch Jr CL, Laws ER Jr: Metastatic tumors of the sella turcica masquerading as primary pituitary tumors. J Clin Endocrinol Metab 65:469–474, 1987.
2. Kaufman B, Arafah B, Selman WR: Advances in neuroradiologic imaging of the pituitary gland: Changing concepts. J Lab Clin Med 109:308–319, 1987.
3. Klibanski A, Zervas NT: Diagnosis and management of hormone-secreting pituitary adenomas. N Engl J Med 324:822–831, 1991.
4. Molitch ME, Russell EJ: The pituitary "incidentaloma." Ann Intern Med 112:925–931, 1990.
5. Mountcastle RB, Roof BS, Mayfield RK, et al: Case report: Pituitary adenocarcinoma in an acromegalic patient: Response to bromocriptine and pituitary testing: A review of the literature on 36 cases of pituitary carcinoma. Am J Med Sci 298(2):109–118, 1989.

17. PROLACTIN-SECRETING PITUITARY TUMORS

Virginia Sarapura, M.D.

1. Describe the normal control of prolactin secretion. How is this altered in prolactin-secreting tumors?

The principal influence on prolactin secretion is tonic inhibition by dopamine input from the hypothalamus. Pituitary stalk interruption leads to increased levels of prolactin. The inhibition is mediated by the interaction of dopamine with receptors of the D2 subtype present on pituitary lactotroph membranes. This interaction activates the inhibitory G-protein, leading to decreased adenylate cyclase activity. In prolactin-secreting pituitary adenomas, a monoclonal population of cells autonomously produces prolactin, escaping the normal physiologic input of dopamine from the hypothalamus. In almost all cases, responsiveness to a pharmacologic dose of dopamine is maintained.

2. What are the normal levels of serum prolactin? Are they different in men and women? What levels are seen in patients with prolactin-secreting tumors?

The normal serum prolactin level is < 15 or 20 ng/ml, depending on the laboratory. Women tend to have slightly higher levels than men, probably because of estrogen stimulation of prolactin secretion. In patients with prolactin-secreting tumors, the levels are usually > 100 ng/ml but may be as low as 30–50 ng/ml if the tumor is small. A level >200 ng/ml is almost always indicative of a prolactin-secreting tumor.

3. What are the physiologic causes of an elevated prolactin level that need to be considered in the differential diagnosis of prolactin-secreting tumors? What levels can be reached under these circumstances?

The most important physiologic states in which prolactin is found to be elevated are pregnancy and lactation. During the third trimester of pregnancy, the prolactin level is usually 200–300 ng/ml and gradually decreases during the first months postpartum in spite of continued lactation. Prolactin levels are also elevated during sleep, strenuous exercise, stress, and nipple stimulation. In these cases, the elevation is mild, below 50 ng/ml.

4. List the abnormal causes of an elevated serum prolactin level other than a prolactin-secreting tumor. State the mechanism underlying the abnormal prolactin production. What are the typical levels of serum prolactin associated with each cause?

Causes of Elevated Levels of Serum Prolactin

CAUSES	MECHANISM	PROLACTIN LEVEL

1. Pituitary stalk interruption
   Trauma
   Surgery
   Pituitary, hypothalamic, or
     parasellar tumors
   Infiltrative disorders of the
     hypothalamus
	Interference with the hypothalamic-pituitary pathways, which usually causes hypopituitarism; prolactin levels increase because the tonic inhibition of prolactin secretion is interrupted	Usually 30–50 ng/ml, rarely above 100 ng/ml

2. Pharmacologic agents
   Phenothiazines
   Tricyclic antidepressants
   Alpha-methyldopa
   Metoclopramide
   Cimetidine
   Estrogens
	Specific interference with dopaminergic input to the pituitary gland	Usually 30–50 ng/ml, rarely above 100 ng/ml

Table continued on following page.

Causes of Elevated Levels of Serum Prolactin (Continued)

CAUSES	MECHANISM	PROLACTIN LEVEL
3. Hypothyroidism	Increased TRH that stimulates prolactin release	Usually 30–50 ng/ml
4. Renal failure Liver cirrhosis	Decreased metabolic clearance of prolactin	Usually 30–50 ng/ml; sometimes as high as 150 ng/ml in chronic renal failure

5. Intercostal nerve stimulation
   Chest wall lesions
   Herpes zoster
	Mimicking of the stimulation caused by suckling	Usually 30–50 ng/ml

TRH = thyrotropin-releasing hormone.

5. What is galactorrhea? Do most patients with prolactin-secreting tumors present with this symptom?

Galactorrhea is the discharge of milk from the breast not associated with pregnancy or lactation. Although a typical symptom of prolactin-secreting tumors, it may be absent in up to 50% of women and is uncommon in men. In men, galactorrhea may be seen in conjunction with gynecomastia when decreased gonadal function results in a low ratio of testosterone to estrogen.

6. Why do men with prolactin-secreting tumors often present with more advanced disease than do women?

The major symptoms of elevated prolactin levels in men are decreased libido and impotence. These symptoms may be ignored or attributed to psychological causes. Many years may go by before an evaluation is sought, often when the patient develops headaches and visual field defects related to the mass effect of the tumor. Women are likely to seek evaluation early in the disease process, when infertility or menstrual irregularities prompt an evaluation of hormonal status.

7. What is the imaging technique of choice when a prolactin-secreting tumor is suspected? Why?

Magnetic resonance imaging (MRI) of the pituitary with a contrast agent such as gadolinium is the imaging technique of choice in the evaluation of pituitary tumors. In particular, discrimination of small tumors is enhanced. Computerized tomographic scanning allows for a better visualization of bone structures, such as the floor of the sella, in cases of large tumors. However, the relationship of the tumor to other soft-tissue structures, such as the cavernous sinus and carotid arteries, is better visualized with MRI. This issue is still somewhat controversial. Skull radiographs and tomograms are not helpful.

8. If a prolactinoma is left untreated, what is the risk of tumor enlargement?

Many longitudinal studies agree that progression of the disease is rare and occurs at a slow pace. This is particularly true of small prolactin-secreting tumors, less than 5% of which will enlarge. There is no reliable way to predict which patients are going to show progression. Spontaneous resolution, attributed to necrosis, has also been described in some patients.

9. Bone metabolism is altered when prolactin levels are elevated. What is the mechanism for this effect?

Elevated prolactin levels suppress the hypothalamic-pituitary-gonadal axis by interference with the secretion of gonadotropin-releasing hormone (GnRH) in the hypothalamus. The resulting decrease in circulating levels of estrogen and testosterone causes a corresponding decrease in osteoblastic function, which becomes uncoupled from normal or increased osteoclastic function.

10. What is the consequence of the altered bone metabolism? Is it reversible?

The consequence is a decrease in bone mineral density and progression to osteoporosis. Studies suggest that normalization of the prolactin level restores bone density in most but not all patients.

11. Is there a medical treatment for prolactin-secreting tumors? What is the mode of action?

Medical treatment with dopamine agonists has been available for about 20 years. The most commonly used is bromocriptine; pergolide is also available. These drugs are highly effective in reducing both the prolactin level and tumor size. The mode of action is as follows: dopamine agonists bind to the pituitary-specific D2 dopamine receptors on the surface membrane of prolactin-secreting cells, decreasing intracellular levels of cyclic adenosine monophosphate (cAMP) and Ca^{2+}. This results in an inhibition of the release and synthesis of prolactin. An increase in cellular lysosomal activity causes involution of the rough endoplasmic reticulum and Golgi apparatus. The action of dopamine agonists on D1 dopamine receptors in the brain causes side effects of nausea and dizziness.

12. How long does it take for medical treatment to reduce the serum prolactin level? To reduce the size of the tumor?

The onset of action of dopamine agonists is rapid, and because prolactin has a serum half-life of 50 minutes, a decrease in the prolactin level may be noted in 1–2 hours. However, normalization of the prolactin level may take weeks or months, with the maximal decrease usually seen by 3 months. A reduction in tumor size may be apparent within the first 48 hours and may be demonstrated by improvement in the visual fields. Tumor shrinkage of at least 50% is usually evident by 3 months. Maximal shrinkage, however, is not usually observed until after 6–12 months of treatment.

13. If a woman with a prolactin-secreting tumor becomes pregnant while on medical treatment, should the treatment be continued? Should she be allowed to breast-feed her infant?

Even though many studies have found that maternal treatment with dopamine agonists is safe to the fetus, it is recommended that the drug be stopped as soon as pregnancy is diagnosed. The risk of reexpansion is low: <5% for small prolactin-secreting tumors and 15–35% for large tumors. Assessment of symptoms, particularly headaches, and visual field tests should be evaluated monthly; any evidence of tumor reexpansion should prompt the reinstitution of treatment. Breast-feeding does not appear to add significant risk to pregnancy, but close follow-up should be continued.

14. How long is medical treatment of prolactin-secreting tumors required? Why?

In general, life-long treatment is required, because prolactin levels rise and tumors reexpand when treatment is interrupted, suggesting that the effect is mostly cytostatic. Recent reports, however, suggest that about 20% of cases may be cured after 2–5 years of treatment, and some evidence suggests a cytolytic effect of dopamine agonists.

15. When is surgical removal of a prolactin-secreting tumor indicated? When is radiotherapy indicated?

With the advent of dopamine agonists, surgery has become a secondary choice in the treatment of prolactin-secreting tumors—particularly large tumors, for which the long-term rate for surgical cure is only 25–50%. The principal indications for surgical treatment of a prolactin-secreting tumor are intolerance or resistance to dopamine agonists and acute hemorrhage into the tumor. Radiotherapy is rarely indicated, because hypopituitarism is a common side effect. This side effect is of critical concern, particularly in patients under treatment for infertility. However, radiotherapy may be a useful adjunct in patients who need additional treatment after surgery and do not tolerate dopamine agonists. Some experts advocate the use of radiotherapy 3 months before attempting pregnancy in women with large tumors to avoid tumor reexpansion during pregnancy.

BIBLIOGRAPHY

1. Bevan JS, Webster J, Burke CW, Scanlon MF: Dopamine agonists and pituitary tumor shrinkage, Endocr Rev 13:220, 1992.
2. Blackwell RE: Hyperprolactinemia: Evaluation and management. Reprod Endocrinol 21:105, 1992.

3. Cunnah D, Besser M: Management of prolactinomas. Clin Endocrinol (Oxf) 34:231, 1991.
4. Effect of dopamine agonist medication on prolactin producing pituitary adenomas: A morphological study including immunocytochemistry, electron microscopy and in situ hybridization. Virchows Archiv A Pathol Anat 418:439, 1991.
5. Faglia G: Should dopamine agonist treatment for prolactinomas be life-long? Clin Endocrinol (Oxf) 34:173, 1991.
6. Gen M. Uozumi T, Ohta M, Ito A, et al: Necrotic changes in prolactinomas after long term administration of bromocriptine. J Clin Endocrinol Metab 59:463, 1984.
7. Klibanski A, Greenspan SL: Increase in bone mass after treatment of hyperprolactinemic amenorrhea. N Engl J Med 315:542, 1986.
8. Klibanski A, Zervas NT: Diagnosis and management of hormone-secreting pituitary adenomas. N Engl J Med 324:822, 1991.
9. March CM, Kletzky OA, Davajan V, et al: Longitudinal evaluation of patients with untreated prolactin-secreting pituitary adenomas. Am J Obstet Gynecol 139:835, 1981.
10. Moseley I: Computed tomography and magnetic resonance imaging of pituitary macroadenomas. Clin Endocrinol (Oxf) 36:333, 1992.
11. Thorner MO, Perryman RL, Rogol AD, et al: Rapid changes of prolactinoma volume after withdrawal and reinstitution of bromocriptine. J Clin Endocrinol Metab 153:480, 1981.
12. Wardlaw SL, Bilezikian JP: Hyperprolactinemia and osteopenia. J Clin Endocinol Metab 75:690, 1992 [editorial].
13. Wood DF, Johnston JM, Johnston DG: Dopamine, the dopamine D2 receptor and pituitary tumours. Clin Endocrinol (Oxf) 35:455, 1991.
14. Wilson JD, Foster DW: Williams' Textbook of Endocrinology, 8th ed. Philadelphia, W.B. Saunders, 1992.

18. GROWTH HORMONE-SECRETING PITUITARY TUMORS

Mary H. Samuels M.D.

1. What is the normal function of growth hormone in children and adults?

In children, growth hormone is responsible for linear growth. In children and adults, growth hormone has many effects on intermediary metabolism, including protein synthesis and nitrogen balance, carbohydrate metabolism, lipolysis, and calcium homeostasis.

2. How are levels of growth hormone normally regulated?

Pituitary secretion of growth hormone is regulated by two hypothalamic hormones: stimulatory growth hormone-releasing hormone (GHRH) and inhibitory somatostatin. Secretion of growth hormone is also affected by adrenergic and dopaminergic hormones as well as by other central nervous system factors.

3. Does growth hormone directly affect peripheral tissues?

No. Many (although not all) effects of growth hormone are mediated by another hormone called somatomedin-C, insulinlike growth factor type 1 (IGF-1). Somatomedin-C is made by the liver and other organs in response to stimulation of growth hormone. Somatomedin-C feeds back to the pituitary gland and suppresses growth hormone levels. Unlike growth hormone, somatomedin-C has a long half-life in plasma, and plasma levels of somatomedin-C are helpful in the diagnosis of growth hormone abnormalities.

4. What are the clinical symptoms of excessive production of growth hormone in children?

In children who have not yet undergone puberty and whose long bones still respond to growth hormone, excessive growth hormone causes accelerated linear growth. The result is gigantism.

5. What are the clinical symptoms of excessive production of growth hormone in adults?

In adults, excessive growth hormone causes acromegaly. The pathologic and metabolic effects include the following:

1. Periosteal formation of new bone, leading to overgrowth of the maxillary and mandibular bones, frontal bossing, and nasal bone and laryngeal hypertrophy (causing deepening of the voice);

2. Hypertrophy of joint cartilage and osseous overgrowth, leading to osteoarthritis and carpal tunnel syndrome;

3. Soft-tissue hypertrophy, leading to enlargement of hands and feet;

4. Cardiac abnormalities, including hypertension and left ventricular hypertrophy;

5. Hypertrophy of other organs, including sweat glands (causing excessive sweating and unpleasant odor), skin (causing skin tags), and tongue and upper airway (causing obstruction and sleep apnea);

6. Hypogonadism;

7. Diabetes mellitus or impaired glucose tolerance; and

8. Colonic polyps and increased risk of colon cancer.

6. What is the single best clue when examining a patient suspected of having acromegaly?

An old driver's license picture or other old photographs provide the best clues. Patients with acromegaly are often unaware of the gradual disfigurement due to the disease or attribute it to aging. Comparing serial photographs can help to establish the diagnosis as well as date its onset.

7. From what do patients with acromegaly die?
The mortality from untreated or inadequately treated acromegaly is about double the expected rate in healthy subjects matched for age. Major causes of death include hypertension, cardiovascular disease, diabetes, pulmonary infections, and cancer.

8. In a patient with acromegaly, are skin tags all over the neck and chest a relevant finding?
There appears to be an association between multiple skin tags and colonic polyps in acromegaly. Therefore, the patient should undergo careful colonoscopic screening for polyps and colon cancer. However, even patients without active disease or skin tags may be at risk for colonic neoplasia and probably should be screened regularly.

9. The husband of the patient with acromegaly complains that he cannot sleep because his wife snores so loudly. Is this relevant?
Sleep apnea occurs in up to 80% of patients with acromegaly. It can be due to soft-tissue overgrowth of the upper airway or to altered central respiratory control. Sleep apnea may contribute to morbidity and mortality in acromegaly by producing hypoxia and pulmonary hypertension.

10. How is the diagnosis of acromegaly or gigantism made?
Two main biochemical tests may confirm excessive secretion of growth hormone:
    1. **Plasma levels of growth hormone in the fasting state and after administration of oral glucose.** Some patients with acromegaly have extremely elevated fasting levels of growth hormone, and further testing is not necessary. Most patients, however, have growth hormone levels that are only mildly elevated or overlap with levels in healthy subjects. Therefore, the diagnosis is usually made by measuring growth hormone levels after a glucose tolerance test. Healthy subjects suppress growth hormone levels after glucose, whereas patients with acromegaly show no suppression or an increase in growth hormone levels.
    2. **Plasma levels of somatomedin-C.** Because plasma levels of somatomedin-C are independent of food intake, samples can be drawn any time of day. In adults, acromegaly is essentially the only condition that causes elevated somatomedin-C levels. In children, somatomedin-C levels are more difficult to interpret, because growing children normally have higher levels than adults.

11. Once the biochemical diagnosis of acromegaly or gigantism is made, what is the next step?
Excessive secretion of growth hormone is almost always due to a benign pituitary tumor. Therefore, the next step is to obtain a radiologic study of the pituitary gland. The optimal study is magnetic resonance imaging (MRI) with special cuts through the pituitary gland. If MRI is not available, the best alternative study is a CT scan with special cuts through the pituitary gland.

12. What causes growth hormone-secreting pituitary tumors?
Recently growth hormone-secreting pituitary tumors have been shown to be monoclonal, suggesting that spontaneous somatic mutation is a key event in neoplastic transformation of somatotrophs. Further studies have clarified the nature of the mutation in some growth hormone tumors which appear to have an altered stimulatory subunit (G_s) of the G proteins that regulate adenylate cyclase activity. In a mutated cell, alterations in the G_s subunit cause autonomous adenylate cyclase activity and elevated secretion of growth hormone. However the mutant G_s is found only in a subset of patients with acromegaly. The mechanism of growth hormone regulation and tumor growth may differ in other patients with acromegaly.

13. Are other endocrine syndromes possible in patients with acromegaly or gigantism?
Of course, otherwise, acromegaly and gigantism would not be endocrine disorders. Three endocrine syndromes include acromegaly:

1. **Multiple endocrine neoplasia type 1 (MEN 1).** This autosomal dominant familial syndrome includes parathyroid hyperplasia (leading to hypercalcemia), pituitary tumors (secreting growth hormone or other pituitary hormones), and gut tumors (secreting gastrin, insulin, or other gut hormones). Therefore, when evaluating patients with acromegaly, check calcium levels (almost all patients with MEN 1 have hypercalcemia) and ask about symptoms of peptic ulcer disease or hypoglycemia.

2. **McCune-Albright syndrome.** McCune-Albright syndrome, which occurs mostly in girls, includes polyostotic fibrous dysplasia, café-au-lait spots, sexual precocity, and hyperfunction of multiple endocrine glands, including at times excessive secretion of growth hormone.

3. **Carney's complex.** Carney's complex is an inherited, autosomal dominant disease of multicentric tumors in many organs. Tumors include cardiac myxomas, pigmented skin lesions, pigmented nodular adrenal dysplasia (causing Cushing's syndrome), myxoid fibroadenomas of the breast, testicular tumors, and growth hormone-secreting pituitary adenomas.

14. Do other tumors besides pituitary tumors make growth hormone and cause acromegaly or gigantism?
Yes. Rare tumors of the pancreas, lung, ovary, and breast may produce growth hormone. However, only one patient has ever been reported to develop clinical acromegaly from ectopic growth hormone production (from a pancreatic tumor).

15. Do tumors ever cause acromegaly or gigantism by making excessive GHRH?
Yes. Over 50 cases of GHRH production by various tumors have been described. These tumors occur in the lung, gastrointestinal tract, pancreas, or adrenal glands and cause acromegaly by stimulating pituitary secretion of growth hormone. The clinical and biochemical features of acromegaly in such patients are indistinguishable from those of acromegaly due to a pituitary adenoma. Pituitary enlargement also occurs as a result of hyperplasia of somatotrophs. Some patients had inadvertent transsphenoidal surgery before the correct diagnosis was made. Therefore, the plasma level of GHRH should be measured in any acromegalic patient with an extrapituitary abnormality or with hyperplasia on pituitary pathology.

16. If MRI of the pituitary confirms a tumor in the acromegalic patient, what issues other than the metabolic effects of excessive growth hormone should be considered?
Three other issues should be considered in any patient with a pituitary tumor:

1. Is the tumor making any other pituitary hormones besides growth hormone? For example, many growth hormone-secreting tumors also produce prolactin; rare tumors also make thyroid-stimulating hormone or other pituitary hormones. In patients with acromegaly prolactin levels should be measured as well as other hormones when clinically indicated.

2. Is the tumor interfering with the normal function of the pituitary gland? Specifically, what is the patient's thyroid, adrenal, and gonadal function? Does the patient have diabetes insipidus? It is important to diagnose and treat pituitary insufficiency before therapy for the excessive secretion of growth hormone, especially if the patient is scheduled for surgery.

3. Is the tumor causing effects due to its size and location? Possible effects include headache, visual field disturbances, and extraocular movement abnormalities. Formal visual field examination should be carried out in patients with large pituitary tumors.

17. How big are growth hormone-secreting pituitary tumors?
Growth hormone-secreting tumors vary considerably in size, but most are larger than 1 cm in diameter when diagnosed (i.e., macroadenomas). Tumor size is an important issue, because it determines success rates of treatment.

18. How should acromegaly or gigantism be treated?
The treatment of choice for growth hormone-secreting tumors is transsphenoidal surgery by an experienced neurosurgeon. The majority of patients with microadenomas are cured, and larger

tumors are debulked. Significant reduction in growth hormone levels and improvement in symptoms typically follow surgery, even when further treatment is required.

19. What if surgery does not cure the patient?
If transsphenoidal surgery is not curative, there are two additional treatment options, often used together.

    1. **Radiotherapy.** Conventional radiation therapy of growth hormone-secreting tumors causes a gradual decline in growth hormone levels over many years. Therefore, although it is not a good initial choice, radiotherapy is often used after surgery for additional control of the tumor. Many patients eventually develop hypopituitarism from radiotherapy.

    2. **Octreotide.** Most growth hormone-secreting tumors have somatostatin receptors and respond to exogenous somatostatin with decreases in growth hormone levels. The development of octreotide, a long-acting analog of somatostatin was a major advance in the treatment of acromegaly. Given as injections 2 or 3 times a day, octreotide leads to markedly decreased levels of growth hormone in most acromegalic patients. It also causes tumor shrinkage in some patients. However, it does not cure acromegaly; stopping the drug usually leads to increases in growth hormone levels and tumor regrowth. Therefore, octreotide must be given indefinitely or while waiting for radiation to take effect.

20. What are the side effects of octreotide?
Gastrointestinal side effects are common, including abdominal bloating, mild diarrhea, nausea, and flatulence. The incidence of gallstones may be increased with octreotide, and patients must be monitored with serial ultrasound examinations of the gallbladder.

21. How can one tell whether a patient has been cured of acromegaly?
The criteria for cure of acromegaly are somewhat controversial. Older studies defined cure as a random growth hormone level below 5 µg/L. More recent studies have shown that this criterion is inadequate, because patients with low levels of growth hormone may still have acromegaly. Therefore, more rigorous criteria have been developed:
    1. Fasting level of growth hormone < 5 µg/L;
    2. Growth hormone levels < 2 µg/L following oral glucose; and
    3. Normal level of somatomedin-C.

22. The patient has undergone transsphenoidal surgery for acromegaly, with normal postoperative fasting levels of growth hormone, suppressed levels of growth hormone following oral glucose, and a normal level of somatomedin-C. How should the patient be followed?
It appears that the patient is cured, but growth hormone tumors can slowly regrow over years. At the least, measurements of growth hormone and/or somatomedin-C should be repeated every 6–12 months. Some physicians also repeat a pituitary MRI at yearly intervals. The patient also needs monitoring for colonic neoplasia at regular intervals. In addition, one needs to assess whether the surgery damaged normal pituitary function by determining the patient's thyroid, adrenal, gonadal, and posterior pituitary function. Finally, the effects of surgery on visual fields should be assessed, especially if she had preoperative defects.

23. The patient asks which symptoms and physical abnormalities will get better after cure is confirmed. What is the appropriate answer?
Most soft-tissue changes improve, including coarsening of facial features, increased size of hands and feet, upper airway hypertrophy, carpel tunnel syndrome, osteoarthritis, and excessive sweating. Hypertension, cardiovascular disease, and diabetes also improve. Unfortunately, bony overgrowth of the facial bones does not regress after treatment.

24. For bonus points, name an actor with acromegaly and the movie in which he starred.
Andre the Giant starred in "The Princess Bride."

BIBLIOGRAPHY

1. Ezzat S, Snyder PJ, Young WF et al: Octreotide treatment of acromegaly. Ann Intern Med 117:711–718, 1992.
2. Ezzat S, Melmed S: Are patients with acromegaly at increased risk for neoplasia? J Clin Endocrinol Metab 72:245–249, 1991.
3. Feek CM, McLelland J, Seth J et al: How effective is external pituitary irradiation for growth hormone-secreting pituitary tumours? Clin Endocrinol 20:401–408, 1984.
4. Frohman LA: Therapeutic options in acromegaly. J Clin Endocrinol Metab 72:1175–1181, 1991.
5. Grunstein RR, Ho KY, Sullivan CE. Sleep apnea in acromegaly. Ann Intern Med 115:527–532, 1991.
6. Hansen I, Tsalikian E, Beaufrere B, et al: Insulin resistance in acromegaly: Defects in both hepatic and extrahepatic insulin action. Am J Physiol 250:E269–E273, 1986.
7. Klibanski A: Further evidence for a somatic mutation theory in the pathogenesis of human pituitary tumors. J Clin Endocrinol Metab 71:1415A–1415C, 1990.
8. Lim MJ, Barkan AL, Buda AJ: Rapid reduction of left ventricular hypertrophy in acromegaly after suppression of growth hormone hypersecretion. Ann Intern Med 117:719–726, 1992.
9. Melmed S: Acromegaly. N Engl J Med 322:966–977, 1990.
10. Sano T, Asa SL, Kovacs K: Growth hormone-releasing hormone-producing tumors: Clinical, biochemical, and morphological manifestations. Endocrinol Rev 9:357–373, 1988.

19. GLYCOPROTEIN-SECRETING PITUITARY TUMORS

Robert C. Smallridge, M.D., COL, MC

1. What are glycoprotein hormones?

Of the four glycoprotein hormones, three are produced in the pituitary gland: luteinizing hormone (LH), follicle-stimulating hormone (FSH), and thyrotropin (TSH). Chorionic gonadotropin (CG) is produced in the placenta. Glycoprotein hormones are composed of two noncovalently bound subunits. The alpha subunit (α-SU) is similar among all four hormones. In contrast, the beta subunit (β-SU) is unique both immunologically and biologically for each hormone; these subunits are identified as LHβ, FSHβ, TSHβ, and βCG.

2. What are the types of glycoprotein hormone-secreting pituitary tumors? What clinical syndromes do they produce?

Gonadotropinomas secrete one or more of the following: LH, FSH, LHβ, FSHβ, or α-SU. They usually do not cause endocrine symptoms but, because of their large size, often produce neurologic symptoms. Thyrotropinomas secrete TSH and cause hyperthyroidism. They also produce α-SU.

3. Do pituitary tumors secrete only a single hormone?

No. Many tumors have been shown to make two or more hormones or subunits. In some circumstances, sufficient quantities of multiple hormones are secreted to produce clinical symptoms characteristic of several syndromes within the same patient.

4. Under what circumstances should a TSH-secreting tumor be considered?

In any patient with suspected hyperthyroidism, an increased serum free T4 or free T4 index, and, most importantly, a detectable serum TSH using a second- or third-generation assay, a TSH-secreting tumor should be considered.

5. Describe the differential diagnosis for a patient who has an increased level of serum total T4 and a detectable or elevated level of serum TSH.

Transient
1. Exogenous
   L-T4 therapy (noncompliance)
   Other drugs (amiodarone, ipodate, amphetamines)
2. Endogenous (subgroup of nonthyroidal illness)
   Acute psychiatric illness
   Acute liver disease

Permanent
1. Binding protein disorders
   Excessive thyroxine-binding globulin (TBG)
   Abnormal thyroxine-binding prealbumin (TBPA) (transthyretin)
   Familial dysalbuminemic hyperthyroxinemia (FDH)
   T4 autoantibody
   TSH heterophile antibody (requires separate cause for T4 elevation)
2. Inappropriate TSH secretion
   Resistance to thyroid hormone
   Pituitary tumor

6. How can one distinguish between the hyperthyroid patient with thyroid hormone resistance and the patient with a pituitary tumor?

TSH tumors secrete α-SU in excess of the whole TSH molecule. The molar ratio of serum α-SU to TSH is greater than unity (i.e., α/TSH > 1.0) in 95% of patients with TSH tumors, but it is

111

normal in persons with resistance. Assessment with thyrotropin-releasing hormone (TRH; protirelin) is also helpful. Fewer than 20% of patients with pituitary tumor have a twofold or greater increase in serum TSH after administration of TRH, whereas all patients with resistance respond to TRH. If a tumor is suspected after both tests are completed, a magnetic resonance imaging (MRI) scan of the pituitary gland should be obtained. Most TSH tumors (about 90%) are macroadenomas (i.e., ≥ 10 mm in size). Most microadenomas (< 10 mm) are also visualized, but on rare occasions it has been necessary to perform sampling of inferior petrosal sinus blood to localize the tumor.

7. How is an α/TSH molar ratio calculated?

TSH values are expressed as μU/mL (or mU/L). One must know the bioactivity and convert these units to ng/ml, the units of α-SU. Furthermore, the molecular weight of the subunit is only half the molecular weight of the whole TSH molecule; this fact also must be considered in calculating the molar ratio. From a practical standpoint, the following formula can be used:

$$\text{Molar ratio} = [\alpha\text{-SU (ng/ml)/TSH (μU/ml)}] \times 10$$

8. Name the various therapeutic options for managing TSH-secreting tumors and their likelihood of success.

Pituitary ablation is the treatment of choice. However, surgery alone has been curative in less than 40% of cases; surgery followed by external beam irradiation has yielded similar results. Now that tumors are identified earlier, surgical cures may improve. Too few patients have been treated with radiation therapy alone to assess its efficacy.

Several medical therapies known to suppress TSH secretion have been tried. Bromocriptine has met with limited success. Dexamethasone reduces serum TSH, but the side effects of steroids make it untenable for long-term treatment. Exciting recent reports indicate that the long-acting somatostatin analogue, octreotide, reduces TSH in more than 90% of cases, reduces T4 in almost all cases, reduces tumor size in 50%, and may improve visual symptoms. Although octreotide is not recommended as primary therapy, it has a promising adjunctive role.

Thyroid gland ablation (with surgery or ^{131}iodine) should never be used as primary therapy. It does nothing to control TSH secretion. In fact, there is theoretical concern that thyroid ablation may enhance pituitary activity and growth.

9. Do all patients with an enlarged pituitary gland and an elevated level of serum TSH have thyrotropinomas?

No. Patients with long-standing hypothyroidism may develop pituitary hyperplasia, producing a pseudotumor (see figure below). The pituitary mass can extend into the suprasellar region and cause visual field defects. Serum T4 is always low, and shrinkage of the enlarged gland usually occurs with L-T4 replacement therapy. No patient should undergo pituitary gland surgery without a preoperative measurement of serum T4.

10. What clinical features raise suspicion of a TSH-secreting pseudotumor?

Of greatest importance, almost all patients have symptoms of hypothyroidism. The underlying abnormality is usually autoimmune thyroiditis, which is predominantly a disease of women. Indeed, approximately 80% of reported cases of pituitary enlargement with hypothyroidism were in women. In contrast, only 52% of true TSH tumors have occurred in women. In children, precocious puberty may occur. Thyroid antibodies are present in 83% of women with pseudotumor, compared to only 14% of women with TSH tumors that produce hyperthyroidism.

11. Does the presence of abnormal visual fields help to distinguish between patients with pituitary hyperplasia due to primary hypothyroidism and patients with TSH-secreting tumors?

No. Abnormal visual fields have been reported in 37% of patients with pituitary hyperplasia compared with 49% of patients with tumors. In contrast, patients with thyroid hormone resistance have normal vision.

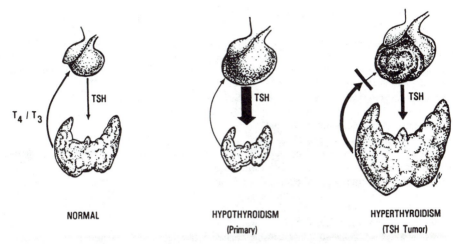

NORMAL	HYPOTHYROIDISM	HYPERTHYROIDISM
	(Primary)	(TSH Tumor)

Schema of the pituitary-thyroid axis in normal persons and in patients with thyrotropin (TSH)-secreting pituitary tumors. On the left is the appropriate feedback loop in euthyroid individuals, with the width of the arrows representing the normal serum concentrations of TSH and thyroxine (T_4). The middle figure depicts a small thyroid gland due to primary hypothyroidism. The low T_4 levels result in markedly increased secretion of TSH and, in some patients, a generalized hyperplasia of the anterior pituitary gland. On the right is an autonomous pituitary tumor secreting TSH. Serum TSH levels may vary greatly but in all cases are sufficiently biologically active to increase levels of serum T_4 above normal. The elevated T_4 level has little, if any, ability to suppress tumor function. (From Smallridge RC: Thyrotropin-secreting tumors. Endocrinol Metab Clin North Am 16:765, 1987, with permission.)

12. Does family history provide any clues in distinguishing these disorders?
In pseudotumor from thyrotroph hyperplasia, the family history may be positive for the presence of autoimmune diseases (e.g., thyroiditis, Graves' disease, diabetes mellitus, rheumatoid arthritis, lupus erythematosus, Sjogren's syndrome, vitiligo, Addison's disease, pernicious anemia). In TSH tumors, family history is of no use. Most cases of generalized thyroid hormone resistance are familial with autosomal dominant inheritance (i.e., 50% of the family have the biochemical abnormalities).

13. Which hormones are elevated in the serum of patients with gonadotroph adenomas?
Serum FSH is increased much more often than LH. An increase in α-SU is not specific for gonadotrophs, because it may also derive from thyrotrophs. Furthermore, an α/LH (or FSH) molar ratio has not been clinically useful.

14. What are the presenting symptoms of patients with gonadotropinomas?
Gonadotropinomas usually do not cause an endocrine disorder from excessive hormone production. They are large, with substantial extrasellar growth. Most patients are identified because of visual impairment due to impingement by the tumor on the optic chiasm. Headaches, diplopia, and pituitary apoplexy also occur. Endocrine symptoms are usually due to deficiencies of other pituitary hormones created by the mass effect of the large tumor.

15. When gonadotropin levels are elevated, how can one distinguish clinically between a gonadotroph adenoma and primary hypogonadism?
This distinction can be difficult, especially in women, because their levels of LH and FSH increase after menopause. This is probably why most gonadotroph adenomas have been recognized in men. Historically, men with such tumors experienced a normal puberty and may have fathered children. On examination, their testicular size may be normal. In contrast, men with hypogonadism may have had abnormal pubertal development or a history of testicular injury; the testes are small.

16. What laboratory tests are helpful?

In primary hypogonadism, both FSH and LH are increased, whereas LH is usually normal in patients with gonadotropinomas. When LH is high in men with gonadotropinomas, testosterone also is high rather than low, as in hypogonadism. Of interest, for unexplained reasons about one-third of patients with tumor have an anomalous rise in serum FSH or LHβ when given a TRH injection. An MRI scan of the pituitary reveals a large tumor. Occasionally, a patient with longstanding hypogonadism may have some degree of pituitary enlargement.

17. How are gonadotropinomas treated?

Pituitary surgery is the treatment of choice. Although complete cure is often impossible, substantial reduction in tumor size and hormone secretion is common. Reduced hormone secretion provides a convenient marker for monitoring recurrence of tumor; an abrupt increase in FSH or subunit should prompt a repeat imaging study. Radiotherapy is often given after surgery with the hope of delaying recurrence of tumor.

18. Is medical therapy effective?

Agonist analogs of gonadotropin-releasing hormone (GnRH) reduce secretion from normal gonadotrophs. Unfortunately, they usually have the opposite effect on gonadotropinomas. Recently an antagonist analog (Nal-Glu GnRH) has effectively reduced serum FSH in a small group of men with gonadotropinomas. More experience is needed with the drug. Bromocriptine has reduced hormone levels in an occasional patient, whereas octreotide has reduced α-SU and improved visual fields in certain patients.

19. Are pituitary tumors malignant?

Pituitary carcinomas are rare, but a small number have been reported for active tumors secreting the following hormones: adrenocorticotropic hormone (ACTH), prolactin, and growth hormone. The first case of a TSH-secreting pituitary carcinoma was reported only recently.

BIBLIOGRAPHY

1. Chanson P, Weintraub BD, Harris AG: Octreotide therapy for thyroid-stimulating hormone-secreting pituitary adenomas: a follow-up of 52 patients. Ann Intern Med 119:236, 1993.
2. Daneshdoost L, Pavlou SN, Molitch ME, et al: Inhibition of follicle-stimulating hormone secretion from gonadotroph adenomas by repetitive administration of a gonadotropin-releasing hormone antagonist. J Clin Endocrinol Metab 71:92, 1990.
3. Frank SJ, Gesundheit N, Doppman JL, et al: Preoperative lateralization of pituitary microadenomas by petrosal sinus sampling: Utility in two patients with non-ACTH-secreting tumors. Am J Med 87:679, 1989.
3a. Gancel A, Vuillermet P, Legrand A, et al: Effects of a slow-release formulation of the new somatostatin analogue lanreotide in TSH-secreting pituitary adenomas. Clin Endocrinol 40:421, 1994.
4. Kaptein EM: Abnormal thyroid function tests in euthyroid persons. In Becker KL (ed): Principles and Practice of Endocrinology and Metabolism. Philadelphia, J.B. Lippincott, 1990.
5. Katznelson L, Oppenheim DS, Coughlin JF, et al: Chronic somatostatin analog administration in patients with α-subunit-secreting pituitary tumors. J Clin Endocrinol Metab 75:1318, 1992.
6. Klibanski A, Zervas NT: Diagnosis and management of hormone-secreting pituitary adenomas. N Engl J Med 324:822, 1991.
7. Lamberts SWJ, Krenning EP, Reubi J-C: The role of somatostatin and its analogs in the diagnosis and treatment of tumors. Endocr Rev 12:450, 1991.
8. Mixson AJ, Friedman TC, Katz DA, et al: Thyrotropin-secreting pituitary carcinoma. J Clin Endocrinol Metab 76:529, 1993.
9. Oppenheim DS, Klibanski A: Medical therapy of glycoprotein hormone-secreting pituitary tumors. Endocrinol Metab Clin North Am 18:339, 1989.
10. Refetoff S, Weiss RE, Usala SJ: The syndromes of resistance to thyroid hormone. Endocr Rev 14:348, 1993.

11. Smallridge RC: Thyrotropin-secreting pituitary tumors. Endocrinol Metab Clin North Am 16:765, 1987.
12. Smallridge RC: Evaluation of thyroid function: Blood tests. In Becker KL (ed): Principles and Practice of Endocrinology and Metabolism. Philadelphia, J.B. Lippincott Company, 1990.
13. Smallridge RC: Thyrotropin-secreting tumors. In Mazzaferri EL, Samaan NA (eds): Endocrine Tumors. Boston, Blackwell, 1993.
14. Snyder PJ: Gonadotroph adenomas. In Mazzaferri EL, Samaan NA (eds): Endocrine Tumors. Boston, Blackwell, 1993.

20. CUSHING'S SYNDROME

Mary H. Samuels M.D.

1. What is the normal function of cortisol in healthy subjects?

Cortisol and other glucocorticoids have many effects as physiologic regulators. They increase glucose production, inhibit protein synthesis and increase protein breakdown, stimulate lipolysis, and affect immunologic and inflammatory responses. Glucocorticoids are important for maintenance of blood pressure and form an essential part of the body's response to stress.

2. How are cortisol levels normally regulated?

Secretion of cortisol from the adrenal glands is stimulated by the pituitary hormone adrenocorticotropin (ACTH). Secretion of ACTH, in turn, is stimulated by the hypothalamic hormones corticotropin-releasing hormone (CRH) and vasopressin (ADH). Cortisol feeds back to the pituitary and hypothalamus to suppress levels of ACTH and CRH. Under basal (nonstress) conditions, cortisol is secreted with a pronounced circadian rhythm, with higher levels early in the morning, and low levels late in the evening. Under stressful conditions, secretion of CRH, ACTH, and cortisol increases, and the circadian variation is blunted. Because of the wide variations in cortisol levels over 24 hours and appropriate elevations during stressful conditions, it may be difficult to distinguish normal from abnormal secretion. Many biochemical tests have been devised to diagnose pathologic hypercortisolemia, but none has proved completely accurate. For this reason, the evaluation of a patient with suspected Cushing's disease is often complex and confusing.

3. What are the clinical symptoms of excessive levels of cortisol?

The manifestations of glucocorticoid excess are as follows:

1. Obesity, especially central (truncal) obesity, with wasting of the extremities, moon facies, supraclavicular fat pads, and buffalo hump;
2. Thinning of the skin, with facial plethora, easy bruising, and violaceous striae;
3. Muscular weakness, especially proximal muscle weakness and atrophy;
4. Hypertension, atherosclerosis, congestive heart failure, and edema;
5. Gonadal dysfunction and menstrual irregularities;
6. Psychological disturbances, including depression, emotional lability, irritability, and sleep disturbances;
7. Osteoporosis and fractures; and
8. Increased rate of infections and poor wound healing.

4. A patient presents with a history of obesity, hypertension, irregular menses, and depression. Does she have excessive production of cortisol?

Excessive cortisol is highly unlikely. Although the listed findings are consistent with glucocorticoid excess, they are nonspecific; most patients with such findings do *not* have Cushing's syndrome. A few symptoms and signs of glucocorticoid excess are more specific, although they do not occur in every patient with Cushing's syndrome: spontaneous ecchymoses, purple (not pale) striae, proximal muscle weakness, osteoporosis, and hypokalemia. Any of these findings should immediately increase suspicion of excessive production of glucocorticoids.

5. The patient also complains of excessive hair growth and has increased terminal hairs on the chin, along the upper lip, and on the upper back. Is this finding relevant?

Hirsutism is a common, nonspecific finding in many female patients. However, it is also consistent with Cushing's syndrome. If it is due to Cushing's syndrome, hirsutism is a complication not of excessive glucocorticoids but of excessive production of androgen by the adrenal glands under ACTH stimulation. Thus, hirsutism in a patient with Cushing's syndrome is a clue that the disorder is due to excessive production of ACTH. (The only other condition associated with excessive production of glucocorticoids and androgen is a malignant adrenal tumor, which is usually obvious on presentation.)

6. The patient also has increased pigmentation of the areolae, palmar creases, and an old surgical scar. Are these findings relevant?

Hyperpigmentation is a sign of elevated production of ACTH and related peptides by the pituitary gland. It is uncommon (but possible) in Cushing's syndrome due to benign pituitary tumors, because levels of ACTH do not usually rise high enough to cause hyperpigmentation. It is more common in the ectopic ACTH syndrome, because ectopic tumors produce more ACTH and other peptides. The combination of Cushing's syndrome and hyperpigmentation may be bad news.

7. What is the cause of death in patients with Cushing's syndrome?

Patients with Cushing's syndrome have a markedly increased mortality rate, usually from cardiovascular disease or infections.

8. What are the causes of Cushing's syndrome?

Cushing's syndrome is a nonspecific name for any source of excessive glucocorticoids. There are four main causes:

1. **Exogenous glucocorticoids.** Patients who receive glucocorticoids for inflammatory or autoimmune diseases (e.g., asthma, rheumatoid arthritis, systemic lupus, dermatitis) invariably develop Cushing's syndrome over time. Other patients surreptitiously ingest glucocorticoids and also develop exogenous Cushing's syndrome. Such patients may be quite difficult to diagnose.

2. **Pituitary Cushing's syndrome.** This entity, called Cushing's disease, is due to a benign pituitary adenoma that secretes excessive ACTH.

3. **Ectopic production of ACTH.** Of the two varieties of ectopic production of ACTH, one is due to malignant tumors, usually of the lung. Patients present with obvious metastatic tumor, weight loss, hypertension, hypokalemia, and hyperpigmentation. The second type is due to more slowly growing tumors called carcinoids. Patients with carcinoid tumors that produce ACTH may appear identical to patients with pituitary Cushing's disease on clinical examination and biochemical testing. Thus, the differential diagnosis between pituitary tumor and carcinoid tumor in a patient with Cushing's syndrome may be difficult.

4. **Adrenal causes of Cushing's syndrome.** Both benign and malignant adrenal tumors can produce excessive glucocorticoids and cause Cushing's syndrome. Benign adrenal adenomas clinically resemble other types of Cushing's syndrome; hirsutism is absent, however, because the tumor produces only cortisol without producing androgens. Malignant adrenal carcinomas causing Cushing's syndrome usually present with obvious widespread tumor in the abdomen and have a poor prognosis. In addition, unusual types of adrenal Cushing's syndrome are associated with multiple adrenal nodules, discussed below.

9. Of various types of Cushing's syndrome, which is the most common?

Overall, exogenous Cushing's syndrome is most common. It rarely presents a diagnostic dilemma, because the physician usually knows that the patient is receiving glucocorticoids. Of the endogenous causes of Cushing's syndrome, pituitary Cushing's disease accounts for at least 70% of cases. Ectopic secretion of ACTH and adrenal tumors cause approximately 15% of cases each.

10. Do age and gender matter in the differential diagnosis of Cushing's syndrome?

Of patients with Cushing's disease (pituitary tumors) 80% are women, whereas the ectopic ACTH syndrome is more common in men. Therefore, in a male patient with Cushing's syndrome, the risk of extrapituitary tumor is increased. The age range in Cushing's disease is most frequently 20–40 years, whereas ectopic ACTH syndrome has a peak incidence at 40–60 years. Therefore, in an older patient with Cushing's syndrome, the risk that he or she has an extrapituitary tumor is increased.

11. The patient with obesity, hypertension, irregular menses, depression, and hirsutism looks like she may have Cushing's syndrome. What should you do?
The single best screening test for excessive production of cortisol is a 24-hour urine collection for urinary free cortisol and creatinine. If the patient can collect her urine for 24 hours, the test should be ordered. Another widely used screening test is the overnight low-dose dexamethasone suppression test. The patient takes 1 mg of dexamethasone at 11 PM and measures her serum cortisol level at 8 AM the next morning. In healthy subjects with intact hypothalamic-pituitary-adrenal function, dexamethasone (a potent glucocorticoid that does not cross-react with the cortisol assay) suppresses production of CRH, ACTH, and cortisol. Patients with Cushing's syndrome of any cause should not suppress cortisol production when given this dose of dexamethasone.

Unfortunately, the overnight dexamethasone suppression test is not foolproof. Occasional patients with Cushing's disease suppress cortisol levels with dexamethasone, and many patients without Cushing's syndrome will not, particularly those with other acute or chronic illnesses, depression, or alcohol abuse. All of these diseases activate the hypothalamic-pituitary-adrenal axis because of stress and make the patient resistant to dexamethasone suppression. Because of such difficulties in the initial screening tests for Cushing's syndrome, patients may require repeated screening and evaluation over time.

12. The patient has an elevated 24-hour urinary level of free cortisol, and serum cortisol levels are not suppressed after overnight 1 mg dexamethasone administration. What do you do?
It looks like the patient has Cushing's syndrome. The next step is to determine whether she has ACTH-dependent or ACTH-independent disease. This distinction is made by measuring plasma levels of ACTH. Measurements should be repeated a number of times, because secretion of ACTH is variable.

13. The patient's ACTH level is "normal." Was the original suspicion of Cushing's syndrome incorrect?
No. Normal levels of ACTH are a common finding in pituitary-dependent Cushing's disease. A normal or slightly elevated ACTH level is the usual finding in ACTH-secreting pituitary adenomas. More marked elevations in ACTH levels suggest ectopic secretion of ACTH, although small carcinoid tumors also may have normal or mildly elevated levels of ACTH. Suppressed levels of ACTH suggest an adrenal tumor.

14. What happened to the 2-day low-dose and high-dose dexamethasone tests for the differential diagnosis of Cushing's syndrome?
The 2-day low- and high-dose dexamethasone suppression tests were once widely used in attempts to distinguish pituitary, ectopic, and adrenal causes of Cushing's syndrome. Although they are still performed, the results are often confusing, and rates of both false-positive and false-negative results are high. Therefore, these tests to some extent have been supplanted by more accurate ACTH assays, the overnight high-dose dexamethasone test, and CRH stimulation tests.

15. After diagnosis of ACTH-dependent Cushing's syndrome, what is the next step?
Because the most common site of excessive secretion of ACTH is a pituitary tumor, radiologic imaging of the pituitary gland is the next step. The best study is high-resolution MRI with thin cuts through the pituitary gland. A chest radiograph should also be obtained at this point in case the patient has a carcinoid tumor large enough to be seen on plain film.

16. The pituitary MRI in the patient with ACTH-dependent Cushing's syndrome is normal. Is the next step a search for carcinoid tumor, under the assumption that the pituitary is not the source of excessive ACTH?
Not so fast. At least one-half of pituitary MRI or CT scans are negative in proven pituitary-dependent Cushing's syndrome, because most corticotroph adenomas are tiny and may not be visible on MRI or CT.

17. The pituitary MRI shows a 3-mm hypodense area in the lateral aspect of the pituitary gland. Is it time to call the neurosurgeon?
Again, not so fast. This finding is nonspecific and occurs in many healthy people. It may or may not be related to Cushing's syndrome. The odds are good that the patient has a pituitary tumor, but the MRI does not prove so. The MRI is helpful in Cushing's syndrome only if it shows a large tumor.

18. So what is the next step?
The best test to distinguish a pituitary source from an ectopic source of ACTH is bilateral simultaneous inferior petrosal sinus sampling for ACTH levels. Catheters are advanced through the femoral veins into the inferior petrosal sinuses, which drain the pituitary gland. Blood samples are obtained through the catheters and assayed for ACTH levels. If ACTH levels in the petrosal sinuses are significantly higher than those in peripheral blood samples, the pituitary gland is the source of excessive ACTH. If there is no gradient between petrosal sinus and peripheral vein levels of ACTH, the patient probably has a carcinoid tumor somewhere else in the body. The accuracy of the test is further increased if ACTH responses to injection of exogenous CRH are measured, because pituitary tumors increase secretion of ACTH in response to CRH. Bilateral inferior petrosal sinus sampling should be performed ideally by experienced invasive radiologists or neuroradiologists at referral centers.

19. Inferior petrosal sinus sampling shows no gradient in ACTH levels. Now what?
Start the search for a carcinoid tumor. Because the most likely location is the lung, a CT scan or MRI of the lung should be ordered. If results are negative, a CT scan or MRI of the abdomen should be ordered, because carcinoids also occur in the pancreas, intestinal tract, and adrenal glands.

20. Inferior petrosal sinus sampling shows a marked central-to-peripheral gradient in ACTH levels. Now what?
Transsphenoidal surgery should be scheduled with an experienced neurosurgeon who is comfortable examining the pituitary gland for small adenomas. ACTH levels from the right and left petrosal sinuses obtained during the sampling study may tell the neurosurgeon in which side of the pituitary gland the tumor is likely to be found, but this information is not 100% accurate.

21. What if surgery is unsuccessful?
If transsphenoidal surgery does not cure a patient with Cushing's disease, alternative therapies must be tried, because patients with inadequately treated hypercortisolism have increased morbidity and mortality rates. Of the various options after failed surgery, none is ideal:
    1. Reevaluate the evidence for a pituitary source for ACTH. If necessary, repeat the petrosal sinus sampling (although this is more difficult after surgery). If the pituitary is in fact the source, repeat surgery should be considered, including the option of total hypophysectomy. Even tumors so tiny that they cannot be seen by the surgeon are removed with total hypophysectomy.
    2. Consider treating the patient with ketoconazole, which blocks adrenal steroidogenesis. It does not cure the underlying tumor but improves the patient's metabolic status and may buy time for further studies or radiation therapy.
    3. Consider pituitary radiotherapy, which eventually leads to control of cortisol levels in many patients with Cushing's disease. Because radiotherapy may take years to work, it is not a good initial option.
    4. Consider bilateral adrenalectomy. This was the preferred treatment for Cushing's syndrome, until transsphenoidal surgery was shown to be effective and much safer. It is still an option in a patient with the devastating clinical consequences of Cushing's syndrome in whom a pituitary tumor cannot be found.

22. What is the main drawback to bilateral adrenalectomy in patients with Cushing's disease?
One drawback is the extensive nature of the surgery, which leads to high levels of morbidity and a lengthy postoperative recuperative period. However, the main drawback is the development of

Nelson's syndrome in up to 30% of patients after adrenalectomy. Nelson's syndrome is the appearance, sometimes years after adrenalectomy, of an aggressive corticotroph pituitary tumor.

23. What are the correct diagnostic and treatment options for patients with ACTH-independent (adrenal) Cushing's syndrome?

Such patients usually have either an adrenal adenoma or an adrenal carcinoma. Once consistent suppression of ACTH levels is confirmed, an adrenal CT scan should be ordered. A mass is almost always present, and surgery should be planned. If the mass is obviously cancer, surgery may still help in debulking the tumor and improving the metabolic consequences of hypercortisolemia.

24. The patient has ACTH-independent Cushing's syndrome, but instead of a solitary adrenal mass, the adrenal glands have multiple nodules. What is the underlying condition?

A number of disease processes cause adrenal Cushing's syndrome with multiple adrenal masses:

1. **Primary pigmented nodular adrenal dysplasia (PPNAD).** In recent years, descriptions of a syndrome of ACTH-independent Cushing's syndrome due to bilateral small pigmented adrenal nodules has appeared. Clinical symptoms usually occur during the second decade of life (earlier than in other causes of Cushing's syndrome). The disease may be sporadic or familial. Careful radiologic and pathologic studies reveal unilateral or bilateral nodularity, with nodule sizes ranging from tiny to 3 cm. Most are deeply pigmented and appear black or brown on cut section. PPNAD may be an autoimmune disease caused by production of adrenal-stimulating immunoglobulins. Patients with PPNAD should undergo bilateral adrenalectomy, which is curative.

2. **Carney complex.** In 1985 Carney at the Mayo Clinic noted an association between PPNAD and cardiac myxomas in a few patients. His resulting description has since been named the Carney complex. This entity is an inherited, autosomal dominant disease of multicentric tumors in many organs, including cardiac myxomas, pigmented skin lesions, PPNAD, myxoid fibroadenomas of the breast, testicular tumors, growth hormone-secreting pituitary adenomas, and peripheral nerve lesions.

3. **Macronodular adrenal hyperplasia.** With the advent of high-resolution CT scans, some patients with Cushing's syndrome are seen to have bilateral adrenal nodules, ranging in size from 0.5–7 cm. This entity, distinct from PPNAD and called macronodular adrenal hyperplasia (MAH), presents with variable biochemical and radiologic findings. MAH probably represents a heterogeneous group of patients with varying degrees of adrenal autonomy. The hypothesis underlying the development of MAH is that long-standing stimulation by ACTH leads to formation of adrenal nodules and that some of the nodules may become autonomous. Treatment must be individualized for each patient with MAH; the most important decision is whether the patient still has ACTH-dependent disease.

4. **McCune-Albright syndrome (polyostotic fibrous dysplasia).** McCune-Albright syndrome is characterized by polyostotic fibrous dysplasia, café-au-lait pigmentation of the skin, and multiple endocrinopathies. The most common endocrine disorders include sexual precocity and pituitary adenomas that secrete growth hormone. In a few cases, autonomous adrenal hyperfunction and Cushing's syndrome have been described; adrenal pathology is characterized by nodular hyperplasia and formation of adenomas.

25. What happens to the hypothalamic-pituitary-adrenal axis after a patient undergoes successful removal of an ACTH-secreting pituitary adenoma or a cortisol-secreting adrenal adenoma?

The axis is suppressed, and the patient develops clinical adrenal insufficiency, unless he or she is given gradually decreasing doses of exogenous glucocorticoids for a time after surgery.

26. What would be the most likely diagnosis if the original patient had all the signs of Cushing's syndrome, but *low* urinary and serum levels of cortisol?

The most likely scenario is that the patient is surreptitiously ingesting a glucocorticoid that gives all the findings of glucocorticoid excess but is not measured in the cortisol assay. The patient and family members should be questioned about possible access to medications.

27. A patient has all the findings of Cushing's syndrome and elevated 24-hour urinary levels of free cortisol. One month later, however, she no longer has clinical signs of Cushing's syndrome. Repeat urine free cortisol is now normal. What is happening?

There are two possibilities: (1) the patient is intermittently ingesting a glucocorticoid that is measured in the cortisol assay (exogenous Cushing's syndrome), or (2) she has a rare corticotroph tumor that is only intermittently active (periodic hormonogenesis).

28. Do tumors ever cause Cushing's syndrome by making excessive CRH?

Yes. Occasionally patients who undergo transsphenoidal surgery for a presumed corticotroph adenoma have corticotroph hyperplasia instead. At least some of these cases are secondary to ectopic production of CRH from a carcinoid tumor in the lung, abdomen, or other location. Therefore, levels of serum CRH should be measured in patients with Cushing's syndrome and corticotroph hyperplasia. If the levels are elevated, a careful search should be performed for possible ectopic sources of CRH.

BIBLIOGRAPHY

1. Carpenter PC: Cushing's syndrome: Update of diagnosis and management. Mayo Clin Proc 61:49–58, 1986.
2. Doppman JL: The search for occult ectopic ACTH-producing tumors. Endocrinologist 2:41–46, 1992.
3. Kaye TB, Crapo L: The Cushing's syndrome: An update on diagnostic tests. Ann Intern Med 112:434–444, 1990.
4. Limper AH, Carpenter PC, Scheithauer B, Staats BA: The Cushing syndrome induced by bronchial carcinoid tumors. Ann Intern Med 117:209–214, 1992.
5. Loli P, Berselli E, Tagliaferri M: Use of ketoconazole in the treatment of Cushing's syndrome. J Clin Endocrinol Metab 63:1365–1371, 1986.
6. Melby JC: Therapy of Cushing disease: A consensus for pituitary microsurgery, Ann Intern Med 109:445–456, 1988.
7. Moore TJ, Dluhy RG, Williams GH, Cain JP: Nelson's syndrome: Frequency, prognosis, and effect of prior pituitary irradiation. Ann Intern Med 85:731–734, 1976.
8. Oldfield EH, Doppman JL, Nieman LK et al: Petrosal sinus sampling with and without corticotropin-releasing hormone for the differential diagnosis of Cushing's syndrome. N Engl J Med 325:897–905, 1991.
9. Orth DN: Differential diagnosis of Cushing's syndrome. N Engl J Med 325:957–959, 1990.
10. Samuels MH: Cushing's syndrome associated with corticotroph hyperplasia. Endocrinologist 3:242–247, 1993.
11. Samuels MH, Loriaux DL: Cushing's syndrome and the nodular adrenal gland. Endocrinol Metab Clin North Am 1994 [in press].

21. DISORDERS OF WATER METABOLISM

Leonard R. Sanders, M.D.

1. List the abbreviations frequently used to discuss disturbances of water metabolism.
Common abbreviations:

P_{Na}	Plasma sodium concentration
U_{Na}	Urine sodium concentration
P_{osm}	Plasma osmolality
U_{osm}	Urine osmolality
TBW	Total body water
ECF	Extracellular fluid
ICF	Intracellular fluid
ADH	Antidiuretic hormone
AVP	Arginine vasopressin
ANP	Atrial natriuretic peptide
SIADH	Syndrome of inappropriate antidiuretic hormone secretion
DI	Diabetes insipidus
ECV	Effective circulating volume

Other abbreviations:

ISF	Interstitial fluid
IVF	Intravascular fluid
PCT	Proximal convoluted tubule
LOH	Loop of Henle
DCT	Distal convoluted tubule
CCT	Cortical collecting tubule

ADH and AVP are the same hormone. As for P_{Na} and U_{Na}, Px or Ux (where X is any substance) represents the plasma or urine **concentration** of that substance.

2. What is the water composition of the human body?
Water composition of the body depends on age, sex, muscle mass, body habitus, and fat content. Various body tissues have the following water percentages: lungs, heart, and kidneys (80%); skeletal muscle and brain (75%); skin and liver (70%); bone (20%); and adipose tissues (10%). Clearly, people with more muscle than fat will have more water. Generally, thin people have less fat and more water. Man is 60% and woman 50% water by weight. Older people have more fat and less muscle. The average man and woman older than 60 years have 50% and 45% water, respectively. Most discussions of TBW consider a man who is 60% water, weights 70 kg, and is 69 inches (175 cm) tall.

Water as a Percent of Body Weight

BODY HABITUS	INFANT	MAN	WOMAN
Thin	80	65	55
Medium	70	60	50
Obese	65	55	45

3. Where is water located within the body?
Total body water (TBW) equals water located inside (ICF) and outside the cells (ECF). TBW is 60% of body weight, and ICF and ECF water are 40% and 20% respectively of body weight. The ECF contains both interstitial (15%) and intravascular water (5%). Thus, in a 70-kg man, TBW = 42 L, ICF water = 28 L, and ECF water = 14 L. The interstitial water is 10.5 L and intravascular

(plasma) water 3.5 L. Therefore, of the TBW, two-thirds is ICF and one-third is ECF. Of the ECF, about one-fourth is IVF and three-fourths is ISF. Tight regulation of the relatively small volume of IVF (plasma) maintains blood pressure and avoids symptomatic hypovolemia, congestive heart failure, and decreased ECV. Normal plasma is 93% water and 7% proteins and lipids.

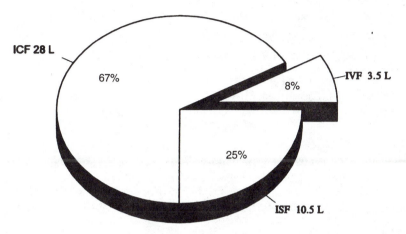

Distribution of body water.

4. What is transcellular water? What is its importance?

Transcellular water (TCW) is that water formed by cellular transport activities and located in various ducts and spaces throughout the body. This water includes cerebrospinal fluid and aqueous humor; secretions in the sweat, salivary, and lacrimal glands; and secretions in the pancreas, liver, biliary, gastrointestinal, and respiratory tracts. Water in the pleural, pericardial, peritoneal, and synovial spaces may also be considered TCW. TCW carries secretions to specific sites for enzymatic and lubricant activity and is normally quite small. In disease states, excess or deficiency of TCW can cause dysfunction. Excess TCW formation may decrease effective circulating volume (ECV), stimulate ADH and aldosterone release, and cause retention of salt and water.

5. What controls distribution of body water?

With few exceptions (e.g., ascending loop of Henle and distal nephron), water moves freely across cell membranes, depending on tonicity. Since tonicity depends on impermeable solutes such as plasma Na, disorders of water metabolism are reflected by changes in solute concentrations. A thorough understanding of disorders of water metabolism requires a clear understanding of changes in plasma Na (P_{Na}) and plasma osmolality (P_{osm}).

6. Define osmolality and tonicity. Outline their effects on water movement.

Osmolality is the **concentration** of active particles in a kilogram of water. Osmolality of a substance is the concentration of the substance in a liter of water divided by its molecular weight. Tonicity = effective osmolality—the osmotic pressure caused by dissolved particles restricted to one side of the cell membrane. Since sodium and glucose (in insulin deficiency) are restricted to the ECF, they account for normal tonicity and are called effective osmols. Mannitol, sorbitol, glycerol, and glycine are also effective osmols. Because urea freely crosses cell membranes and distributes evenly in TBW, changes in urea change osmolality but not tonicity. Therefore, urea is an ineffective osmol. Ethanol and methanol are other ineffective osmols. Water will always move across cell membranes from higher to lower osmolality until osmolality on both sides is equal. Accordingly, **ICF osmolality will always equal ECF osmolality.** Since plasma is part of the ECF, the following is always true: **ICF osmolality = ECF osmolality = P$_{osm}$.** Clinical changes in osmolality are usually due to changes in TBW or the movement of water between the ICF and ECF.

7. What formulas are useful in evaluating osmolality and tonicity?

ECF osmolality = 2 P$_{Na}$ + Glucose/18 + BUN/2.8

Normal osmolality = 2(140) + 90/18 + 14/2.8 = 280 + 5 + 5 = 290 mOsm/kg.

ECF tonicity (effective osmolality) = 2 P$_{Na}$ + Glucose/18

Normal tonicity = 2(140) + 90/18 = 280 + 5 = 285 mOsm/kg.

However, the normal range for P$_{Na}$ is 135–145 mEq/L. When substituted, the normal range for P$_{osm}$ is 280–295 mOsm/kg and normal tonicity is 275–290 mOsm/kg. Correction factors for other effective solutes (osmols) are mannitol/18, sorbitol/18, and glycerol/9. Correction factors for other ineffective solutes (osmols) are ethanol/4.6 and methanol/3.2.

8. A 75-year-old woman presents with confusion but no focal neurologic signs. She has type II diabetes. BP is 110/54 mm Hg. Pulse is 96 per min. Neck veins are not visualized in the supine position. P$_{Glucose}$ = 900 mg/dl, P$_{Na}$=135 mEq/L, P$_{Cr}$=3.0 mg/dl, BUN=50 mg/dl, U$_{Na}$=40mEq/L, urine SG=1.012, and ketones 3+. Describe her fluid and volume status.

Glucose remains in the ECF due to insulin deficiency. This increases ECF tonicity and pulls water from the ICF to the ECF, concentrating the ICF and diluting the ECF until ICF and ECF osmolalities are equal. The osmotic pressure of 900 mg/dl glucose (900/18 = 50 mOsm/kg) is the driving force for water movement from ICF to ECF. Water movement from the ICF to ECF dilutes the ECF and decreases P$_{Na}$. Each 100 mg/dl rise in P$_{Glucose}$ above 100 mg/dl decreases the P$_{Na}$ 1.6 mEq/L. In this patient, the predicted decrease in P$_{Na}$ = [(900-100)/100 × 1.6] = 13 mEq/L. The predicted P$_{Na}$ would be 140–13 = 127 mEq/L. P$_{Na}$ of 135 suggests further water loss from osmotic diuresis. The P$_{osm}$ of [2(135) + 900/18 + 56/2.8] 340 mOsm/kg is compatible with hyperosmolar coma. Since she has decreased TBW and volume, you might expect the U$_{Na}$ to be low and U$_{osm}$ high. However, osmotic diuresis caused by urine glucose, ketones, and urea increases urinary Na and water, making U$_{Na}$ and U$_{osm}$ less useful markers of dehydration. **A good rule of thumb is U$_{osm}$ approximates 35 × the last two digits of the urine specific gravity.** By this, her U$_{osm}$ approximates [12 × 35] 420 mOsm/kg. Postural vital signs are not given, but **almost nothing will give flat neck veins in the supine position except intravascular volume depletion.** Rapid lowering of her glucose to 100 mg/dl will rapidly decrease P$_{osm}$, shift water to the ICF, increase P$_{Na}$ by 13 mEq/L, and potentially cause cardiovascular collapse. Thus, therapy is normal saline to replace volume and judicious lowering of P$_{Glucose}$ with IV insulin.

9. How do plasma sodium and total body potassium relate to TBW?

The following formulas are useful in understanding the relationship of plasma Na (P$_{Na}$), plasma K, total body sodium and potassium [Na$^+$ + K$^+$], and TBW. [Na$^+$ + K$^+$] estimates total body solute.

1. P$_{Na}$ ≅ Total body [Na$^+$ + K$^+$]/TBW

2. TBW ∝ [Na$^+$ + K$^+$]/P$_{Na}$

3. P$_{Na}$ ∝ P$_{osm}$ ∝ [total body osmolality] ∝ [total body solutes] ∝ 1/TBW

Thus P$_{Na}$ is proportional to total body sodium and potassium and inversely proportional to TBW. From these equations and factors outlined in questions 6 and 7, P$_{Na}$ is a convenient estimate of plasma water, TBW, P$_{osm}$, total body osmolality, and total body solute. An increase or decrease in plasma Na particles can proportionately change the P$_{Na}$. However, in clinical medicine, **changes in P$_{Na}$ usually reflect changes in plasma water.** When P$_{Na}$ is high, plasma water is low. When P$_{Na}$ is low, plasma water is high. Although 98% of K$^+$ is intracellular, P$_{Na}$ is proportional to total body K$^+$, and infusions of Na$^+$ or K$^+$ will increase P$_{Na}$. This occurs as follows. In hypokalemia, the infused K$^+$ enters cells. To preserve electroneutrality, Na$^+$ leaves cells or Cl$^-$ enters. ECF water follows K^+ and Cl^- into cells due to increased osmolality. Either mechanism increases P_{Na} because of KCl infusion. Hypokalemic patients infused with equal amounts of KCl or NaCl will have equal increases in P_{Na}. Thus, addition of KCl to isotonic saline makes hypertonic saline, and infusion of saline with too much KCl may correct hyponatremia too rapidly (see question 31).

10. Describe the input and output of water.
TBW is a balance of input (including endogenous production) and output. In an average adult, input approximates 1600 ml (liquids), 700 ml (foods), and 200 ml (metabolic oxidation of carbohydrate and fat) for a total of 2500 ml/d. Average water losses are 1500 ml (kidneys), 500 ml (skin [400 ml evaporation and 100 ml perspiration]), 300 ml (lung – respiration), and 200 ml from the GI tract (stool) for a total of 2500 ml/d. Large losses of water (increased output) occur with excessive sweating, respiration (exercise), burns, diarrhea, vomiting, and diuresis. Decreased input occurs with defects in thirst or altered mental or physical function (especially in the elderly) preventing access to water.

11. A 35-year-old schizophrenic is admitted to the hospital because of excessive urine output. U_{osm} = 70 mOsm/kg. Posm = 290 mOsm/kg. 24-hour urine output = 12 L/d. How much free water is being excreted each day?
Free water clearance (C_{H2O}) is the amount of solute free water excreted per day. Osmolar clearance is the amount of urine excreted per day that contains all the solute that is isosmotic to plasma. When the urine is hypotonic to plasma, the total urine volume consists of two components. One part is free of solute (C_{H2O}) and the other contains all the solution that is isosmotic to plasma (C_{osm}). To measure how much of the urine is pure (free) water, calculate the free water clearance. To do that, you need to know the osmolar clearance (C_{osm}) and the urine volume (V). The calculations follow.

1. $V = C_{osm} + C_{H2O}$

2. $C_{H2O} = V - C_{osm}$

3. $C_{osm} = U_{osm} V/P_{osm}$

4. $C_{H2O} = V [1 - U_{osm}/P_{osm}]$

5. $C_{H2O} = 12 L [1 - 70/290] = 9 L$

6. $C_{osm} = (70 \text{ mOsm/kg} \times 12 \text{ L/d}) / 290 \text{ mOsm/kg} = 2.9 \text{ L/d or about 3L/d}$

So, this patient's daily urine output contains 9 L/d of pure (free) water and 3 L/d that is isotonic to plasma. This information does not distinguish primary polydipsia from diabetes insipidus (DI). However, the relatively high P_{osm} of 290 suggests DI.

12. Another patient has P_{osm} = 280 mOsm/kg, U_{osm} = 600 mOsm/kg, and a urine volume = 1 L/d. How much free water is being excreted each day?
Urine hypertonic to plasma contains two parts. That volume that contains all solute that is isosmotic to plasma is the osmolar clearance (C_{osm}). The volume of free water removed from the isotonic glomerular filtrate that made $U_{osm} > P_{osm}$ is T^c_{H2O} (negative free water clearance). The calculations follow.

1. $V = C_{osm} - T^c_{H2O}$

2. $T^c_{H2O} = C_{osm} - V$

3. $T^c_{H2O} = V [U_{osm}/P_{osm} -1]$

4. $T^c_{H2O} = 1 L/d [600/280 -1] = 1.14 L/d.$

Thus, this patient's kidneys add 1 L of free water to plasma each day. With a low P_{osm}, it is usually inappropriate to retain water in excess of output. This suggests SIADH. Always exclude glucocorticoid deficiency and hypothyroidism by history, physical examination, and laboratory tests before diagnosing SIADH. Conditions such as hemorrhagic shock and volume depletion stimulate ADH release by effects on central-circulation baroreceptors. Here, increased ADH secretion is appropriate to help restore volume.

13. What are the normal limits of urine output?
Water intake and osmotic products of metabolism determine the usual daily output of urine. On a normal diet a normal adult must excrete about 800–1000 mOsm of solute per day. The range of normal renal concentrating function is 50–1200 mOsm/kg. Based on this fact, the obligate water excretion is 0.8–20 L/d. The calculations are: 1000 mOsm/1200 mOsm/kg = 0.8 L/d at the maximum concentration and 1000 mOsm/50 mOsm/kg = 20 L/d at maximum dilution. Note that higher solute loads (e.g., dietary) allow more water excretion. Thus, low solute intake (starvation) with high water intake predispose to water retention and water intoxication. This combination exists in binge beer drinkers where the solute load may be only 300 mOsm/kg. By similar calculations, the range of urine output would drop to 0.25–6 L/d in these patients. As a consequence of aging, elderly patients lose GFR, concentrating ability, and diluting ability. Thus, an 80-year-old woman may have a normal (for age) renal-concentrating range of 100–700 mOsm/kg. However, maximum U_{osm} in the elderly may be as low as 350 mOsm/kg. Her average diet may generate only 600 mOsm/d. Her normal range of urine output would then be 0.9–6 L/d. If her dietary intake fell to 300 mOsm/d, her maximum urine output would fall to 3L/d. Given free access to water and a thiazide diuretic, which impairs urinary dilution, she could easily become water intoxicated and hyponatremic.

14. What are the main factors controlling water metabolism?
Thirst, hormonal, and renal mechanisms are tightly integrated for control of water metabolism.

15. What are the stimuli of thirst?
Osmoreceptors in the organum vasculosum of the anterior hypothalamus control thirst. Increasing tonicity stimulates thirst at a threshold about 5 mOsm/kg higher than that for ADH release. However, oropharyngeal receptors are also important in thirst regulation. A dry mouth increases thirst. Drinking and swallowing water decrease thirst even without changing P_{osm}. As with ADH release, volume depletion and resulting afferent baroreceptor input increase thirst. Increased angiotensin II from volume depletion is also an important stimulus.

16. What hormonal mechanisms are involved in control of body water?
Supraoptic and paraventricular nuclei respond to changes in osmolality and volume to increase or decrease ADH secretion. ADH and other hormones, including ANP, aldosterone, prostaglandins, and angiotensin II, as well as neurohumoral influences control renal excretion and retention of salt and water. The kidney also produces its own ANP-like hormone called urodilatin. However, ADH remains the most important influence on water retention and excretion. The kidney has such a great capacity to excrete water that hyponatremia rarely develops without impaired renal water excretion. ADH has a short half-life of 15–20 minutes and is metabolized in the kidney and the liver. It attaches to its V_2 receptors on the basolateral membrane of the principal cells of the cortical and medullary collecting tubules and activates cAMP. The increased cAMP activates protein kinase, causing water channels within the cell to insert into the luminal membrane. Water moves from the lumen through these channels down an osmotic gradient and into the cell and interstitium (reabsorption). However, 20% of ADH receptors in the collecting tubular cells are V_1 receptors. When ADH activates V_1 receptors, it stimulates prostaglandin E_2 and prostacyclin synthesis. These prostaglandins oppose the antidiuretic effects of ADH. Since the ADH-stimulated V_1 receptors are activated only at very high ADH levels, this short negative feedback loop opposes excessive ADH action.

17. What are the major conditions that influence ADH secretion?
ADH functions to maintain osmotic and volume homeostasis. Secretion starts at an osmotic threshold of 280 mOsm/kg and increases proportionate to further rises in tonicity. A 1–2%

increase in osmolality and a 10% drop in vascular volume stimulate ADH secretion. By effects on carotid sinus, aortic, and atrial baroreceptors, increased ECV (effective circulating volume) raises the osmotic threshold for secretion, whereas decreased ECV lowers the threshold. Severe volume depletion and hypotension override the hypoosmotic inhibition of ADH secretion. This has been called **the law of circulating volume.** In these states, ADH secretion continues with worsening hyponatremia. Nausea, pain, and stress, as seen postoperatively, are very potent stimuli of ADH release that can produce life-threatening hyponatremia if excess free water is given. This is especially important if drugs that potentiate release or action of ADH are given.

Major causes of ADH secretion: hyperosmolality, hypovolemia, nausea, pain and stress, human chorionic gonadotropin (HCG) as in pregnancy, nicotine (possibly by nausea), hypoglycemia (CRH/ADH release), bacterial and viral CNS infections, CNS tumors or vascular catastrophes (thrombosis, hemorrhage), and ectopic ADH of malignancy (carcinomas of lung [oat cell and bronchogenic], duodenum, pancreas, ureter, bladder, and prostate, and lymphoma). ADH secretion may be increased by any major pulmonary disorder, including pneumonia, tuberculosis, asthma, atelectasis, cystic fibrosis, positive pressure ventilation, and ARDS. HIV infection may have the multifactorial role of CNS dysfunction, pulmonary disease, and malignancy. Excess exogenous ADH or desmopressin acetate (DDAVP) in patients with diabetes insipidus directly increases ADH effect. Oxytocin also has significant ADH activity in the large doses used to induce labor.

Drugs that stimulate ADH secretion: morphine, carbamazepine, clofibrate, intravenous cyclophosphamide, vincristine, vinblastine, haloperidol, amitriptyline, thioridazine, and bromocriptine. Since psychosis itself may cause SIADH, one must question the true ADH stimulatory effect of the listed antipsychotic drugs.

Drugs that enhance ADH effect: chlorpropamide, tolbutamide, carbamazepine, acetaminophen, nonsteroidal anti-inflammatory drugs, and intravenous cyclophosphamide.

Major inhibitors of ADH secretion: hypoosmolality, hypervolemia, ethanol, phenytoin, and vasoconstrictors (baroreceptor effect).

Drugs that decrease ADH effect: demeclocycline, lithium, acetohexamide, tolazamide, glyburide, propoxyphene, amphotericin, methoxyflurane, colchicine, vinblastine, prostaglandin E_2, and prostacyclin.

18. How does the kidney handle salt and water?

In order for the kidney to control for excess or deficiency of water intake, there must be a normal GFR allowing the delivery of isotonic fluid to the loop of Henle (LOH); separation of solute from water in the ascending limb of the LOH, distal convoluted tubule (DCT), and cortical connecting segment; and normal action of ADH to allow controlled reabsorption or excretion of water in the cortical and medullary collecting tubules (CCT and MCT). Since normal GFR is 125 ml/min, the normal kidneys filter 180 L of plasma each day. Since the normal urine output is 1.5–2 L per day, the kidneys reabsorb 99% of the water and salt. The $3Na^+$–$2K^+$-ATPase pump located on the basolateral membrane provides the energy for solute reabsorption **throughout the nephron.** Solute is usually reabsorbed from the tubular lumen by carrier proteins that do not require additional active transport processes. However, active transport of Na and K by the $3Na^+$–$2K^+$-ATPase pump establishes osmotic, electrical, and chemical gradients necessary for solute reabsorption. For this reason, solute reabsorption may be said to occur by secondary active transport. The kidneys reabsorb water passively along an osmotic concentration gradient established by solute reabsorption. The proximal convoluted tubule (PCT) reabsorbs **65%** of filtered Na and water isotonically. The loop of Henle (LOH) receives 35% of the glomerular filtrate and reabsorbs **25%** of this filtrate. Since the ascending limb is impermeable to water, the descending limb of the LOH reabsorbs the water (25%) isotonically. The Na^+–K^+-2Cl carrier on the luminal membrane of the thick ascending limb removes Na, K, and Cl from the tubular lumen.

This causes net reabsorption of Na and Cl, but K recycles to the lumen for reuse. As in the proximal tubule, the $3Na^+-2K^+$-ATPase active pump on the basolateral membrane transports intracellular Na and Cl to the medullary interstitium. This forms the osmotic gradient for passive Na^+-K^+-2Cl carrier transport. The overall process **directly dilutes the urine and forms a hypertonic medullary interstitium necessary for ADH-induced urinary concentration.** Urea reabsorption from the medullary collecting tubule (MCT) further increases the interstitial tonicity. The osmolality of the filtrate leaving the ascending limb is about 100–150 mOsm/kg. **Ten percent** of filtered Na and water enters the distal convoluted tubule (DCT). The DCT and connecting segment reabsorb about 5% of the filtered NaCl, further diluting the urine. However, like the ascending LOH, the distal tubule and connecting segment are impermeable to water. The final volume delivered to the cortical collecting tubule (CCT) is about **10%** of the initial glomerular filtrate with an osmolality of 100 mOsm/kg. The collecting tubule reabsorbs all but **1%** of the remaining filtrate leaving a final urine output of 1.5–2 liters per day. In the absence of ADH, this fluid (about 18 L/d) would be lost in the urine and cause marked dehydration.

19. What are the consequences and causes of decreased renal excretion of water?
Any reduction in water excretion predisposes to **hyponatremia** and **hypoosmolality.** Conditions that impair GFR, delivery of tubular fluid to the distal nephron, or action of the distal nephron to separate solute from water, or increase the permeability of the collecting tubule to water will impair water excretion. Such conditions include renal failure, decreased ECV, diuretics (thiazides >> loop), and excess ADH.

20. How do hypothyroidism and adrenal insufficiency cause hyponatremia?
Hypothyroidism decreases cardiac output and ECV (effective circulating volume). Adrenal insufficiency causes volume depletion, decreased blood pressure, and decreased cardiac output, all of which decreases ECV. The decreased ECV decreases GFR, which reduces delivery of filtrate to the distal nephron and enhances proximal tubular water reabsorption. Decreased ECV also stimulates secretion of ADH. Corticotropin releasing hormone (CRH) and ADH are co-secreted from the same neurons in the paraventricular nuclei of the hypothalamus. Both hormones work synergistically to release ACTH from the anterior pituitary. Since cortisol feeds back negatively at the hypothalamus and pituitary, inhibition of CRH also inhibits ADH release. Therefore, absence of cortisol increases ADH levels, which enhance water reabsorption. These events all predispose to hyponatremia.

21. What plasma sodium concentrations (P_{Na}) are a cause for concern?
The severity of hyponatremia depends on the rapidity of development. Patients with a P_{Na} of 115 mEq/L or 165 mEq/L may not show any clinical abnormalities if they develop the problem over days to weeks. However, both conditions may produce major neurologic dysfunction if they develop over hours to days. As a rule, however, sodium concentrations of 120 to 155 mEq/L are not usually associated with symptoms. P_{Na} outside these limits and occasionally rapidly developing disturbances within these limits may be of major concern.

22. What are and what causes the symptoms and signs of increased or decreased TBW?
The main symptoms and signs of too much (decreased P_{Na}) or too little (increased P_{Na}) TBW result from brain swelling or contraction. If changes in TBW occur more rapidly than the brain can adapt, symptoms and signs will occur. The severity of the symptoms and signs depends on the degree and rapidity of the TBW change. Once the adaptation occurs, correcting the disturbance in body water too rapidly may be more deleterious than the initial disturbance.

Symptoms and signs of hyponatremia include headache, confusion, muscle cramps, weakness, lethargy, apathy, agitation, nausea, vomiting, anorexia, altered levels of consciousness, seizures, depressed deep tendon reflexes, hypothermia, Cheyne-Stokes respiration, respiratory depression, and death.

Symptoms and signs of hypernatremia include weakness, irritability, lethargy, confusion, somnolence, muscle twitching, seizures, respiratory depression, paralysis, and death.

23. How does the brain adapt to changes in TBW?

Brain adaptation to hyponatremia: Since ICF and ECF osmolality must always be equal, developing hyponatremia immediately shifts water into the brain increasing intracranial pressure. The increased intracerebral pressure (ICP) causes loss of NaCl into the CSF. Over the next several hours there is loss of intracellular potassium and over the next few days loss of organic solute. These changes return the brain volume to normal. However, if severe hyponatremia occurs too rapidly, there is not enough time for cerebral adaptation. Brain edema occurs further increasing intracranial pressure; the brain herniates; and the patient dies.

Brain adaptation to hypernatremia: Since brain water is part of TBW, it immediately adapts to changes in P_{osm}. With acute hypernatremia and increased P_{osm}, there is an immediate shift of water out of the brain, decreasing ICP (intracerebral pressure). The decreased ICP promotes movement of CSF fluid with NaCl into the brain ECF, partially correcting volume. Within hours, further brain adaptation occurs, increasing ICF K^+, Na^+, and Cl^-. The resulting increased osmolality pulls water from the ECF and restores about 60% of the brain volume. Over the next several days, the brain accumulates organic solutes (osmolytes), previously called idiogenic osmoles, that return the brain volume to a near-normal level. These solutes include glutamine, taurine, glutamate, myoinositol, and phosphocreatine. If the brain has no time to adapt to rapidly developing hypernatremia, it will shrink, retract from the dura, and tear vessels, causing intracranial hemorrhage, increased ICP, compressive injury, herniation, and death.

24. How would you approach the patient with hyponatremia?

Hyponatremia occurs in > 3% of hospitalized patients. Hyponatremia always means too much ECF water relative to sodium. Since total body volume $\propto$ total body Na, thorough assessment of the patient's volume will allow rational selection of therapy. Patients with flat neck veins and postural BP and pulse changes (standing BP decreases > 20/10 mm Hg and pulse increases > 20 per min) are invariably saline (isotonic NaCl) depleted. Those with distended neck veins and edema are saline overloaded. Always direct treatment at correcting the underlying disorder (see table). If patients have lost saline, give them saline. If they have retained too much water, restrict their water. If they have retained too much salt and water but more water than salt, restrict their salt and water but water more than salt. Sounds simple and it is. However, the difficulty is remembering the importance of and performing an **initial thorough volume assessment.** Assess the patient's volume by looking at neck veins, postural signs, and edema. At times, the best clinician cannot get a good assessment of ECV (effective circulating volume), and central monitoring with a Swan-Ganz catheter is sometimes necessary. Get an initial weight and continue daily weights. Continue assessment of postural signs as needed. Initially, obtain P_{osm}, SMA-10 (Na, K, Cl, CO_2, Cr, BUN, glucose, albumin, Ca, Mg), and urinary Na, Cl, Cr and FENa. Approach therapy as outlined below.

Approach to Hyponatremia

CONDITION	POSTURAL SIGNS	EDEMA	U_{Na}	TREATMENT
Renal saline loss	Yes	No	>20	Give isotonic saline
Nonrenal saline loss	Yes	No	<10	Give isotonic saline
Water excess	No	No	>20	Restrict water
Na and water excess	No	Yes	<10	Restrict water > salt
Na and water excess	No	Yes	>20	Restrict water > salt

Some hyponatremic conditions include: **Renal saline loss:** diuretics, salt-losing nephritis, primary adrenal insufficiency (mineralocorticoid deficit), and renal tubular acidosis. **Nonrenal saline loss:** vomiting, diarrhea, pancreatitis, burns, rhabdomyolysis, peritonitis, and third spacing.

Water excess: SIADH, secondary adrenal insufficiency (glucocorticoid deficit), and hypothyroidism. **Na and water excess:** cirrhosis, nephrosis, and cardiac failure (U_{Na} < 10 mEq/L), and acute and chronic renal failure (U_{Na} >20 mEq/L). Marked hyperglycemia may lower the P_{Na} (true hypertonic hyponatremia). Since P_{Na} is usually measured with ion-selective electrodes, artifactual lowering of the P_{Na} is now unusual. If your lab does not use ion-selective electrodes, marked hyperlipidemia or hyperproteinemia could produce pseudohyponatremia. Notwithstanding, measured P_{osm} will differentiate these disorders. Because P_{osm} measures the osmotic activity of plasma water, plasma water excludes lipids, and protein contributes very little to P_{osm}, the measured P_{osm} will be essentially normal in pseudohyponatremia.

25. How would you characterize, diagnose, and manage the patient with the syndrome of inappropriate antidiuretic hormone secretion (SIADH)?

Hyponatremia is the tipoff to SIADH. Approach the patient as in question 24 and its accompanying table. It is important to establish "normovolemia" with water excess by excluding other conditions in the table. Then measure the P_{osm}, U_{osm}, P_{Na}, U_{Na}, and U_K. Finally, exclude pituitary, adrenal, and thyroid dysfunction prior to diagnosis. Confirmatory criteria of SIADH include low P_{Na} (< 135 mEq/L), low P_{osm} (<280 mOsm/kg), U_{osm} > 100 mOsm/kg, U_{Na} > 40 mEq/L, and $[U_{Na} + U_K]>P_{Na}$. Patients with SIADH are usually said to have normal volume status. However, they actually have excess TBW. Unlike excess saline that is limited to the ECF, excess water distributes two-thirds ICF and one-third ECF. Thus, the ECF excess is minor and not usually perceptible by clinical examination. Nonetheless, patients with SIADH have increased ECV that is sensed by the kidney. This increases GFR, which causes a low uric acid, BUN, and creatinine. The increased ECV also increases ANP which, with the increased GFR, promotes natriuresis. These are the classic findings in SIADH. Obviously, SIADH does not protect against dehydration and other conditions that can obscure the classic presentation. For example, a patient with ectopic ADH from lung cancer may present with dehydration from diarrhea and lack of water intake from debilitation. In this instance, the U_{Na} and U_{Cl} may be less than 10 mEq/L. Initially, treat SIADH with water restriction. If the patient has marked symptoms, treat for symptomatic hyponatremia (question 31). Attempt to correct the underlying abnormality (question 17). If the patient has unresectable cancer and water restriction (500–1500 ml/d) is not tolerated, give demeclocycline 600–1200 mg/d or lithium carbonate 600–1200 mg/d in 2–4 divided doses. Since lithium carbonate can cause neurologic, cardiovascular, and other toxicites, avoid it unless demeclocycline is contraindicated.

26. What are the four patterns of SIADH?

The table below summarizes the four SIADH patterns according to responses of ADH to P_{osm}.

Patterns of ADH Secretion in SIADH

PATTERN	CHARACTERISTICS	FREQUENCY
Type A	**Erratic ADH secretion** with no predictable relationship to P_{osm}	20%
Type B	**Reset osmostat** with normal relationship of ADH to P_{osm} but a lower threshold for ADH release (e.g., 250–260 mOsm/kg)	35%
Type C	**ADH leak with selective loss of ADH suppression** and continued secretion when P_{osm} is low but normal suppression and secretion when P_{osm} is normal	35%
Type D	**ADH-dissociated antidiuresis** at low P_{osm} with appropriately low or undetectable ADH (possibly from increased renal sensitivity to ADH or unknown ADH-like substance)	10%

27. Define polyuria and list the main causes.

Polyuria is a urine output greater than 2.5–3 L/d. Four main defects cause polyuria: psychogenic polydipsia (psychosis), dipsogenic diabetes insipidus (defect in thirst center), central neurogenic DI (defect in ADH secretion), and nephrogenic DI (defect in ADH action on the kidney). All forms of DI may be partial or complete. Polyuria may also occur from osmotic diuresis in such conditions as diabetes (glucose), recovery from renal failure (urea), and intravenous infusions (saline, mannitol). See question 17 for drugs and conditions that decrease ADH secretion and action. Causes of acquired nephrogenic DI include chronic renal disease, electrolyte abnormalities (hypokalemia and hypercalcemia), drugs (lithium, demeclocycline), sickle cell disease (damaged medullary interstitium), diet (increased water and decreased solute—beer, starvation), inflammatory or infiltrative renal disease (multiple myeloma, amyloidosis, sarcoidosis), and others.

28. How would you distinguish polyuric patients with the various forms of diabetes insipidus (DI) from excessive water drinking?

If the diagnosis of polyuria is not clear from the history and initial lab tests, perform a water restriction test (WRT). Other names for the WRT are dehydration test and water deprivation test. The test may take 6–18 hours depending on the state of hydration. Perform the WRT as follows. Admit mildly polyuric patients to the ward and more severely polyuric patients to the ICU. Start the test at 10:00–11:00 PM for mildly polyuric patients and at 6:00 AM for more severely polyuric patients. Measure **baseline** weight, P_{osm}, P_{Na}, P_{BUN}, $P_{glucose}$, U_{volume}, U_{osm}, U_{Na}, and U_K. Measure hourly weight and U_{osm}. Allow no food or water. Watch these patients closely for signs of dehydration and surreptitious water drinking. End the WRT when U_{osm} has not increased more than 30 mOsm/kg for 3 consecutive hours and P_{osm} has reached 295–300 mOsm/Kg or the patient has lost 3–5% of body weight. At 295–300 mOsm/kg endogenous ADH levels should be 3–5 pg/mL and the kidney should respond with maximum urinary concentration. If weight loss exceeds 5% of body weight, further dehydration is unsafe. Repeat all baseline tests toward and at the end of the WRT. Then give 5 units of aqueous AVP or 1 μg of desmopressin acetate (DDAVP) SC. Repeat the baseline tests at 30, 60, and 120 minutes. Calculate U_{osm}/P_{osm} and $[U_{Na} + U_K]/P_{Na}$ as a check on measured U_{osm}/P_{osm}. The table below summarizes the expected results of the WRT. The WRT stimulates maximum endogenous release of ADH by increasing P_{osm} and evaluates the concentrating ability of the kidney by measuring U_{osm}. Giving exogenous ADH allows evaluation of the renal concentrating response to ADH if dehydration-induced endogenous ADH production was impaired. Save frozen baseline and end-test plasma to measure plasma ADH if results are equivocal. Expected values for P_{ADH} are ≤ 0.5 pg/mL for $P_{osm} \leq 280$ mOsm/kg and ≥ 5 pg/mL for $P_{osm} \geq 295$ mOsm/kg.

Values Before and After Water Restriction

	PRE P_{osm}	PRE P_{Na}	POST U_{osm}/P_{osm}	POST U_{osm}/P_{osm} + ADH	POST P_{ADH}
Normals	NL	NL	>1	>1 (<10%)	↑
PPD/DDI	↓	↓	>1	>1 (<10%)	↑
CCDI	↑	↑	<1	>1 (>50%)	–
PCDI	↑	↑	>1	>1 (10–50%)	↓
CNDI	↑	↑	<1	<1 (<10%)	↑↑
PNDI	↑	↑	>1	>1 (<10%)	↑↑

PPD/DDI = psychogenic polydipsia/dipsogenic DI; **CCDI** = complete central DI; **PCDI** = partial central DI; **CNDI** = complete nephrogenic DI; and **PNDI** = partial nephrogenic DI. Relative to the normal range, the down and up arrows respectively mean low or low normal and high or high normal values for P_{osm}, P_{Na}, and P_{ADH}. Recall that when $U_{osm} > P_{osm}$, there is antidiuresis and the kidney is retaining free water. The same is true when $[U_{Na} + U_K] > P_{Na}$, and these tests are more easily obtainable. When $U_{osm} < P_{osm}$ or $[U_{Na} + U_K] < P_{Na}$, there is net loss of free water and little net clinical ADH effect. The % in parentheses indicates the percentage change in U_{osm} (not the U_{osm}/P_{osm} ratio) after 5 units of aqueous vasopressin SC.

29. How would you approach the patient with hypernatremia?

Problems of hypernatremia are uncommon compared to hyponatremia and occur in < 1% of hospitalized patients. Loss of water and not gain of sodium usually causes hypernatremia. However, unless patients have an abnormality of thirst or don't have access to water, they usually maintain near-normal P_{Na} by drinking water in proportion to losses. As in question 24, assess the patient's volume status. Once lab studies are obtained, approach the patient per the following table. If the patient has polyuria, also include the approach in questions 27 and 28.

Approach to Hypernatremia

CONDITION CAUSING HYPERNATREMIA	POSTURAL SIGNS	EDEMA	U_{Na}	U_{osm}	TREATMENT
Renal Na and H_2O loss	Yes	No	>20	$\downarrow-$	Hypotonic saline
Non-renal Na and H_2O loss	Yes	No	<10	$\uparrow$	Hypotonic saline
Sodium Excess	No	No	>20	$\uparrow-$	Diuretics and water
Renal H_2O loss	No	No	VAR	$\downarrow\uparrow-$	Water
Non-renal H_2O loss	No	No	VAR	$\uparrow$	Water

VAR = variable; $\uparrow$ = hypertonic; $\downarrow$ = hypotonic; and -= isoosmotic.
Representative conditions: **1. Conditions with low total body sodium but with water loss > sodium loss include** (a) renal sodium and water loss (osmotic and loop diuretics, postobstructive diuresis, and renal disease) and (b) nonrenal sodium and water loss (sweating, burns, diarrhea). **2. Conditions with high total body sodium include** primary hyperaldosteronism, Cushing's syndrome, excess NaCl or $NaHCO_3$ input, and hypertonic dialysis. **3. Conditions with normal total body sodium but with water loss include** (a) renal water losses (central or nephrogenic diabetes insipidus) and (b) nonrenal water loss: increased insensible losses from respiration and skin. With access to water, the rise in P_{Na} is mild (usually in upper normal range) due to thirst-induced water replacement.

30. How would you diagnose and manage the patient with diabetes insipidus (DI)?

DI is a syndrome of excessive water loss by the kidney due to decreased ADH (central DI) or renal resistance to ADH effect (nephrogenic DI). Therefore, the hallmark of DI is polyuria. As in questions 27 and 28, first distinguish primary polydipsia from DI and identify the DI as central or nephrogenic. Then give water to prevent dehydration until the evaluation suggests definitive therapy. A patient with DI will probably self-treat with water unless there is a thirst deficit or the patient has no access to water. An example is a 70-year-old woman who noted the onset of polyuria and polydipsia a week before admission. She increased water intake but then developed the flu and could not hold down liquids. Family brought her to the hospital. Her P_{Na} was 150 mEq/L. Her weight was 60 kg. Her evaluation showed breast cancer metastatic to the brain. Her water deficit is as follows.

$$\text{Water deficit} = [(\text{Observed } P_{Na} - \text{Normal } P_{Na})/\text{Normal } P_{Na}] \times \text{TBW}$$
$$= [(P_{Na} - 140)/140] \times \text{TBW}$$
$$= [(150 - 140) / 140] \times 0.5 \times 60 \text{ kg}$$
$$= 2 \text{ L deficit in TBW}$$

Treat the polyuria and the underlying cause if possible. If not, just treat the polyuria. If the diagnosis is central DI, as in this case, desmopressin acetate is the therapy of choice. DDAVP has an antidiuretic to pressor ratio of 2000:1 compared to AVP's ratio of 1:1. The usual dose is 5–20 μg intranasally in 2 divided doses. Some important causes of central DI include idiopathic (autoimmune), primary tumors (craniopharyngioma), metastatic tumors (breast, lung, leukemia), infections (viral), vascular disorders (aneurysm),·granulomas (sarcoidosis), drugs (clonidine), head trauma, and cranial or pituitary surgery. Treat nephrogenic DI with 12.5–25 mg hydrochlorothiazide qd to bid to decrease ECV, enhance proximal nephron water reabsorption, and increase medullary interstitial osmolality. Other therapies that increase U_{osm} by ADH-independent mechanisms include low sodium and protein diet, amiloride, and NSAIDs (e.g., indomethacin). By preventing sodium and lithium entry into the tubular cell, amiloride is particularly useful in lithium carbonate-induced DI.

CONTROVERSIES

31. How quickly should you correct states of water excess or deficiency?

The main concern of therapy is to prevent devastating neurologic complications. Understanding brain adaptation to changes in TBW, as outlined in question 23, emphasizes the need for urgent therapy in the symptomatic patient. There are three useful rules in treating disturbances of water (measured by changes in P_{Na}):

1. Return the plasma P_{Na} to normal at the relative **speed** that it became abnormal. If the change in P_{Na} was slow (days), then correct it slowly (days). If the change was rapid (minutes to hours) then correct it rapidly (minutes to hours).

2. If there are no **symptoms** of water or sodium imbalance (question 22), there is no immediate urgency. If there are symptoms, there is an urgency. Question 23 outlines the brain adaptations to altered tonicity that may cause devastating changes in brain volume. These adaptations also cause the patient's symptoms. Thus, symptoms should drive the clinician to rapidly correct the altered tonicity.

3. The **degree of P_{Na} correction** should be **toward normal** not to normal (until symptoms abate). An example is a 34 year-old woman presenting 12 hours post discharge after cholecystectomy. She had headache, confusion, muscle cramps, weakness, lethargy, agitation, nausea, and vomiting but had been asymptomatic at discharge. **P_{Na} was 110 mEq/L.** By this history hyponatremia developed rapidly and was symptomatic. Treatment is ICU admission and administration of 3% saline and furosemide at rates sufficient to increase P_{Na} 1.5–2 mEq/L/h for 2–4 hours based on symptom resolution. Measure hourly P_{Na}, U_{Na}, and U_K to follow progress and guide therapy. Once serious signs and symptoms improve, decrease the rate of correction to 0.5–1 mEq/L/h until symptoms further improve or the P_{Na} is 120 mEq/L. Unless patient symptoms dictate otherwise, attempt to avoid a net increase in P_{Na} > 12 mEq/L/d and 18–20 mEq/L over 2 days. For chronic hyponatremia without symptoms, the appropriate rate of correction would be 0.5 mEq/L/h with similar net daily increases in P_{Na}. Acute symptomatic hyponatremia requires expeditious correction of the P_{Na} because the symptomatic patient has cerebral edema caused by "normal" brain-cell solute content that pulls water into the brain. Acutely raising P_{Na} increases ECF tonicity, pulls water out of the swollen brain, and reduces the brain volume toward normal. Conversely, the patient with chronic asymptomatic hyponatremia has adapted by loss of brain solute and has near-normal brain volume. Increasing this patient's P_{Na} too rapidly (> 0.5 mEq/L/h) will shrink the brain and predispose to the osmotic demyelination syndrome (previously called central pontine myelinolysis). The risk of not correcting a patient with acute symptomatic hyponatremia is increased cerebral edema, seizures, coma, and death. Outlined below are calculations of this patient's water excess and how much NaCl would correct her P_{Na} to 120 mEq/L.

$$\text{Water excess} = [(\text{Normal } P_{Na} - \text{Observed } P_{Na})/\text{Normal } P_{Na}] \times \text{TBW}$$
$$= [(140 - 110) / 140] \times 0.5 \times 60 \text{ kg}$$
$$= 0.21 \times 30 \text{ L}$$
$$= 6.3 \text{ L excess in TBW}$$

$$\text{Na}^+ \text{ deficit} = (\text{Desired } P_{Na} - \text{Observed } P_{Na}) \times \text{TBW}$$
$$= (120 - 110) \times 0.5 \times 60 \text{ kg}$$
$$= 10 \text{ mEq/L} \times 30 \text{ L}$$
$$= 300 \text{ mEq Na}$$

Knowing the sodium deficient is useful clinically since the deficit can be replaced at a controlled rate to improve the hyponatremia. The Na^+ in 3% saline is 513 mEq/L. 300 mEq Na^+/513 mEq/L = 0.585 L. Thus, assuming no Na or water loss, giving 585 ml of 3% saline would correct the P_{Na} to 120 mEq/L. Make a similar calculation for the amount of 3% saline to infuse over 3–4 hours to increase the P_{Na} by 6 mEq/L. The answer is 350 ml. Use P_{Na}, U_{Na}, and U_K to estimate loss and gain of sodium and water during therapy.

The same concepts of **speed, symptoms, and degree of P_{Na} correction** apply in opposite osmotic directions for hypernatremia.

BIBLIOGRAPHY

1. Arroyo V, Gines P, Planas R: Treatment of ascites in cirrhosis: Diuretics, peritoneovenous shunt, and large-volume paracentesis. Gastroenterol Clin North Am 21:237–256, 1992.
2. Ayus JC, Arieff AI: Pathogenesis and prevention of hyponatremic encephalopathy. Endocrinol Metab Clin North Am 22:425–446, 1993.

3. Berl T, Schrier RW: Disorders of water metabolism. In Schrier RW (ed): Renal and Electrolyte Disorders, 4th ed. Boston, Little, Brown, 1992, pp 1–87.
4. Brown RG: Disorders of water and sodium balance. Postgrad Med 93:227–228, 231–334, 239–240, 1993.
5. Buonocore CM, Robinson AG: The diagnosis and management of diabetes insipidus during medical emergencies. Endocrinol Metab Clin North Am 22:411–423, 1993.
6. Cheng JC, Zikos D, Skopicki HA, et al: Long-term neurologic outcome in psychogenic water drinkers with severe symptomatic hyponatremia: The effect of rapid correction [see comments]. Am J Med 88:561–566, 1990.
7. Davis PJ, Davis FB: Water excretion in the elderly. Endocrinol Metab Clin North Am 16:867–875, 1987.
8. Gruskin AB, Sarnaik A: Hyponatremia: Pathophysiology and treatment, a pediatric perspective. Pediatr Nephrol 6:280–286, 1992.
9. Gullans SR, Verbalis JG: Control of brain volume during hyperosmolar and hypoosmolar conditions. Annu Rev Med 44:289–301, 1993.
10. Kamel KS, Bear RA: Treatment of hyponatremia: A quantitative analysis. Am J Kidney Dis 21:439–443, 1993.
11. Kovacs L, Robertson GL: Syndrome of inappropriate antidiuresis. Endocrinol Metab Clin North Am 21:859–875, 1992.
12. Kovacs L, Robertson GL: Disorders of water balance—hyponatraemia and hypernatraemia. Baillieres Clin Endocrinol Metab 6:107–127, 1992.
13. Morrison G, Singer I: Hyperosmolal states. In Narins RG (ed): Maxwell & Kleeman's Clinical Disorders of Fluid and Electrolyte Metabolism, 5th ed. New York, McGraw-Hill, 1994, pp 617–658.
14. Oster JR, Materson BJ: Renal and electrolyte complications of congestive heart failure and effects of therapy with angiotensin-covering enzyme inhibitors. Arch Intern Med 152:704–710, 1992.
15. Rose BD: Clinical Physiology of Acid-Base and Electrolyte Disorders, 4th ed. New York, McGraw-Hall, 1994.
16. Sonnenblick M, Friedlander Y, Rosin AJ: Diuretic-induced severe hyponatremia: Review and analysis of 129 reported patients. Chest 103:601–606, 1993.
17. Sterns RH: Severe hyponatremia: The case for conservative management. Crit Care Med 20:534–539, 1992.
18. Sterns RH: The management of hyponatremic emergencies. Crit Care Clin 7:127–142, 1991.
19. Strange K: Maintenance of cell volume in the central nervous system. Pediatr Nephrol 7:689–697, 1993.
20. Tyrrell JB, Finding JW, Aron DC: Hypothalamus and pituitary. In Greenspan FS, Baxter JD (eds): Basic and Clinical Endocrinology, 4th ed. Norwalk, Appleton & Lange, 1994, pp 64–127.

22. DISORDERS OF GROWTH

Robert H. Slover, M.D.

1. What is a normal growth velocity for children?

The normal growth increment in the first 6 months of life is 16–17 cm and in the second 6 months about 8 cm. Growth in the second year of life is just over 10 cm, whereas it is about 8 cm in the third year and 7 cm in the fourth year. During the fifth through tenth year (until puberty) growth averages 5–6 cm/year.

2. What are the tools used to define growth in children?

First and most essential is the ability to obtain accurate measurements. In infants and children up to age 2 years, supine length is measured, ideally using a boxlike structure with a movable foot plate. In children 2 years of age and older, standing height is measured, most accurately by a stadiometer, which allows the measurer to exert upward pressure on the patient at the angle of the jaw while a balanced platform touches the top of the head and a counter reads the measurement. If this device is not available, the child should stand against a wall with heels, buttocks, thoracic spine, and head touching the wall. A right angle is moved downward to touch the top of the head, and a mark is made and measured. Scales with height sticks are notoriously unreliable. Weight and (when appropriate) head circumference also are needed.

The second tool is the growth curve. Clearly the more points that are plotted on a curve, the greater the understanding of the child's growth. A point is just a point—at least two are needed to define a line!

Finally, a bone-age film gives important information about skeletal (and by implication) physical maturity. This study is obtained with a radiograph of the left hand and wrist in children over 2 years of age and by counting epiphyseal centers in the upper and lower extremities in infants.

The combination of accurate heights and weights, a well-plotted growth curve, and bone-age studies often leads quickly to diagnosis of the cause of short stature and direct further evaluations.

3. Using the tools of growth curve, bone age, and height, how does one distinguish between familial (genetic) short stature and other causes?

Children with familial short stature grow at a normal velocity but below the curve. In such children, bone age approximately equals chronologic age. For example, a 5-year-old who is below the third percentile, but whose growth has traced a line parallel to the third percentile and whose bone age is also 5 years may reasonably be expected to have familial short stature. A simple formula helps to determine whether a child's size is explained by parental heights: add the parents' heights in cm; add 13 cm if the child is male, or subtract 13 cm if the child is a female; divide by two. The resulting height ± 5 cm gives a rough range for predicted adult height. If the child's projected height (by extrapolation of the curve) falls within this range, the likelihood is high that current height may be explained by genetic factors. Conversely, if the projected height falls below the predicted range, other factors *may be* involved in the short stature. See examples 1 and 2 on p. 136.

4. Other than familial short stature, what is the most common etiology of short stature?

Constitutional delay of growth (constitutional short stature), which affects up to 2% of children, is characterized by short stature and delayed bone age. Affected children typically have a period of subnormal growth between 18 and 30 months of age followed by normal growth velocity throughout the remainder of childhood. At any given chronologic age, bone age is delayed. The continuing growth delay results in a delay in pubertal development as well as physical maturity. Such children (usually boys) often have a positive family history and may have a more dramatic deceleration of growth velocity before entering puberty than normal children. Growth, including dental, skeletal, and pubertal development, is simply physiologically delayed. They complete their growth at a later age, ending at a normal adult height within expected genetic potential. See examples at top of p. 137.

Example 1: 7-year-old girl with height of 110 cm

> Height age = 5 years, 3 months
> Bone age = 7 years
>
> Father's height 65 in (165 cm)
> Mother's height 62 in (157 cm)
>
> Corrected midparental height (± 1 SD) = 155 ± 5 cm
>
> Predicted adult height = 60 in
>
> The child has a predicted adult height within genetic potential, a bone age equal to chronologic age, and genetic short stature.

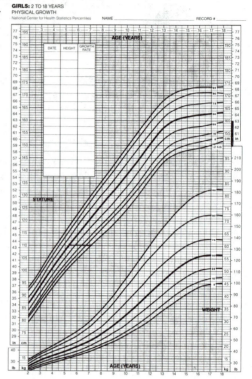

Example 2: 7-year-old girl with height of 110 cm

> Height age = 5 years, 3 months
> Bone age = 5 years
>
> Father's height 70 in (718 cm)
> Mother's height 66 in (168 cm)
>
> Corrected midparental height (± 1 SD) + 167 ± 5 cm
>
> The child is growing below the fifth percentile, but extrapolation of her growth to adult height gives a final height below genetic potential. Clearly her height cannot be attributed to genetic short stature alone.

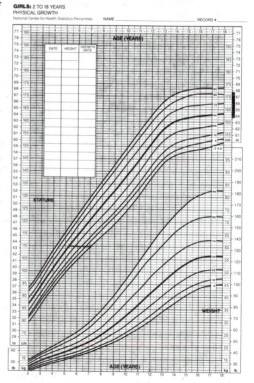

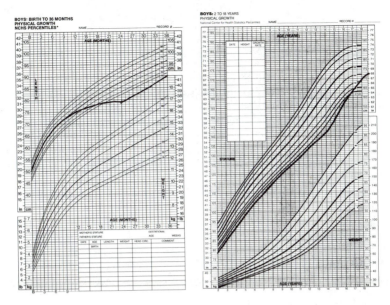

Constitutional delay of growth. Subnormal velocity during second year of life followed by normal velocity through childhood and a prolonged growth period.

5. How is the diagnosis of constitutional delay of growth made?

These elements may allow one to feel comfortable with the diagnosis of constitutional delay of growth:

    1. Short stature;

    2. A period of poor growth in the second year of life followed by a normal growth velocity;

    3. Delayed bone age (bone age is often roughly equivalent to "height age"—a point determined by extrapolating height backward to the 50% on the height curve); and

    4. Positive family history, delayed dentition, and delayed puberty in adolescnce.

The diagnosis of constitutional delay of growth based on the above criteria does not need further laboratory support.

Example: 6-year-old boy

Height age = 3 years, 6 months
Bone age = 3 years, 9 months
Normal velocity
Predicted adult height 68 1/2 in

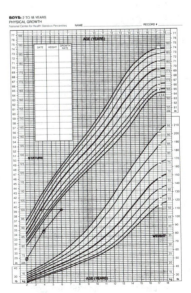

6. What is the effect of testosterone therapy on boys with constitutional delay of growth?
Short-term testosterone therapy for boys with constitutional delay accelerates growth and
stimulates pubertal development without compromising final adult height or advancing bone age.
In European studies, doses of 100–250 mg/month of long-acting testosterone esters given for 6
months, starting at bone age 12 1/2 years, brought positive psychosocial effects without negative
somatic effects or reduction in final adult height. Furthermore, testosterone therapy improves
secretion of growth hormone contributing to the observable acceleration of growth. Clinically the
boys experience pubertal changes, including genital enlargement (but not testicular growth),
growth of pubic and axillary hair, deepening of voice, body odor, and acne. Not surprisingly, there
are fairly typical personality changes as well!

7. Name the endocrine causes for short stature in children.
Nonendocrine causes account for over 90% of short children. Important endocrine causes,
however, include the following:

- Deficiency of growth hormone
- Excess of glucocorticoids
- Congenital hypothyroidism
- Acquired hypothyroidism
- Pseudohypoparathyroidism
- Poorly controlled diabetes mellitus
- Rickets and other metabolic bone diseases

8. Describe the etiologies of growth hormone deficiency.
Idiopathic growth hormone deficiency affects as many as 1 of 10,000–15,000 children and is by
far the most common etiology. It is sporadic in the great majority of cases, but a handful of
hereditary cases have been reported, some with specific deletions of genes for growth hormone.
The other important underlying causes are listed below:

1. Congenital
    Septooptic dysplasia
    Midline facial or skull defects
    Congenital absence of the pituitary
2. Trauma
    Accidental, including birth injuries
    Nonaccidental (child abuse)
3. Iatrogenic, after therapy
    Surgery
    Radiation
    Chemotherapy
4. Infectious
5. Vascular diseases
6. Psychosocial disorders
7. Tumors of hypothalamus and pituitary
    (craniopharygioma, glioma, pinealoma,
    hamartoma, neurofibroma)
8. Histiocytosis
9. End-organ resistance
    Laron dwarfism
    Biologically inactive growth hormone
    Malnutrition

9. How is growth hormone deficiency diagnosed?
Children with subnormal growth should be evaluated for growth hormone deficiency after a
thorough search fails to reveal any other etiology for growth delay. Because secretion of growth
hormone is episodic, random levels are meaningless. Instead, growth hormone is measured in
response to a series of physiologic or pharamacologic stimuli.

Normal children typically respond to stimulation with growth hormone levels 8–10 ng/ml
and may have levels as high as 30 ng/ml. For results to have meaning, the child must be euthyroid,
with no underlying chronic disease or psychosocial deprivation. Concurrent testing for other
pituitary functions should include studies of thyroid-stimulating hormone (TSH) and thyroid
function, adrenocorticotropic hormone (ACTH) and cortisol, and gonadotropins, because growth
hormone deficiency may be associated with broader pituitary deficiency.

Physiologic stimuli include sleep induction and exercise. Most nonaffected children secrete
growth hormone shortly after sleep and within 20–40 minutes after 20 minutes of vigorous
exercise. These tests are useful as screening measures only.

More commonly, pharmacologic stimulation is used to make the diagnosis of growth
hormone deficiency. Various agents are used. At least two tests are required, because a patient

may fail to respond to one agent on a given day but respond to another. All tests require an overnight fast.

Drugs Used to Test Adequacy of Growth Hormone Secretion

	ARGININE	L-DOPA	CLONIDINE	INSULIN
Dosage	0.5 g/kg of 5–10% solution intravenously	0.5 g/1.73 m² orally (125 mg if <10kg 250 mg if 10–30 kg 500 mg if >30 kg)	0.15 mg/m² orally	.05–0.10 U/kg regular insulin intravenously
Sample times	0, 30, 60, 90, 120 min	0, 30, 60, 90, 120 min	0, 30, 60, 90, 120 min	45, 60, 90 min

Failure to respond to pharmalogic stimulation with growth hormone levels above 8–10 ng/ml in all studies is definitive of classic growth hormone deficiency.

10. Is there a role for levels of somatomedin-C in making the diagnosis of growth hormone deficiency?

Somatomedin-C (insulin-like growth factor - 1 [IGF-1]) is one of a class of peptides in serum at levels mediated by growth hormone. IGF-1 is currently under intense investigation, and its role in promoting growth promises to be extremely important. As a tool for diagnosis of growth hormone deficiency, it is suggestive but not diagnostic. In general, concentrations of somatomedin-C are reduced in hypopituitarism and elevated in acromegaly. Normal levels of somatomedin-C usually indicate growth hormone sufficiency and may be used as a screen, but they do not replace provocative, stimulated growth hormone levels in diagnosis. Low levels of somatomedin-C may indicate growth hormone deficiency, but they also are influenced by poor nutrition, chronic disease, and hypothyroidism.

The fact that levels of somatomedin-C remain constant through the day, unlike levels of growth hormone, make them an attractive screen. However, they vary with age (quite low under 6 years) and are subject to the limitations mentioned above.

Normal Ranges of Somatomedin-C

AGE (yrs)	MALES (U/ml)	FEMALES (U/ml)
Birth–3	0.08–1.1	0.11–2.2
3–6	0.12–1.6	0.18–2.4
6–11	0.22–2.8	0.41–4.5
11–13	0.28–3.7	0.99–6.8
13–15	0.9–5.6	1.2–5.9
15–18	0.91–3.1	0.71–4.1
18–64	0.34–1.9	0.45–2.3

Source: Nichols Institute, San Juan Capistrano, CA.

11. How is idiopathic growth hormone deficiency treated?

Children with classic growth hormone deficiency have been successfully treated for nearly 30 years. Currently, growth hormone is available through recombinant DNA technology and is not derived from human pituitary sources. Many questions remain about dose-response relationships, but the majority of children are now treated with 6–7 daily shots/week, with a total weekly dose of approximately 0.30 mg/kg/week. The injections are administered subcutaneously. Because the effect of growth hormone wanes after several years of therapy, it is common to see dramatic catch-up growth (velocities ≥ 10–12 cm/year) in the first year or two of therapy, followed by velocities ranging from normal to 1 1/2 times normal in subsequent years of therapy. Throughout therapy, levels of thyroid hormone as well as other pituitary hormones must be monitored closely. Yearly bone age studies help to update height predictions and to predict the timing of puberty.

Example: 14½-year-old boy with growth hormone deficiency treated from age 9.

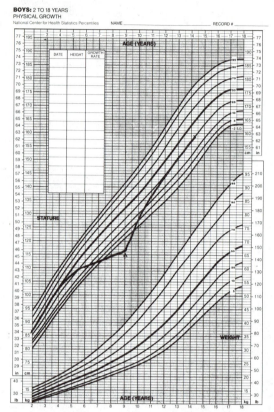

BOYS: 2 TO 18 YEARS
PHYSICAL GROWTH
National Center for Health Statistics Percentiles   NAME _____ RECORD # _____

12. What is the prognosis for adult height in treated children with idiopathic growth hormone deficiency?

Growth hormone therapy advances both linear growth and skeletal maturity proportionally. However, whereas most treated children reach the third percentile on the growth curve and have an adult height significantly better than predicted before therapy is initiated, most do not reach their predicted genetic potential. Older reports indicate that treated children may expect a final adult height 2.0 SD below calculated midparental mean height as opposed to 6.0 SD below mean without treatment. This expectation seems to have improved with shorter dose intervals and more aggressive dosing. In addition, children diagnosed and treated at an earlier age have a better height prognosis than children whose therapy is initiated later. The more mature the skeleton at diagnosis, the poorer the final outcome. Children with idiopathic growth hormone deficiency respond better than children with Turner syndrome or underlying renal disease.

13. When is growth hormone therapy discontinued?

In children with idiopathic growth hormone deficiency, the point of diminishing benefit of therapy correlates to skeletal maturity rather than chronologic age or duration of therapy. Therapy often is discontinued at a bone age of 15 years (96% of growth) to 16 years (98% of growth) in boys and 14 years (98% of growth) in girls.

14. What syndrome is most commonly treated with human growth hormone?

Turner syndrome (45 XO or mosaic variants) in girls is commonly associated with short stature that seems to be independent of the reduction in height caused by failure in estrogen production. It has become common practice to treat affected girls with growth hormone or with combinations of growth hormone and estrogen or oxandrolone.

15. What is the prognosis for girls with Turner syndrome treated with human growth hormone?

The treatment of Turner syndrome with growth hormone has been studied carefully for over 6 years. Girls treated for this period demonstrated an increase in predicted adult height of 14 cm. In a cohort of women who completed therapy, the average increase was 8.8 cm. It seems clear that growth hormone increases actual height by accelerating growth velocity without accelerating bone age. Such therapy may be enhanced by the addition of low doses of estradiol or oxandrolone. Therapy may result not only in improved adult height but also in normalization of childhood growth velocity.

16. What other syndromes associated with short stature are now treated with growth hormone?

Because human growth hormone is readily available, several of the short-stature syndromes are under study. The largest numbers of patients so far are children with Noonan's syndrome. Russell-Silver dwarfism, Prader-Willi syndrome, and Down syndrome. In addition, several hundred children with renal failure and transplant are being treated.

17. What are the potential risks of human growth hormone therapy?

Although glucose intolerance or hyperglycemia is often mentioned as a potential risk of human growth hormone therapy, in actual clinical management with standard doses (up to 0.35 mg/kg/week) neither has proved to be a problem. In 1982 a few patients who had been treated with human pituitary-derived growth hormone died of Jacob-Creutzfeldt disease, a prion-caused degenerative neurologic disease with a latency of decades. This previral particle was assumed to hve been a contaminant of the pituitary extract. As a result, the use of pituitary-derived growth hormone was discontinued; since 1983 all growth hormone given in the United States has been made by recombinant DNA technology.

Most recently the question of an association between growth hormone and leukemia has been raised. Worldwide about 35 patients receiving human growth hormone have developed leukemia. In North America none of the children affected was being treated for idiopathic growth hormone deficiency. Instead, the risk seemed to be present in children with underlying lesions or previous treatment with chemotherapy or radiation. The overall increase in risk for leukemia in North America (based on these small numbers) is about fourfold.

Finally, about 25 children treated with growth hormone have developed pseudotumor cerebri. Of these, a disporportionately large number were being treated for growth failure associated with severa renal disease or transplant.

18. Should short children without growth hormone deficiency be treated with growth hormone?

At present, this question is intensely controversial among pediatric endocrinologists. Certainly this group represents by far the largest number of short children. Several short-term studies involving small cohorts have demonstrated a consistent increase in growth velocity with growth hormone therapy in children in whom no secretary abnormality could be demonstrated. Bone ages did not advance disproportionately. Again, growth response was greatest in the first year of therapy and declined in the second year. Because no study has followed children to final height, the question remains: will therapy with growth hormone make a difference in adult height?

On the one hand, a small subset of children with normal growth hormone responses may grow at a subnormal rate and fail to achieve adult heights consistent with family-based predictions. Such children may produce biologically inactive hormone or may have inadequate daily production. At this time no conclusive evidence proves that growth hormone increases adult height, but perhaps affected children should not be required to wait until data are available, because treatment may be of substantial benefit.

On the other hand, enormous numbers of short children grow at a normal rate. Growth hormone increases velocity in many such children in the short term but no data show that adult height is enhanced by treatment. Expense, potential risks, and uncertain benefit make such treatment problematic.

19. How does the pattern of growth in children with excessive glucocorticoids differ from the pattern in children with exogenous obesity?

Excess of steroids, whether iatrogenic (common) or intrinsic (rare), results in impairment of linear growth. The mechanism relates to direct metabolic actions, including increased protein catabolism for energy, decreased lipoloysis, and decline in collagen synthesis. Glucocorticoids also suppress growth hormone response by increasing somatostatin and by suppressing pulsatile release of growth hormone. They also suppress production of IGF-1. The net result is that children with steroid excess are frequently short. Typically they have an increased weight-to-height ratio and appear obese. Unlike adults with Cushing's features, children are usually proportionally obese; in addition, muscle weakness is an important feature of their disease.

Children with exogenous obesity, on the other hand, frequently show accelerated linear growth; thus they seem not only obese but also tall for their age.

Corticosteroid excess.   Exogenous obesity

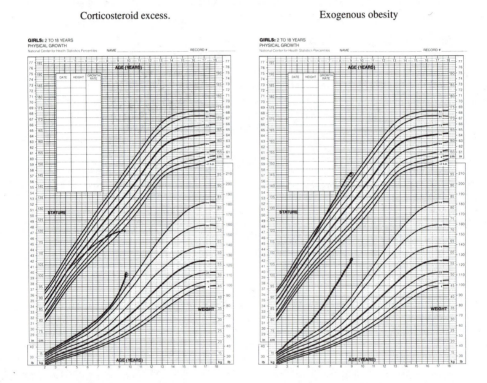

20. What conditions are associated with excessive growth in childhood?

In contrast to the large number of conditions that delay or suppress growth, relatively few conditions result in overgrowth. The most common, other than genetic tall stature, is constitutional advanced growth. As expected, affected children have advanced bone age, accelerated growth, and early puberty.

Excess of growth hormone is rare in children but causes tall stature rather than bony overgrowth, because the growth plates are open. Excessive growth hormone is associated with elevated, random levels of growth hormone and extremely high levels of somatomedin-C. Syndromes associated with large size and rapid growth include the following:

1. Genetic factors
2. Constitutional advanced growth
3. Klinefelter's syndrome (47 XXY)—tall stature, small testes, delay of puberty.

4. Connective tissue disorders:
   Marfan's syndrome—tall stature, arachnodactyly, joint laxity, lens displacement
   Sticklers
5. Excess of growth hormone (pituitary gigantism)
6. Soto's syndrome (cerebral gigantism)—macrocephaly, progressive macrosomia, dilated ventricles, retardation, advanced bone age
7. Hyperthyroidism
8. Excess of androgen
   Precocious puberty
   Congenital adrenal hyperplasia
   Androgen-producing tumor
9. Excess of estrogen
   Precocious puberty
   Congenital adrenal hyperplasia
   Estrogen-producing tumor
10. Obesity
11. Beckwith-Wiedemann syndrome—macroglossia, umbilical hernia, hypoglycemia, macrosomia in infancy
12. Homocystinuria—arachnodactyly, retardation, homocystine in urine

BIBLIOGRAPHY

1. Allen DB, Fost NC: Growth hormone therapy for short stature: Panacea or Pandora's box? J Pediatr 117:16, 1990.
2. Frasier SD: Human pituitary growth hormone (hGH) therapy in growth hormone deficiency. Endocr Rev 4:155, 1983.
3. Frasier SD, Lippe B: Clinical review 11: The rational use of growth hormone during childhood. J Clin Endocrinol Metab 71:269, 1990.
4. Kaplan S (ed): Clinical Pediatric Endocrinology. Philadelphia, W.B. Saunders, 1990.
5. Lifshitz F (ed): Pediatric Endocrinology. New York, Marcel Dekker, 1990.
6. Lippe B: Short stature in children. Evaluation and management. J Pediatr Heath Care 1:313, 1987.
7. Rosenfeld RG, et al: Six-year results of a randomized, prospective trial of human growth hormone and oxandrolone in Turner syndrome. J Pediatr 121:49, 1992.
8. Underwood LE, Rosenfel RG, Hinz RL: Human growth and growth disorders: An update. Stanford Genentech, 1989.
9. Zachmann SS, Prader A: Short term testosterone treatment at bone age of 12 to 13 years does not reduce adult height in boys with constitutional delay of growth and adolescence. Helv Pediatr Acta 42:21, 1987.

IV. Adrenal Disorders

23. PRIMARY ALDOSTERONISM

Arnold A. Asp, M.D.

1. What is primary aldosteronism?

Primary aldosteronism is a generic term for a group of disorders in which excessive production of aldosterone by the zona glomerulosa of the adrenal cortex occurs independently of normal renin-angiotensin stimulation. These primary disorders of the adrenal system are distinct from forms of hyperaldosteronism due to excessive renin, such as renal artery stenosis. The five clinical entities comprising primary aldosteronism include solitary aldosterone-producing adenoma (APA), bilateral hyperplasia of the zona golmerulosa (also known as idiopathic hyperaldosteronism or IHA), primary adrenal hyperplasia, adrenal carcinoma, and glucocorticoid-remediable aldosteronism.

The terms ''aldosteronism'' and ''hyperaldosteronism'' are used interchangeably in the literature. This chapter uses the most common designation for each disorder.

2. How common are these disorders?

The most common manifestation of hyperaldosteronism is hypertension. It is estimated that 0.05–2.0% of the hypertensive population may have primary aldosteronism.

3. What are the common clinical manifestations of primary aldosteronism?

Aldosterone acts at the distal convoluted tubule to stimulate reabsorption of sodium ions (Na^+) as well as secretion of potassium (K^+) and hydrogen ions (H^+) and at the cortical and medullary collecting ducts to cause direct secretion of H^+. These effects result in hypertension, hypokalemia, hypomagnesemia and metabolic alkalosis. Spontaneous hypokalemia (<3.5 mEq/L) occurs in 80% of cases of primary aldosteronism; the remaining patients develop hypokalemia within 3–5 days of initiation of liberal sodium intake (150 mEq/day). Most symptoms cited by patients are manifestations of hypokalemia: weakness, muscle cramping, paresthesias, headaches, palpitations, polyuria, and polydipsia. Glucose intolerance due to insulinopenia occurs in approximately 25% of patients. This group of disorders affects more women then men and occurs most commonly in the third through fifth decades of life.

4. What is the most common form of primary aldosteronism?

Of the five causes mentioned in question 1, solitary aldosterone-producing adenomas (APAs) are most common, comprising up to 65% of cases in most series. These tumors are small (<2 cm), occur more commonly in the left adrenal gland, and are composed of zona golmerulosa cells, zona reticularis cells, and hybrid cells with characteristics of both layers. Adenomas produce greater amounts of aldosterone than do other forms of aldosteronism; consequently, the degree of hypertension and the extent of biochemical abnormalities tend to be more severe. APAs also produce an excess of 18-hydroxycorticosterone (18-OHB), an immediate precursor of aldosterone produced by hydroxylation of corticosterone, that facilitates the biochemical diagnosis. Unlike other forms of primary aldosteronism APAs demonstrate only partial autonomy of function and produce aldosterone in response to stimulation by corticotropin (ACTH). Aldosterone synthesis, therefore, parallels the normal circadian rhythm of ACTH secretion, with the highest concentrations occurring in the morning and the lowest in the evening. APAs are also know as Conn's syndrome.

5. What is the second most common cause of primary aldosteronism?

Idiopathic hyperaldosteronism (IHA), also known as bilateral adrenal glomerulosa hyperplasia, makes up approximately 30% of cases of primary aldosteronism. This clinical entity is marked by bilateral hyperplasia (diffuse and focal) of the zona glomerulosa layer of both adrenal glands. Because both glands appear to be hyperstimulated, a circulating secretagogue has been postulated. Candidates include a glycoprotein aldosterone-stimulating factor. Another, more likely cause is a supranormal sensitivity of the zona glomerulosa in affected adrenal glands to physiologic concentrations of angiotensin II. Aldosterone is produced in smaller amounts in IHA than in APA; therefore, the degree of hypertension, hypokalemia, hypomagnesemia, and metabolic alkalosis is less dramatic. Serum aldosterone levels tend to increase during upright posture, perhaps due to increased sensitivity to angiotensin II.

6. How common does adrenal cancer cause primary aldosteronism?

The literature reports fewer than 20 cases. The tumors are very large (>6 cm) and usually have metastasized by the time of diagnosis.

7. What is primary adrenal hyperplasia?

In this seemingly rare clinical entity (which may be more commonly recognized in the future) the zona glomerulosa of one adrenal gland becomes hyperplastic and histopathologically resembles unilateral IHA. Biochemically, however, such cases more closely resemble APA and respond to surgical resection.

8. What is glucocorticoid-remediable aldosteronism?

In this rare cause of aldosteronism, production of mineralocorticoid is stimulated solely by ACTH. The literature reports fewer than 100 cases. The disorder is inherited in an autosomal dominant fashion and results from a heritable mutation that causes the fusion of genes encoding steroid 11-beta hydroxylase and aldosterone synthetase. Normal secretion of ACTH causes overproduction not only of aldosterone but also of 18-hydroxycortisol and 18-oxocortisol. These metabolities of the cortisol C-18 oxidation pathway are biochemical markers that facilitate identification of affected kindreds. Excessive secretion of aldosterone may be inhibited by administration of glucocorticoids that suppress secretion of ACTH by the pituitary.

9. How are patients screened for primary aldosteronism?

The diagnosis of primary aldosteronism is based on the demonstration of inappropriately elevated levels of plasma aldosterone (PA) with concomitantly suppressed plasma renin activity (PRA). Unfortunately, there is no single specific and sensitive screening test.

One method of screening the hypertensive, hypokalemic patient is to discontinue diuretics, beta blockers, and inhibitors of angiotension-converting enzyme (ACE) for at least 2 weeks. Prazosin may be used to control hypertension. The patient is allowed to consume at least 150 mEq of sodium daily, and potassium supplements are administered to maintain the serum potassium >3.5 mEq/L. Then, while the patient assumes an upright posture, blood samples for assessment of PA and PRA are drawn. A 24-hour urine collection for aldosterone also should be collected. A ratio of PA (in ng/dl) to PRA (in ng/ml/hr) that exceeds 20 raises the possibility of primary aldosteronism. Because 12% of patients may have PA:PRA ratios lower than 20, review of the urinary aldosterone value is helpful. Urinary excretion of aldosterone (18-monogluconide) that exceeds 20 μg/day is also suggestive of primary aldosteronism.

10. How is the diagnosis of primary aldosteronism confirmed?

Several diagnostic schema may be used to confirm the diagnosis of primary aldosteronism.The following protocol not only confirms the diagnosis but also aids in identification of the specific disorder.

The patient is instructed to consume at least 150 mEq of sodium each day of the week prior to testing. Ample potassium supplements are given to ensure a serum potassium level greater than 3.5 mEq/L. The patient is then admitted in the evening and remains recumbent overnight. At 8:00 AM, levels of PA, PRA, 18-OHB are determined while the patient is supine. The patient then assumes an upright posture and/or ambulates for 4 hours, after which levels of PA and PRA are again determined.

In normal and essential hypertensive individuals, a high sodium diet suppresses PA, whereas upright posture for 4 hours stimulates PRA. In patients with primary aldosteronism, excessive sodium does not suppress synthesis of aldosterone; supine levels of PA at 8:00 AM exceed 15 ng/dl. Because excessive aldosterone in such patients causes intravascular expansion, PRA is undetectable (<1 ng/ml/hr) and remains suppressed despite 4 hours of upright posture. An unsuppressed PA with a concomitant unstimulated PRA confirms the diagnosis of primary aldosteronism.

Some centers rely on a saline-loading procedure rather than a high-salt diet to assess suppression of aldosterone. In this test 2 liters of saline solution are administered intravenously over 4 hours. PRA, PA, and 18-OHB are determined at the beginning and PRA and PA at the conclusion of the test. As in the previous test, patients with primary aldosteronism should demonstrate undetectable levels of PRA, whereas PA should exceed 15 ng/dl before and after saline loading.

Differentiation of APA from IHA is also possible with the above data. APAs produce greater amounts of aldosterone and are stimulated by ACTH. Patients with APA, therefore, have greater PA levels at 8:00 AM, that decrease over the ensuing 4 hours as normal secretion of ACTH diminishes. Patients with IHA, on the other hand, have lower levels of PA at 8:00 AM which then increase with upright ambulation. Finally APAs produce large amounts of 18-OHB; levels >100 μg/dl occur in APA and primary adrenal hyperplasia.

11. Is it important to differentiate APA from IHA?
Yes. APA is amenable to surgical resection of the involved adrenal gland, whereas IHA is usually treated medically.

12. Does computed tomography (CT) or magnetic resonance imaging (MRI) aid in differentiation?
To a limited extent, both localizing procedures may aid in identifying the cause of primary aldosteronism. Adrenal carcinoma, a rare cause of excessive aldosterone, is easily identified with either modality. A large APA may be discernible on high-resolution CT, which at some institutions can identify adenomas as small as 7 mm in size. MRI presently performs as well as CT in identifying APA but involves higher cost and longer scan time. The diagnostic accuracy of MRI or CT in preoperatively localizing an APA is approximately 70%. Neither modality is able to differentiate IHA from a small APA.

13. Are other localizing tests of help if CT or MRI fails to identify an APA when biochemical data indicate the presence of an adenoma?
Yes. The least invasive is a radionuclide test with NP-59 (6β-[131] I-iodomethyl-19-norcholesterol). In this procedure, supraphysiologic doses of dexamethasone are administered to the patient for 7 days in an attempt to suppress adrenal cortical activity. NP-59, which is incorporated into steroid molecules by the adrenal cortex, is then administered to the patient on the fourth day of the procedure. The patient is imaged under a γ-camera. If an APA is present, NP-59 is concentrated within the tumor, which becomes visible on the scan. IHA does not visualize. Accuracy of the procedure is approximately 70%.

A more accurate, but hazardous, localizing procedure to differentiate a normal adrenal gland from one containing an adenoma is adrenal venous sampling. In this procedure, catheters are introduced into the left and right adrenal veins and the inferior vena cava. Levels of PA are determined from these sites, along with concomitant levels of cortisol. APAs produce large amounts of aldosterone; the normal concentration of PA is 100–400 ng/dl whereas APA may generate concentrations of 1,000–10,000 ng/dl. The ratio of PA produced on the affected side vs.

the unaffected side always exceeds 10:1. Cortisol levels are determined to ensure that the adrenal veins are properly catheterized. Therein is the difficulty with adrenal venous sampling. Collection of aldosterone and cortisol from the left adrenal gland is relatively simple, because the venous effluent drains directly into the left renal vein. The venous flow from the right adrenal, however, flows directly into the inferior vena cava. Catheterization of the right adrenal vein is difficult because of the few angiographic landmarks. Contrast material used to localize the right adrenal gland can cause corticomedullary hemorrhage during the procedure (10% incidence). Overall, the procedure is 90% accurate in localizing APA.

14. How is the patient with APA managed?
The patient undergoes screening tests, as described above in question 9. The diagnosis of primary aldosteronism is confirmed with salt loading, as described in question 10. Levels of aldosterone are elevated but decline during the course of ambulation. 18-OHB exceeds 100 μg/dl. All such findings indicate the possibility of APA. If the patient is fortunate, CT scan reveals a unilateral adenoma. If an APA is not visible on CT or if the physician is concerned about a concomitant incidental nonfunctioning adenoma, NP-59 radionuclide imaging is appropriate, or adrenal venous sampling may be performed by an experienced angiographer. After the APA is localized, unilateral adrenalectomy is performed using a posterior approach. One year postoperatively, 70% of patients are normotensive. By the fifth postoperative year, only 53% remain normotensive. Normal potassium balance is permanent.

15. How is a patient with IHA managed?
The patient undergoes screening and confirmatory tests, as described in questions 9 and 10. Concentrations of aldosterone are elevated but continue to rise with ambulation over 4 hours. Levels of 18-OHB are less than 100 μg/dl. CT fails to reveal unilateral enlargement of the adrenals. NP-59 imaging fails to visualize an adenoma. Adrenal venous sampling fails to lateralize. After the diagnosis of IHA is made, the patient is scrupulously sequestered from surgical colleagues.

Pharmacologic therapy is quite effective. The agent of choice is spironolactone (50–200 mg twice daily), a competitive inhibitor of aldosterone. Hypokalemia corrects dramatically, whereas hypertension responds after 4–8 weeks. Unfortunately, spironolactone also inhibits synthesis of testosterone and peripheral action of androgen, causing decreased libido, impotence, and gynecomastia in men. In patients intolerant of spironolactone, amiloride (5–15 mg twice daily) corrects hypokalemia within several days. A concomitant antihypertensive agent is usually necessary to reduce blood pressure. Success also has been reported in cases of IHA treated with calcium channel blockers (calcium is involved in the final common pathway for production of aldosterone) and ACE inhibitors (IHA appears to be sensitive to low concentrations of angiotensin II).

16. How is a patient with primary adrenal hyperplasia (PAH) managed?
During evaluation, these rare cases appear to be APA. Screening and confirmatory tests, as described in questions 9 and 10, seemingly indicate an APA. Levels of 18-OHB exceed 100 μg/dl. Localizing tests are consistent with APA, and patients usually undergo surgical resection of a nodular hyperplastic gland. The diagnosis is made retrospectively, but surgery is curative.

17. How is a patient with glucocorticoid-remediable aldosteronism managed?
This disorder is discussed in question 8. Therapy with low doses of dexamethasone (0.75 mg/day) or any of the agents used for therapy of IHA (question 15) may be effective.

BIBLIOGRAPHY

1. Arterga E, Klein R, Biglieri EG: Use of the saline infusion test to diagnose the cause of primary aldosteronism. Am J Med 79:722–728, 1985.
2. Biglieri EG, Schambelin M, Hirai J, et al: The significance of elevated levels of plasma 18-hydroxycorticosterone in patients with primary aldosteronism. J Clin Endocrinol Metab 49:87–91, 1979.

3. Blevins LS, Wand GS: Primary aldosteronism: An endocrine perspective. Radiology 184:599–600, 1992.
4. Liftin RP, Dluhy RG, Powers M, et al: A chimaeric 11β hydroxylase/aldosterone synthetase gene causes glucocorticoid-remediable aldosteronism and human hypertension. Nature 355:262–265, 1992.
5. Melby JC: Primary aldosteronism. Kidney Int 26:769–778, 1984.
6. Melby JC: Diagnosis of hyperaldosteronism. Endocrinol Metabol Clin North Am 20:247–255, 1991.
7. Rich GM, Ulick S, Cook S, et al: Glucocorticoid-remediable aldosteronism in a large kindred: Clinical spectrum and diagnosis using characteristic biochemical phenotype. N Engl J Med 116:813–820, 1992.
8. Young WF, Hogan MJ, Klee GG, et al: Primary aldosteronism: Diagnosis and treatment. Mayo Clin Proc 65:96–110, 1990.

24. PHEOCHROMOCYTOMA

Arnold A. Asp, M.D.

1. What is pheochromocytoma?

Pheochromocytoma is an adrenal medullary tumor composed of chromaffin cells and capable of secreting biogenic amines and peptides, including epinephrine, norepinephrine, and dopamine. Such tumors arise from neural crest cells, which also give rise to portions of the central nervous system and the sympathetic (paraganglion) system. Because of this common origin, neoplasms of the sympathetic ganglia, such as neuroblastomas, paragangliomas, and ganglioneuromas, may produce similar amines and peptides.

2. How common are pheochromocytomas?

Pheochromocytomas are relatively rare. Data from the Mayo Clinic indicate that pheochromocytomas occur in 1–2/100,000 adults/year; autopsy data from the same institution reflect an incidence of 0.3%. The incidence of pheochromocytoma from other countries, such as Japan, is lower: 0.4 cases/1 million/year.

3. Where are the tumors located?

Nearly 90% of tumors arise within the adrenal glands, whereas approximately 10% are extraadrenal and therefore classified as paragangliomas. Sporadic, solitary pheochromocytomas are located more commonly in the right adrenal gland, whereas familial forms (10% of all pheochromocytomas) are bilateral and multicentric. Bilateral adrenal tumors raise the possibility of multiple endocrine neoplasia syndromes 2A or 2B (MEN-2A or MEN-2B) syndromes (see chapter 46). Paragangliomas occur most commonly within the abdomen but also have been described along the entire sympathetic paraganglia chain from the base of the brain to the testicles. The most common locations for paragangliomas are the organ of Zuckerkandl, the aortic bifucation, and the bladder wall; the mediastinum, heart, carotid arteries and glomus jugulare bodies are less common locations.

4. Can pheochromocytomas metastasize?

Yes. Demonstration of a metastatic focus in tissue normally devoid of chromaffin cells is the only accepted indication that pheochromocytoma is malignant. Metastasis occurs in 3–14% of cases. The most common sites of metastases include regional lymph nodes, liver, bone, lung, and muscle.

5. What are the common clinical features of a pheochromocytoma?

The signs and symptoms of a pheochromocytoma are variable. The classic triad of sudden severe headache, diaphoresis, and palpitations carries a high degree of specificity (94%) and sensitivity (91%) for pheochromocytoma in a hypertensive population. The absence of all three symptoms reliably excludes the condition. Hypertension occurs in 90–95% of cases and is paroxysmal in 25–50% of these. Orthostatic hypotension occurs in 40% because of hypovolemia and impaired arterial and venous constriction responses. Tremor and pallor also may be accompanying signs, whereas flushing is uncommonly encountered. Other symptoms include anxiety and constipation.

6. What are some of the nonclassic manifestations of pheochromocytoma?

Signs and symptoms of other endocrine disorders may dominate the presentation of pheochromocytoma. Tumors have been reported to elaborate corticotropin (ACTH) with resultant manifestations of Cushing's syndrome and hypokalemic alkalosis. Vasoactive intestinal peptide has been produced in several cases, resulting in severe diarrhea. Hyperglycemia, due to catecholamine-associated antagonism of insulin release, and hypercalcemia, due to adrenergic stimulation of the parathyroid glands or elaboration of parathyroid hormone-related peptide (PTH-rP) also have been encountered. Lactic acidosis may be observed as a result of epinephrine-associated decrements in oxygen delivery with concomitant increases in oxygen utilization.

Cardiovascular manifestations of pheochromocytoma include arrhythmias and catecholamine-induced dilated, congestive cardiomyopathy. Atrial and ventricular fibrillation commonly result from precipitous release of catecholamines during surgical induction or from therapy with tricyclic antidepressants, phenothiazines, metoclopramide, and naloxone. Although cardiogenic pulmonary edema may result from cardiomyopathy, noncardiogenic pulmonary edema also may occur as a result of transient pulmonary vasoconstriction and increased capillary permeability. Finally, seizure, altered mental status, and cerebral infarction may occur as a result of intracerebral hemorrhage or embolization.

7. What do pheochromocytomas elaborate?

Most pheochromocytomas secrete norepinephrine. Tumors that produce epinephrine are more commonly intraadrenal, because the sympathetic ganglia do not contain phenylethanolamine-N-methyltransferase (PNMT), which converts norepinephrine to epinephrine. Dopamine is most commonly associated with malignant tumors.

8. Why is the blood pressure response among patients with pheochromocytoma so variable?

Blood pressures vary so widely among pheochromocytoma patients for several reasons. First, the tumors elaborate different biogenic amines. Intraadrenal tumors secrete epinephrine (EPI), which possesses beta-stimulatory vasodilation properties that cause hypotension, whereas most intraadrenal and all extraadrenal tumors produce norepinephrine (NE) with predominantly alpha-stimulatory vasoconstrictive effects. Second, tumor size indirectly correlates with concentrations of plasma catecholamines. Large tumors (>50-g) manifest slow turnover rates and release catecholamine degradation product, whereas small tumors (<50 g) with rapid turnover rates elaborate active catecholamines. Finally, tissue responsiveness to ambient concentrations of catecholamines does not remain constant. Prolonged exposure of tissue to increased plasma catecholamines causes downregulation of $alpha_1$-receptors and tachyphylaxis. Plasma catecholamine levels, therefore, do not correlate with mean arterial pressure.

9. How is pheochromocytoma diagnosed?

The diagnosis depends on the demonstration of excessive amounts of catecholamines in plasma or urine or degradation products in urine. The most widely used tests involve measurement of urinary metanephrine (MN), normetanephrine (NMN), vanillylmandelic acid (VMA), and free catecholamines produced in a 24-hour period. The ability of such tests to differentiate pheochromocytoma from essential hypertension varies among institutions: for VMA, sensitivity is 28–56% and specificity is 98%; for MN and NMN, sensitivity is 67–91% and specificity is 100%; and for free catecholamines, sensitivity is 100% and specificity is 98%. Many groups advocate 24-hour urinary levels of MN as good screening test, usually combined with 24-hour urinary levels of catecholamines. Yield is improved when urine is collected after a paroxysmal episode.

Direct measurement of plasma catecholamines (NE and EPI), collected from an indwelling venous catheter at rest, may contribute to diagnostic accuracy of timed urine assays. Levels greater than 2,000 pg/ml are abnormal and suggestive of pheochromocytoma, whereas levels less than 500 pg/ml are normal and levels of 500–2,000 pg/ml are equivocal.

10. What conditions may alter the above diagnostic tests?

Older assays for VMA were sensitive to dietary vanillin and phenolic acids, requiring patients to restrict their intake of such substances. High-pressure liquid chromatography assays have eliminated most false-positive results due to diet and drugs. The following list includes some of the more common drugs and conditions that may obfuscate the diagnosis of pheochromocytoma:

Drugs that alter metabolism of catecholamines:

Reduce plasma and urine catecholamines: alpha$_2$ agonists, calcium channel blockers (chronic), angiotensin-converting enzyme inhibitors, bromocriptine

Decrease VMA and increase catecholamines and MN: methyldopa, monoamine oxidase inhibitors.

Increase plasma or urine catecholamines: alpha$_1$ blockers, beta blockers, labetalol

Produce variable changes in any test: phenothiazines, tricyclic antidepressants, levodopa

Interfering medications:

Decrease MN: methylglucamine in radiocontrast agents

Decrease urinary catecholamines: methenamine mandelate

Decrease VMA: clofibrate

Increase VMA: nalidixic acid

Miscellaneous conditions

Stimulation of endogenous catecholamines: physiologic stress (ischemia, exercise), drug withdrawal (alcohol, clonidine), vasodilator therapy (nitroglycerin, acute administration of calcium channel blockers)

Exogenous catecholamines: appetite suppressants, decongestants

11. What other biochemical tests are available?

Cases in which screening tests are equivocal may warrant a clonidine suppression test. This test employs a centrally acting alpha$_2$ agonist that, in patients without pheochromocytoma, suppresses neurogenically mediated release of catecholamines through the sympathetic nervous system. Blood samples to assess plasma catecholamines (NE and EPI) are drawn through an indwelling venous catheter, clonidine 0.3 mg is administered orally, and plasma catecholamines are sampled again at 1, 2, and 3 hours. Plasma catecholamines decrease to less than 500 pg/ml in patients with essential hypertension but exceed this level in patients with pheochromocytomas.

The glucagon stimulation test has been proposed for patients in whom clinical results are highly suggestive of pheochromocytoma, but plasma catecholamines are <1,000 pg/ml. After an intravenous bolus of 1–2 mg of glucagon, patients with pheochromocytomas manifest a threefold increase in levels of plasma catecholamines (at least >2,000 pg/ml) and a rise in blood pressure of at least 20/15 mmHg. The hazard associated with increased blood pressure can be attenuated by pretreatment with calcium channel or alpha-adrenergic blockade. This test is used less frequently than the clonidine suppression test.

Chromogranin A is a soluble protein stored with NE and released from catecholamine storage vesicles. Chromogranin A may be elevated by pheochromocytomas as well as by other neuroendocrine tumors.

12. How are pheochromocytomas localized?

The majority of tumors are greater than 3 cm in size, rendering them detectable by computed tomographic (CT) or magnetic resonance imaging (MRI) studies. CT, with special attention to the adrenal glands and pelvis, is advocated as the initial localizing procedure (97% are intraabdominal). Many also recommend MRI as an adjunctive localizing modality. Advantages of MRI include the lack of radiation exposure and the characteristic hyperintense image on T_2-weighted scans. The hyperintense image allows definition of tumor size, differentiation from vascular structures, and identification of unsuspected metastases. Scintigraphic localization with m-(^{131})iodobenzylguanidine (MIBG) may also reveal unsuspected metastases. This compound is actively concentrated by sympathomedullary tissue and is subject to interference by drugs that block reuptake of catecholamines (tricyclic antidepressants, guanethidine, labetalol). Performance criteria of each localizing procedure are depicted below:

	CT (%)	MRI (%)	MIBG (%)
Sensitivity	98	100	78
Specificity	70	67	100
Positive predictive value	69	83	100
Negative predictive value	98	100	87

13. How is pheochromocytoma treated?

Surgical resection is the only definitive therapy. Preoperative preparation with alpha blockade reduces the incidence of intraoperative hypertensive crisis and postoperative hypotension. The most commonly used agents are phenoxybenzamine, a long-acting, noncompetitive antagonist

(10–20 mg 2–3 ×/day, advanced to 80–100 mg/day), or prazosin, a short-acting antagonist (1 mg 3 ×/day advanced to 5 mg 3 ×/day). Therapy may be limited by hypotension, tachycardia, and dizziness. Goals of therapy include blood pressure <160/90, an electrocardiogram free of ST- or T-wave changes over 2 weeks before surgery, and no more than one premature ventricular contraction/15 min. Opinions about the duration of preparation vary between 7 and 28 days before surgery. Beta blockade to control tachycardia is added only after alpha-adrenergic blockade has been instituted to prevent unopposed alpha stimulation. Other agents used in the preoperative period include labetalol or calcium channel blockers. Intraoperative hypertension associated with tumor manipulation may be controlled with either phentolamine or nitroprusside. Postoperative hypotension may be minimized by preoperative volume expansion with crystalloid.

14. How is malignant pheochromocytoma treated?

Although evidence of malignancy may be discovered at the time of surgery, metastases from slow-growing pheochromocytomas may remain unapparent for several years. Therapy is rarely curative, because the tumors respond poorly to radiotherapy and chemotherapy; treatment is therefore palliative. Surgical debulking is the therapy of choice, followed by use of alpha-methyltyrosine. This drug is a "false" catecholamine precursor that inhibits tyrosine hydroxylase (the rate-limiting enzyme in catecholamine synthesis) and reduces excessive production of catecholamines. Combination chemotherapy with cyclophosphamide, vincristine, and adriamycin may slow tumor growth, as may ablation with MIBG. Unfortunately, neither of these therapeutic measures has resulted in prolonged survival. Prognosis, however, is not dismal: cases of 20-year survival have been reported, and the 5-year survival rate with malignant pheochromocytoma is 44%.

15. Which medical conditions are associated with pheochromocytoma?

MEN-2A: hyperparathyroidism, medullary carcinoma of the thyroid, pheochromocytoma

MEN-2B: medullary carcinoma of the thyroid, marfanoid habitus, pheochromocytoma

Carney's triad: paragangliomas, gastric epithelioid leiomyosarcoma, benign pulmonary chondromas (females), and Leydig-cell tumors (males)

Neurofibromatosis: café-au-lait spots in 5% of patients with pheochromocytoma; 1% of patients with neurofibromatosis have pheochromocytomas

Von Hippel–Lindau syndrome: retinal and cerebellar hemangioblastomas; as many as 10% may have pheochromocytomas

BIBLIOGRAPHY

1. Bravo EL, Tarazi RC, Fouad FM, et al: Clonidine-suppression test. A useful aid in the diagnosis of pheochromocytoma. N Engl J Med 305:623–626, 1981.
2. Bravo EL. Pheochromocytoma: New concepts and future trends. Kidney Int 40:544–556, 1991.
3. Francis IR, Gross MD, Shapiro B, et al: Integrated imaging of adrenal disease. Radiology 187:1–13, 1992.
4. Golub MS, Tuck ML: Diagnostic and therapeutic strategies in pheochromocytoma. Endocrinologist 2:101–105, 1992.
5. Krane NK: Clinically unsuspected pheochromocytoma: Experience at Henry Ford Hospital and a review of the literature. Arch Intern Med 146:54–57, 1986.
6. Sheps SG, Jiang N, Klee GG, van Heerden JA: Recent developments in the diagnosis and treatment of pheochromocytoma. Mayo Clin Proc 65:88–95, 1990.
7. Sjoberg RS, Simcic KJ, Kidd GS: The clonidine suppression test for pheochromocytoma. A review of its utility and pitfalls. Arch Intern Med 152:1193–1197, 1992.

25. ADRENAL MALIGNANCIES

Michael T. McDermott, M.D.

1. What types of cancer occur in the adrenal glands?
The adrenal glands may be the site of adrenal cortical carcinomas, malignant pheochromocytomas, and carcinomas metastatic from other sites.

2. Do adrenocortical carcinomas produce hormones?
Approximately 50–70% of adrenocortical carcinomas secrete steroid hormones, whereas 30–50% do not.

3. What are the clinical features of functioning adrenocortical carcinomas?
Functioning adrenocortical carcinomas secrete aldosterone, cortisol, or androgens—alone or in combination. Excessive aldosterone (Conn's syndrome) causes hypertension and hypokalemia. Overproduction of cortisol results in the development of Cushing's syndrome. Excessive androgen causes hirsutism and virilization in women and abnormal precocious puberty in children.

4. What are the clinical features of nonfunctioning adrenocortical carcinomas?
Nonfunctioning adrenocortical carcinomas present clinically as abdominal or flank pain or as an incidentally discovered adrenal mass. They are locally invasive and metastasize most commonly to liver and lung.

5. What clues are most suggestive that an adrenocortical tumor is malignant?
Malignancy is most strongly suggested by elevated urinary excretion of 17-ketosteroids, tumor size greater than 6 cm, and evidence of locally invasive or distant metastatic disease. However, the diagnosis of malignancy is frequently not suspected until the tumor is examined histologically after its removal.

6. What is the treatment for an adrenocortical carcinoma?
The treatment of choice is surgery. Mitotane has produced partial or complete tumor regression, reduced production of adrenal hormones, and improved survival in nonrandomized, noncontrolled trials. Other chemotherapeutic agents and radiation therapy do not appear to be effective.

7. What is the prognosis for patients with adrenocortical carcinoma?
The mean survival is about 15 months. The 5-year survival rate is approximately 20%.

8. How often are pheochromocytomas malignant?
Approximately 10–15% of pheochromocytomas are malignant.

9. What are the clinical features of a malignant pheochromocytoma?
Most pheochromocytomas cause hypertension, headaches, sweating, and palpitations and are diagnosed by increased urinary excretion of vanillylmandelic acid (VMA), metanephrine, or catecholamines or by elevated levels of plasma catecholamines. Malignant pheochromocytomas usually do not differ, except that they eventually metastasize to lymph nodes, liver, lungs, and bones.

10. What clues suggest that a pheochromocytoma is malignant?
Malignancy is most strongly suggested by disproportionately increased urinary excretion of dopamine and/or homovanillic acid, tumor size greater than 6 cm, and evidence of extraadrenal

spread. The malignant character of such tumors may be missed even histologically and not become apparent until metastatic disease appears.

11. What is the treatment for a malignant pheochromocytoma?
Surgery is the treatment of choice. Alpha-adrenergic blocking agents, such as phenoxybenzamine and prazosin, are given preoperatively to control blood pressure and to replete intravascular volume. These drugs and alpha methyl tyrosine, an inhibitor of catecholamine synthesis, are also effective long-term therapy for patients with unresectable tumors. Cyclophosphamide, vincristine, dacarbazine, and I^{131} metaiodobenzylguanidine (MIBG) may cause partial regression of residual tumors.

12. What is the prognosis for malignant pheochromocytoma?
The 5-year survival rate for malignant pheochromocytoma is 40–45%.

13. What tumors metastasize to the adrenal glands?
The vascular adrenal glands are a frequent site of bilateral metastatic spread from cancers of the lung, breast, stomach, pancreas, colon, and kidney and from melanomas and lymphomas.

14. What is the clinical significance of metastatic disease to the adrenal glands?
Acute adrenal crisis is rare. However, up to 33% of patients may have subtle adrenal insufficiency manifested by nonspecific symptoms and an inadequate cortisol response to the ACTH (Cortrosyn) stimulation test. Patients often experience improvement in well-being when given physiologic corticosteroid replacement.

15. How should the incidentally discovered adrenal mass be evaluated?
Incidental adrenal masses should be evaluated for evidence of hormone secretion and malignancy. Plasma aldosterone and renin, serum testosterone and dehydroepiandrosterone sulfate (DHEA-SO_4), and 24-hour urinary excretion of cortisol, VMA, metanephrine, and catecholamines should be measured. Size is the greatest predictor of cancer; masses less than 6 cm are rarely malignant.

16. How should the incidentally discovered adrenal mass be managed?
Nonfunctioning masses ≥ 6.0 cm and all hormone-secreting tumors should be removed surgically. Some experts recommend a size cutoff of 4.5 cm for surgery. Smaller masses should be reassessed in 3–6 months, then annually, and removed if growth occurs or if hormone secretion develops.

BIBLIOGRAPHY

1. Brennan MF: Adrenocortical carcinoma. Cancer 37:348–365, 1987.
2. Copeland PM: The incidentally discovered adrenal mass. Ann Intern Med 98:940–945, 1983.
3. Luton J-P, Cerdas S, Billaud L, et al: Clinical features of adrenocortical carcinoma, prognostic factors, and the effect of mitotane therapy. N Engl J Med 322:1195–1201, 1990.
4. Schteingart, DE: Treating adrenal cancer. Endocrinologist 2:149–257, 1992.

26. ADRENAL INSUFFICIENCY

Robert E. Jones, M.D.

1. How is adrenal insufficiency classified?

The clinical classification of adrenal insufficiency follows the functional organization of the hypothalamic-pituitary-adrenal axis. Primary adrenal insufficiency is defined as the loss of adrenocortical hormones due to destruction or impairment of the adrenal cortex. Secondary adrenal insufficiency is due to reduced secretion by the pituitary gland of adrenocorticotropic hormone (ACTH), whereas tertiary adrenal insufficiency is caused by failure of the hypothalamus to produce corticotropin-releasing hormone (CRH).

2. What are the causes of primary adrenal insufficiency?

The most common cause of primary adrenal insufficiency is autoimmune adrenalitis, which may be either confined to the adrenal gland or part of a polyglandular autoimmune syndrome. Infectious adrenalitis due to tuberculosis or disseminated fungal infections also may result in adrenal insufficiency. In patients infected with the human immunodeficiency virus (HIV), cytomegalovirus- or HIV-induced adrenalitis results on rare occasions in reduced synthesis of glucocorticoids or mineralocorticoids. Acute, fulminant adrenal insufficiency due to bilateral adrenal hemorrhage may occur in the settings of sepsis or anticoagulant therapy. Although bilateral metastatic disease from lung, breast, or enteric carcinomas is common, the metastases rarely result in adrenal insufficiency, because greater than 90% of the glandular tissue must be replaced by tumor before clinical insufficiency is seen. Lastly, several different medications may reduce circulating levels of adrenal steroids, either by inhibiting one or more steroidogenic enzymes or by enhancing the metabolic clearance rate of steroids. Ketoconazole and aminoglutethimide are examples of the former, whereas rifampin is an example of the latter. Typically, however, adrenal insufficiency does not result, unless the medications are given in high doses or the patient has an underlying adrenal condition that limits adrenal secretory reserve.

3. What are the causes of secondary or tertiary adrenal insufficiency?

Secondary adrenal insufficiency typically results from either a loss of anterior pituitary corticotrophs or a disruption of the pituitary stalk. Secondary adrenal insufficiency usually occurs in association with panhypopituitarism, but selective ACTH deficiency, either inherited or due to autoimmunity, also has been reported. Most commonly, panhypopituitarism results from space-occupying lesions of the sella turcica. Primary pituitary tumors, craniopharyngiomas, or, on rare occasion, metastatic lesions from breast, prostate, or lung carcinomas may infiltrate and destroy corticotrophs. Aneurysms of the internal carotid artery may erode into the sella, and infiltrative diseases such as histiocytosis X or sarcoidosis have been associated with secondary adrenal insufficiency. Infections due to tuberculosis and histoplasmosis have resulted in a loss of anterior pituitary function. Severe head trauma that disrupts the pituitary stalk and either excessive blood loss that causes shock during delivery (Sheehan syndrome) or hemorrhage into a pituitary adenoma (pituitary apoplexy) may result in panhypopituitarism. Lymphocytic hypophysitis, another autoimmune disorder, also causes secondary adrenal insufficiency. Loss of corticotrophs also may occur after pituitary surgery or 5–10 years after the delivery of 4,800–5,200 R to the pituitary fossa as radiation therapy for a pituitary tumor. The most common cause of tertiary adrenal insufficiency is the long-term use of suppressive doses of glucocorticoids; for example, the use of prednisone in the treatment of rheumatic disease or inflammatory disease. Suppression of CRH with resultant adrenal insufficiency is a paradoxical concomitant of successful therapy for Cushing syndrome. Loss of hypothalamic function also may result from various tumors, infiltrative diseases, and cranial radiotherapy.

4. Which symptoms are frequently encountered in adrenal insufficiency?

Most of the symptoms of adrenal insufficiency are relatively nonspecific. Weakness, fatigue, and anorexia are almost universal complaints. Most patients also report minor gastrointestinal symptoms, such as nausea, vomiting, ill-defined abdominal pain, or constipation. On occasion, the gastrointestinal symptoms may be the predominant complaint and, as a result, may divert the physician into a long and fruitless evaluation. Symptoms of orthostatic hypotension, arthralgias, myalgias and salt-craving are also encountered. Psychiatric symptoms may range from mild memory impairment to overt psychosis.

5. Describe the signs of adrenal insufficiency.

Weight loss occurs in all patients with adrenal insufficiency. Hyperpigmentation, presumably caused by elevated levels of ACTH or related peptide fragments, is noted in over 90% of patients with primary adrenal insufficiency. Hyperpigmentation may be generalized or localized to regions subjected to repeated trauma, such as elbows, knees, knuckles, and buccal mucosa. New scars are also frequently hyperpigmented, and preexisting freckles may increase in number. Vitiligo, areas of cutaneous pigment loss, may coexist in 10–20% of patients with autoimmune adrenalitis. Hypotension is also common in both primary and secondary adrenal insufficiency. Loss of axillary and pubic hair is more pronounced in women because of the loss of adrenal androgen secretion. A peculiar finding—auricular cartilage calcification—may be seen in long-standing adrenal insufficiency from any cause.

6. What laboratory abnormalities are encountered in adrenal insufficiency?

Hyponatremia and hyperkalemia are the most common abnormalities. Patients also may have a mild normocytic, normochromic anemia and may demonstrate eosinophilia and lymphocytosis on a peripheral blood smear. Prerenal azotemia secondary to volume depletion is encountered more frequently in primary adrenal insufficiency, whereas hypoglycemia is more common in secondary insufficiency. Modest hypercalcemia is present in less than 10% of patients. Moderate elevations of thyroid-stimulating hormone (TSH) (usually <15 µU/ml) are also common. Whether the elevation is due to underlying autoimmune thyroid disease, to loss of TSH suppression by endogenous steroids, or to the euthyroid sick syndrome is unclear.

7. How do the presentations of primary and secondary adrenal insufficiency differ?

The features of primary and secondary adrenal insufficiency have many similarities and two major differences: hyperpigmentation and hyperkalemia are not seen in secondary adrenal insufficiency. Due to the loss of ACTH secretion, hyperpigmentation does not occur in secondary adrenal insufficiency. Similarly, the adrenal zona glomerulosa remains responsive to the renin-angiotensin system in secondary adrenal insufficiency, and secretion of aldosterone is not compromised. Consequently, severe volume depletion is uncommon, and hyperkalemia is not encountered with the loss of ACTH. Cortisol is important in clearance of free water; thus a deficiency of cortisol from any cause may result in hyponatremia.

8. What other autoimmune diseases may be associated with autoimmune adrenalitis?

Both type I and type II polyglandular autoimmune syndromes are associated with primary adrenal insufficiency. In type II, the more common syndrome, adrenal insufficiency is universally present. Both syndromes are discussed in greater detail in chapter 47. On rare occasions, patients with other autoimmune endocrinopathies, such as chronic lymphocytic thyroiditis or insulin-dependent diabetes mellitus, may develop adrenal insufficiency.

9. How is the diagnosis of adrenal insufficiency confirmed?

A low plasma cortisol (<5 µg/dl) in the face of severe physiologic stress provides reasonably solid evidence for adrenal insufficiency. Conversely, a random plasma cortisol >20 µg/dl virtually excludes the diagnosis. In the basal or nonstressed state, a morning cortisol >10 µg/dl generally correlates well with an intact hypothalamic-pituitary-adrenal axis, but cortisol values in this range also may be seen in patients with limited functional reserve of the axis. Additional testing is frequently required (see below).

10. Which tests can differentiate primary from secondary or tertiary adrenal insufficiency?

If a reliable assay is available and if the blood sample has been obtained and handled correctly (these are very big ifs), measurement of ACTH clearly differentiates primary adrenal insufficiency from other causes. A short ACTH (Cortrosyn) stimulation test confirms the diagnosis of adrenal insufficiency; however, it does not discriminate the level of the lesion in the axis. A prolonged ACTH infusion (2–5 days) distinguishes between hypocortisolemia due to adrenal destruction and adrenal atrophy due to the loss of the trophic effects of ACTH on the adrenal gland. An infusion of corticotropin-releasing hormone (CRH) discriminates between pituitary and hypothalamic etiologies, but CRH testing is performed in only a few specialized centers because of the limited availability of the compound. On occasion, the patient is overlooked during the diagnostic evaluation. Do not forget to give replacement doses of glucocorticoids during metabolic testing, and do not forget that endogenous ACTH may be suppressed by exogenous steroids. Dexamethasone is the recommended supplement, because it can be used in low doses and does not interfere with the measurement of cortisol.

11. How is adrenal crisis managed?

The five S's of management are salt, sugar, steroids, support, and search for a precipitating illness. Volume should be restored with several liters of 0.9% saline with 5% dextrose. After a sample of blood has been obtained for measurement of cortisol and ACTH, 100 mg of hydrocortisone (cortisol) should be immediately administered intravenously. When hydrocortisone is given in the recommended dose of 100 mg every 6 hours, additional mineralocorticoid is unnecessary. Some authors also advocate the administration of a single dose of dexamethasone (4 mg) during the initial resuscitation of the patient. If the precipitating event or complicating illness has been controlled, the glucocorticoids should be tapered to maintenance levels after 1–3 days.

12. How urgently should a patient with suspected adrenal crisis to be treated?

Left untreated, adrenal crisis is fatal. If adrenal crisis is suspected, it must be aggressively treated; stress doses of glucocorticoids carry virtually no morbidity when used in the short term. A formal diagnostic evaluation can be performed at a later date, after the patient has been stabilized.

13. What is the management of chronic adrenal insufficiency?

Maintenance therapy of adrenal insufficiency involves replacement of both glucocorticoid and, if necessary, mineralocorticoid. Hydrocortisone may be given in doses of 15–20 mg on arising in the morning and 5–10 mg in the early afternoon. Alternatively, prednisone (2.5–7.5 mg) or dexamethasone (0.25–0.75 mg) may be given as a single evening dose. With any of these regimens a midafternoon supplement of hydrocortisone (5–10 mg) is occasionally needed. Fludrocortisone (Florinef), given as a daily dose of 0.05–0.2 mg, is used as a replacement for aldosterone. The response to replacement therapy may be monitored simply and inexpensively by careful attention to serial weights, blood pressure, electrolytes, and a directed history to assess general health status and well-being.

14. Do patients with adrenal insufficiency require additional hormone supplementation during times of stress?

Any stress that includes febrile illness, trauma, or diagnostic/surgical procedures may precipitate an acute adrenal crisis. Therefore, the judicious use of supplemental steroids prevents possible tragedy. Doubling or tripling the glucocorticoid dose is sufficient for mild-to-moderate infections. If vomiting is a feature of the illness or if symptoms consistent with adrenal crisis supervene, the patient should be hospitalized for therapy. More severe infections or surgical procedures involving general anesthesia usually require the intravenous administration of hydrocortisone (100 mg every 8 hours). The stress doses of glucocorticoids may be tapered rapidly over 1 or 2 days after resolution of the underlying stress. Additional steroid coverage also should be given in the presence of moderate-to-severe trauma.

15. Describe the nonpharmacologic interventions necessary for effective management of patients with adrenal insufficiency.
Education of the patient is paramount. The patient must know what to do during an intercurrent illness. An injectable glucocorticoid, such as dexamethasone, should always be readily available for emergency use. Likewise, a warning tag may prove to be providential in alerting a health care team to the presence of adrenal insufficiency if the patient is incapable of providing an appropriate history.

16. What are the relative potencies of available steroids?
The biologic potency of steroids depends on various factors, including absorption, affinity to corticosteroid-binding globulin (CBG), hepatic metabolism, and affinity to the intracellular glucocorticoid receptor. As a general rule, synthetic steroids are poorly bound to CBG and more slowly metabolized; they also have a greater affinity for the glucocorticoid receptor than cortisol. The following table gives the approximate potencies of available preparations.

Relative Potencies of Steroid Hormones

COMPOUND	GLUCOCORTICOID ACTIVITY	MINERALOCORTICOID ACTIVITY	DURATION
Hydrocortisone	1	1	Short
Cortisone	0.7	0.7	Short
Prednisone	4	0.7	Short
Methylprednisolone	5	0.5	Short
Dexamethasone	30	0	Long
Fludrocortisone	10	400	Long

17. When is diagnostic imaging helpful in the evaluation of adrenal insufficiency?
Pituitary and hypothalamic imaging is absolutely essential to assess the regional anatomy in all patients with newly diagnosed secondary or tertiary adrenal insufficiency. By contrast, adrenal imaging in patients with primary adrenal insufficiency is rarely helpful. The only exception is when the diagnosis of bilateral adrenal hemorrhage is entertained. In this circumstance, an adrenal computed tomographic (CT) scan is virtually diagnostic.

18. What is the prognosis for patients with adrenal insufficiency?
Before isolation of glucocorticoids, the life expectancy of patients with adrenal insufficiency was less than 6 months. With prompt diagnosis and appropriate replacement therapy, patients with autoimmune adrenalitis now enjoy a normal life span. The prognosis of adrenal insufficiency due to other causes depends on the underlying disorder.

19. When patients are given pharmacologic doses of corticosteroids for nonadrenal diseases, how should tapering from steroids be handled?
There are as many suggested regimens of steroid tapering as there are authors who write on the subject. However, certain universal concepts are common to all approaches. The initial tapering of glucocorticoids from pharmacologic to physiologic doses is limited by the behavior of the treated illness. If the illness flares, the higher dose of steroids should be reinstituted, and continued until the symptoms stabilize. Later a more gradual tapering should be reinitiated. When near physiologic doses of glucocorticoids are reached, the patient may be switched either to hydrocortisone or to alternate-day therapy, with tapering continued. Reestablishment of a normal hypothalamic-pituitary-adrenal axis is heralded by a return of the plasma cortisol to >10 µg/dl 24 hours after the last dose of steroid and normal adrenal responsiveness to exogenous ACTH (short ACTH stimulation). Full recovery of the complete axis may take 6–9 months; the adrenal

responsiveness to ACTH is the last limb of the axis to recover. Some patients may develop steroid withdrawal syndrome during rapid tapering or after steroids have been discontinued. This syndrome is characterized by the typical features of adrenal insufficiency; however, arthralgias, myalgias and, on rare occasions, desquamation may be the predominating symptoms.

20. When should a patient on exogenous glucocorticoids be considered functionally suppressed?

Any patient who has received more than 20 mg of daily prednisone (or glucocorticoid equivalent) for more than 1 month in the preceding year or greater-than-replacement doses of glucorticoids for more than 1 year should be considered to have a potentially suppressed axis and, therefore, should be given stress doses of glucocorticoids during intercurrent illnesses.

BIBLIOGRAPHY

1. Dahlberg PJ, Goellner MH, Pehling GB: Adrenal insufficiency secondary to adrenal hemorrhage: Two case reports and a review of cases confirmed by computed tomography. Arch Intern Med 150:905–909, 1990.
2. Grinspoon SK, Bilezikian JP: Current concepts: HIV disease and the endocrine system. N Engl J Med 327:1360–1365, 1992.
3. Kamilaris TC, Chrousos GP: Adrenal diseases. In Moore WT, Eastman RC (eds): Diagnostic Endocrinology. Philadelphia, B.C. Decker, 1990, pp 79–109.
4. Khosla S, Wolfson JS, Demerjian Z, Godine JE: Adrenal crisis in the setting of high-dose ketoconazole therapy. Arch Intern Med 149:802–804, 1989.
5. Merenich JA, McDermott MT, Asp AA, et al: Evidence of endocrine involvement early in the course of human immunodeficiency virus infection. J Clin Endocrinol Metab 70:572–577, 1990.
6. Nerup J: Addison's disease-clinical studies: A report of 108 cases. Acta Endocrinol 76:127–141, 1974.
7. Oelkers W: Hyponatremia and inappropriate secretion of vasopressin (antiduretic hormone) in patients with hypopituitarism. N Engl J Med 321:492–496, 1989.
8. Oelkers W, Diederich S, Bähr V: Diagnosis and therapy surveillance in Addison's disease: Rapid adrenocorticotropin (ACTH) test and measurement of plasma ACTH, renin activity and aldosterone. J Clin Endocrinol Metab 75:259–264, 1992.
9. Orth DN, Kovacs WJ, DeBold CR: The adrenal cortex. In Wilson JD, Foster DW (eds): Williams' Textbook of Endocrinology, 8th ed. Philadelphia, W.B. Saunders, 1992, pp 489–619.
10. Penrice J, Nussey SS: Recovery of adrenocortical function following treatment of tuberculous Addison's disease. Postgrad Med J 68:204–205, 1992.
11. Seidenwurm DJ, Elmer EB, Kaplan LM, et al: Metastases to the adrenal glands and the development of Addison's disease. Cancer 54:522–557, 1984.
12. Webel SS, Ober KP: Acute adrenal insufficiency. Endocrinol Metab Clin North Am 22:303–328, 1993.

27. CONGENITAL ADRENAL HYPERPLASIA

Allan R. Glass, M.D.

1. What is congenital adrenal hyperplasia?
Congenital adrenal hyperplasia (CAH) is a disorder that results from a decrease in the activity of one of the various enzymes required for the biosynthesis of cortisol. These defects are genetic in nature and are manifested during both prenatal and postnatal life.

2. What enzyme defects can lead to CAH?
Defects in any of the enzymes required for the synthesis of cortisol from cholesterol can lead to CAH, including the cholesterol side-chain cleavage enzyme; 3-beta-ol isomerase-dehydrogenase; and three hydroxylases: 17-hydroxylase, 21-hydroxylase, and 11-hydroxylase (see figure, next page).

3. What are the genetics of CAH?
All of the enzyme defects leading to CAH are autosomal recessive disorders; that is, both copies of the gene involved must be abnormal for the condition to occur. The gene for 21-hydroxylase, the enzyme most commonly affected in CAH, is located on the long arm of chromosome 6 close to the HLA (histocompatibility) gene complex. Modern techniques of molecular biology have determined that the defective enzyme activity may reflect a wide variety of different genetic defects in different families, including gene deletions, point mutations, and gene conversions.

4. How common is CAH?
The most common variant of CAH is 21-hydroxylase deficiency, which occurs in about 1 of 12,000 newborns. The prevalence of this disorder varies greatly among different ethnic populations. CAH due to deficiency of 11-hydroxylase is about one-tenth as common as deficiency of 21-hydroxylase, and CAH due to defects of the other enzyme defects listed above is extremely uncommon. About 1–2% of the population at large are heterozygote carriers of the 21-hydroxylase defect; that is, one of the two copies of the 21-hydroxylase gene is abnormal. Such heterozygote carriers appear normal in all respects.

5. Why does adrenal hyperplasia develop?
The process of adrenal hyperplasia begins in utero. Reduced production of cortisol in the fetus, which results from the decreased activity of one of the enzymes needed for cortisol synthesis, results in lowered levels of serum cortisol. Cortisol inhibits the pituitary output of adrenocorticotropic hormone ACTH (part of the normal feedback loop of cortisol regulation); thus, as serum cortisol drops in an individual with CAH, serum ACTH rises in an attempt to stimulate the adrenal glands to overcome the enzyme block and to return the level of serum cortisol to normal. As this process continues over time, the elevated levels of serum ACTH stimulate growth of the adrenal glands, leading to hyperplasia.

6. What is the most serious clinical consequence of CAH?
As a result of a congenital enzyme defect, production of cortisol is impaired. In some cases, depending on the precise nature of the enzyme defect, production of aldosterone also may be impaired (see figure, next page). Deficient production of cortisol and/or aldosterone may lead to salt loss, hypovolemia, and fatal adrenal crisis in the newborn period. The degree of residual activity of the defective enzyme, which affects the ability to produce glucocorticoids and mineralocorticoids and consequently the corresponding clinical manifestations, varies greatly from one affected family to another, depending on the specific genetic alteration. Adrenal crisis in the newborn period usually occurs with genetic defects that result in severe reduction in enzyme activity and steroid biosynthesis, a condition often termed salt-losing CAH.

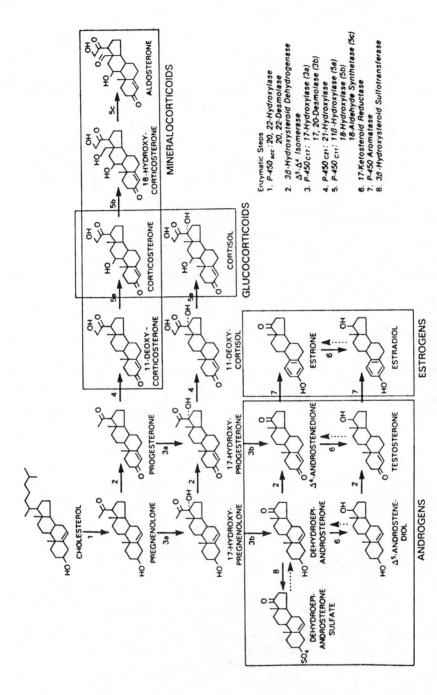

The pathway for steroid biosynthesis, with individual enzymatic steps indicated by number. Deficiencies in enzymes numbered 1, 2, 3a, 4, or 5a can lead to congenital adrenal hyperplasia. (From Becker KL (ed): Principles and Practice of Endocrinology and Metabolism. Philadelphia, J.B. Lippincott, 1990, with permission.)

7. What are other clinical consequences of CAH?
Another important consequence of CAH relates to the cortisol precursors (and their metabolites) that build up behind the blocked enzyme. Build-up of enzyme precursors is enhanced by the high levels of ACTH (see above), which stimulate production of adrenal steroids. Many of these precursors and metabolities are androgens; thus overproduction during fetal development in CAH due to defects in 21-hydroxylase, 11-hydroxylase, or 3-beta-ol isomerase-dehydrogenase may masculinize the external genitalia of a female fetus, leading to ambiguous genitalia at birth. By contrast, in the female fetus with CAH due to deficient activity of 17-hydroxylase or cholesterol side-chain cleavage enzyme, the enzyme defect also blocks synthesis of androgens (see figure, p. 162); thus masculinization of the external genitalia does not occur and ambiguous genitalia are not seen.

8. How do the manifestations of CAH in males differ from those in females?
Like female newborn infants with CAH, newborn males with CAH may also develop adrenal crisis related to salt loss and deficient production of glucocorticoid and mineralocorticoid. However, newborn males with CAH due to deficiency of 21-hydroxylase or 11-hydroxylase, the most common forms of CAH, do not manifest ambiguous genitalia; overproduction of androgen in male fetuses seems to have minimal effect on development of normal male external genitalia. Males with CAH due to deficient activity of 17-hydroxylase, 3-beta-ol isomerase-dehydrogenase, or cholesterol side-chain cleavage enzymes, all of which are rare, are unable to produce androgens such as testosterone in a normal fashion because of the enzyme block (see figure on p. 162). Because adequate production of androgen during fetal development is necessary for the formation of male external genitalia, the external genitalia at birth are only partially masculinized or, in severe cases, may have a normal female appearance.

9. What clinical features suggest the possibility of CAH?
Adrenal crisis or severe salt-wasting in the newborn period suggests the possibility of CAH. CAH also must be considered prominently in the differential diagnosis of any newborn with ambiguous genitalia. Because adrenal crisis and salt loss in CAH may be fatal if not treated, the finding of ambiguous genitalia in a newborn should trigger a rapid attempt to confirm or exclude CAH. Most males with CAH do not have ambiguous genitalia; consequently, many cases go unrecognized at birth, unless there is a previously documented family history of the disorder.

10. What clinical clues help to support or refute the diagnosis of CAH in a newborn with ambiguous genitalia?
The overwhelming majority of genetic males with CAH have unambiguous external genitalia at birth; conversely, CAH is an uncommon cause of ambiguous genitalia in a genetic male. Thus, determination that the infant with ambiguous genitalia is a genetic male makes CAH unlikely and decreases the diagnostic urgency, because the disorders giving rise to ambiguous genitalia in genetic males are rarely associated with fatal outcome. For example, the finding of palpable gonads in the scrotal or inguinal area suggests that the infant is a genetic male, because such palpable gonads are almost always testes. Conversely, the detection of a uterus in an infant with ambiguous genitalia, either by physical examination or by ultrasound, strongly suggests that the infant is a genetic female, thus heightening the possibility of CAH. Modern techniques of molecular biology rapidly confirm the genetic sex of the newborn without the prolonged wait for a traditional chromosome analysis. Because of the potentially severe consequences, it is probably prudent to assume that any genetic female with ambiguous genitalia has CAH until proved otherwise.

11. How is the diagnosis of CAH confirmed?
The most reliable way to confirm the diagnosis of CAH is to measure the blood levels of the cortisol precursor immediately proximal to the deficient enzyme. For example, in 21-hydroxylase deficiency, one measures the serum levels of the precursor of the 21-hydroxylase enzyme, namely 17-hydroxyprogesterone. In infants with classic 21-hydroxylase deficiency, serum levels of

17-hydroxyprogesterone are several orders of magnitude above normal. Blood levels of compounds that follow the blocked enzyme in the synthetic pathway, such as cortisol and aldosterone, may be low normal or frankly reduced. In practice, because one does not know a priori which enzyme is deficient in a newborn with suspected CAH (unless there is a documented family history of a particular enzyme defect), serum levels of all steroids that may be in the affected biosynthetic pathway must be measured. Determination of which steroid levels are supranormal and which are low facilitates localization of the specific enzyme block. Specific genetic defects may be confirmed with modern techniques of gene isolation and sequencing.

12. How is CAH treated?
The most important goal of treatment is to prevent salt loss and adrenal crisis in the newborn period. This goal requires administration of cortisol and, in many cases, mineralocorticoids, as well as careful monitoring of salt intake. This treatment not only replaces any deficient hormones but also suppresses the elevated levels of serum ACTH, thereby reducing the output of androgenic cortisol precursors and metabolites. Such treatment may be given presumptively while awaiting the results of definitive laboratory tests and then discontinued if such tests are not confirmatory. Surgical correction of ambiguous genitalia, such as repair of labioscrotal fusion, usually is carried out at a later time. Like all patients with deficient adrenal reserve, patients with CAH need increased cortisol replacement during times of stress.

13. How is treatment monitored?
The goals of treatment with steroids are to prevent adrenal insufficiency and to suppress ACTH and production of adrenal androgens. For the second goal, it is usually most appropriate to monitor the levels of the key precursor immediately behind the blocked enzyme (e.g., 17-hydroxyprogesterone in the case of 21-hydroxylase deficiency), with the ultimate aim of normalizing its level by adjusting the dosage of cortisol. However, such suppression of adrenal androgen production often can be achieved only with cortisol doses higher than average replacement levels (6.8 mg/m^2/day). If cortisol dosages are too high, growth and development may be irreversibly impaired, and it is sometimes extremely difficult or impossible to find a dosage of glucocorticoid that normalizes production of androgen without impairing growth. In such situations, mineralocorticoids (9-fluorocortisol) and antiandrogens (spironolactone or flutamide) may be useful adjunctive therapy in combination with nonsuppressive replacement doses of glucocorticoids.

14. What happens to children with untreated CAH?
As noted above, the degree of deficiency of cortisol and aldosterone may vary greatly from one affected family to another, depending on the precise nature of the genetic enzyme alteration. In untreated children with CAH—especially boys, who do not have ambiguous genitalia as a clue to the disorder—severe enzyme defects may lead to fatal adrenal crisis. If the enzyme defect is milder, death from adrenal crisis in the perinatal period can be averted, but overproduction of androgen continues unabated during childhood, leading to enhanced growth rate and masculinization. However, production of excessive androgen ultimately leads to premature closure of epiphyses and short stature in adulthood. Individuals with CAH due to enzyme deficiencies that also impair production of gonadal steroids, such as 17-hydroxylase deficiency, may not show signs of excessive androgen during childhood but may present in early adolescence with impaired sexual maturation. Patients with CAH due to deficiency of 11-hydroxylase or 17-hydroxylase may overproduce the steroid deoxycorticosterone, which is proximal to the enzyme block (see figure, p. 162); because this steroid has mineralocorticoid effects, patients may have hypertension and hypokalemia. Adult women with untreated CAH often have menstrual irregularity and infertility. Adult men with untreated CAH are often short but otherwise normal; many are fertile.

15. What is nonclassic CAH?
Nonclassic CAH, also termed late-onset CAH, has the same pathophysiology as classic CAH (congenital defect in one of the enzymes needed for biosynthesis of cortisol); in nonclassic CAH,

however, the specific nature of the genetic defect results in a much milder reduction of enzyme activity. Consequently, individuals with nonclassic CAH—which, like classic CAH, is most often due to a defect in 21-hydroxylase—do not have ambiguous genitalia at birth and are not at risk for adrenal crisis in the newborn period. Girls with nonclassic CAH generally do not become symptomatic until adolescence, at which time the overproduction of androgen may be manifested by acne, hirsutism, or menstrual irregularity. Boys with nonclassic CAH are generally asymptomatic. Nonclassic CAH may be treated with exogenous glucocorticoid to suppress levels of ACTH and thus to decrease the overproduction of androgen. Nonclassic CAH due to 21-hydroxylase deficiency is extremely common, affecting perhaps 1% or more of the population.

16. What genetic counseling is appropriate for a couple who previously had a child with CAH?

Because all forms of CAH are autosomal recessive disorders, both parents of a child with CAH are obligate heterozygote carriers of the gene defect. Consequently, the chance that another child of the same couple also will have CAH is 1 in 4; 50% of the children will be heterozygote carriers. Modern genetic techniques and chorionic villus sampling of fetal DNA allow the diagnosis of CAH during the first trimester of pregnancy. Preliminary evidence suggests that prenatal treatment of female fetuses with 21-hydroxylase deficiency by giving relatively high doses of dexamethasone to the mother, beginning in early gestation, may ameliorate the masculinization of genitalia. By contrast, male fetuses with 21-hydroxylase deficiency do not develop ambiguous genitalia and do not require steroid treatment until after birth.

BIBLIOGRAPHY

1. Cassorla FG, Chrousos GP: Congenital adrenal hyperplasia. In Becker KL (ed): Principles and Practice of Endocrinology and Metabolism. Philadelphia, J.B. Lippincott, 1990, p 604.
2. Chrousos GP, Loriaux DL, Mann DL, et al: Late-onset 21-hydroxylase deficiency mimicking idiopathic hirsutism or polycystic ovarian disease: An allelic variant of congenital virilizing adrenal hyperplasia with a milder enzymatic defect. Ann Intern Med 96:143, 1982.
3. Forest MG, Betuel H, David M: Prenatal treatment in congenital adrenal hyperplasia due to 21-hydroxylase deficiency: Update 88 of the French multicenter study. Endocr Res 15:277, 1989.
4. Linder B, Esteban NV, Yergey AL, et al: Cortisol production rate in childhood and adolescence. J Pediatr 117:892, 1991.
5. Miller WL: Congenital adrenal hyperplasias. Endocrinol Metab Clin North Am 20:721, 1991.
6. Miller WL, Levine LS: Molecular and clinical advances in congenital adrenal hyperplasia. J Pediatr 111:1, 1987.
7. Morel Y, Miller WL: Clinical and molecular genetics of congenital adrenal hyerplasia due to 21-hydroxylase deficiency. Adv Hum Genet 20:1, 1991.
8. Mulaikal RM, Migeon CJ, Rock JA: Fertility rates in female patients with congenital adrenal hyperplasia due to 21-hydroxylase deficiency. N Engl J Med 316:178, 1987.
9. Pang S, Pollack MS, Marshall RN, et al: Prenatal treatment of congenital adrenal hyperplasia due to 21-hydroxylase deficiency. N Engl J Med 322:111, 1990.
10. Sherman SL, Aston CE, Morton NE, et al: A segregation and linkage study of classical and nonclassical 21-hydroxylase deficiency. Am J Hum Genet 42:830, 1988.
11. Urban MD, Lee PA, Migeon CJ: Adult height and fertility in men with congenital virilizing adrenal hyperplasia. N Engl J Med 299:1392, 1978.
12. White PC, New MI, Dupont B: Structure of the human 21-hydroxylase gene. Proc Nat Acad Sci USA 83:5111, 1986.
13. White PC, New MI, Dupont B: Congenital adrenal hyperplasia (Part 1). N Engl J Med 316:1519, 1987.
14. White PC, New MI, Dupont B: Congenital adrenal hyperplasia (Part 2). N Engl J Med 316:1580, 1987.
15. Winter JSD, Couch RM: Modern medical therapy of congenital adrenal hyperplasia. Ann NY Acad Sci 458:165, 1985.

V. *Thyroid Disorders*

28. THYROID FUNCTION TESTS AND METHODS OF IMAGING THE THYROID GLAND

William L. Lasswell, Jr., M.D., Ph.D., and Kenneth D. Burman, M.D.

1. What are the essential steps in production of thyroid hormone?

Iodide is absorbed from the gut and actively transported into follicular cells of the thyroid gland. The thyroid gland also concentrates other monovalent anions, such as pertechnetate; this process forms the basis of a thyroid-imaging technique discussed below. Once transported into cells, iodide is subsequently oxidized by a thyroid peroxidase enzyme. Iodide is then incorporated into tyrosine residues of thyroglobulin (organification), where multiple processing steps take place to result in the formation of thyroid hormones, thyroxine (T_4) and triiodothyronine (T_3). Thyroglobulin is stored in the form of colloid, which later is processed to allow release of active thyroid hormone.

2. What are the end products of thyroid hormone synthesis and their mode of transport through the bloodstream?

Once formed and secreted, the thyroid hormones bind in the serum to thyroid-binding globulin (75%), thyroid-binding prealbumin (15%), and albumin (10%). Changes in levels of binding proteins (as in pregnancy and liver disease) affect the levels of total thyroid hormones in blood and result in abnormal measurements.

T_4 is the major hormonal product of the thyroid gland. It has a half-life of about 2–3 days and is converted to T_3 in peripheral tissues. Approximately 20% of T_3 is formed in the thyroid gland, but about 80% is produced by conversion of T_4 in peripheral tissues. This conversion occurs by way of a 5'-deiodinase enzyme. T_3 has a half-life of about 1 day. Once it is produced, T_3 enters the nuclei of cells in target tissues. Reverse T_3, or rT_3 is also formed from T_4. Levels of this inactive metabolite are increased in nonthyroidal illness, because production of T_3 is controlled for homeostatic reasons.

3. How do homeostatic mechanisms regulate production of thyroid hormone?

Under normal circumstances thyroid-stimulating hormone (TSH) controls the activity of the thyroid gland. The pituitary gland responds to the need for additional thyroid hormone by secreting TSH, which stimulates production and secretion of thyroid hormone. Excessive T_4 and T_3, in turn, suppress secretion of TSH. As a result, primary hyperthyroidism is characterized by elevated levels of thyroid hormone and suppressed TSH, whereas primary hypothyroidism is characterized by reciprocal alterations. Secondary hypothyroidism (pituitary or hypothalamic disease) is characterized by subnormal concentration of thyroid hormone and a subnormal or inappropriately normal level of TSH. Secondary hyperthyroidism is characterized by elevated levels of thyroid hormone and elevated or inappropriately normal levels of TSH.

4. Which thyroid function tests are most useful in assessing the status of thyroid hormone?

Thyroid function tests include assays for TSH, T_4 and T_3 as well as rT_3 and thyroglobulin. The most sensitive and accurate measurements of thyroid function are third-generation TSH assays and assays for the free levels of T_4 and T_3. Newer third-generation TSH assays use two different antibodies and provide more sensitive and accurate measures. The normal range of these assays is about 0.5–5.0 µU/ml; they have a sensitivity of about 0.01 µU/ml. Assays for free T_4 and T_3 measure the pool of hormone that is not protein-bound and thus is available to tissues.

5. Does the TSH assay play an important role in assessing the status of thyroid hormone?
TSH is thought to be the most sensitive indicator of thyroid function. Newer double-antibody assays provide the most useful reflection of the present level of peripheral thyroid hormone in the body. An elevation of TSH is the first laboratory abnormality seen in primary hypothyroidism. Similarly, suppressed or undetectable TSH is the most sensitive indicator of primary hyperthyroidism.

6. How is the TSH assay useful in guiding therapy of thyroid disorders?
The dose of thyroid hormone supplement used to treat hypothyroidism is adjusted according to the TSH level, with a normal value indicating adequate supplementation. TSH levels are not useful in assessing adequacy of treatment of hypothyroidism due to pituitary insufficiency, because production of TSH is impaired or absent in this situation. Assays of free T_4 and free T_3 are useful alternatives for monitoring therapy in such cases. A laboratory value is, of course, taken in the context of the history and physical exam.

7. What role does measurement of free T_4 play in assessing the status of thyroid hormone?
Free T_4 is best measured either by dialysis or ultrafiltration. Measurement of T_4 is a useful tool in patients with suspected protein-binding abnormalities and the most useful assay in assessing the true status of T_4 in the body. Abnormalities in binding proteins may change the amount of total and bound T_4, but in a euthyroid individual, homeostatic mechanisms should maintain a constant concentration of free T_4. Levels of free T_4 are especially useful in monitoring therapy of hyperthyroidism because 4–6 months may be required for the pituitary gland to recover from the suppressive effects of longstanding excess of thyroid hormone. During this recovery phase levels of TSH may be suppressed despite the fact that free T_4 is normal or low and hyperthyroidism is adequately treated.

8. What other tests are used to assess the function of thyroid hormone?
As implied above, it is possible to measure total serum levels of T_4. In fact, this was the only clinical T_4 assay available for many years. Use of the total T_4 assay has fallen into disfavor because of the advent of the ability to measure free hormone levels and because the total T_4 level is altered by perturbations of serum binding proteins.

In the T_3 resin uptake (T3RU) measurement, a known amount of radiolabeled T_3 is mixed with the patient's serum and a binding matrix is added. The matrix binds the free labeled T_3 that remains after labeled T_3 occupies all available binding sites on the patient's thyroid-binding globulin (TBG). An isotope-counting device records the amount of matrix-bound labeled T_3. When serum binding proteins are increased, more radiolabeled T_3 binds to the proteins and less to the matrix, thus decreasing the T3RU measurement. Thus, the T3RU test is not a measure of thyroid function but only an indirect measure of hormone binding sites. It can be interpreted only in conjunction with a total T_4 level. Total levels of T_3 are measured by radioimmunoassay (T3 RIA). Again, because total T_3 levels are affected by the levels of binding proteins, an even more accurate assessment of T_3 status is the free T_3 assay. Free T_3 or total T_3 levels are especially useful in patients with recurrent Graves' disease or solitary autonomous nodules, in which T_3 may be produced preferentially to T_4 (T_3 toxicosis).

Whenever T3RU and T_4 are abnormal but divergent and the free thyroxine index (FTI) is normal, the cause is likely to be a disorder in hormone binding proteins. Free T_4 in such cases agrees well with the calculated FTI values. The FTI is an artifactual adjustment of the total T_4 and T3RU measurements designed to assess free hormone levels. It is preferable to measure free T_4 directly rather than to use this estimate.

9. Does measurement of levels of various thyroid antibodies have any usefulness?
Elevated levels of thyroid antibodies provide circumstantial evidence but not proof of autoimmune thyroid disease, i.e., Graves' disease and Hashimoto's thyroiditis. Thyroid-binding

immunoglobulins (thyroid-binding inhibitory immunoglobulins [TBII] and thyroid stimulatory immunoglobulins [TSI]) are elevated in most patients with Graves' disease and occasionally in patients with Hashimoto's thyroiditis. Antimicrosomal antibodies and thyroglobulin antibodies are found most often in patients with Hashimoto's disease. In fact, elevated titers of antimicrosomal antibodies (>1:1,600) in a person with hypothyroidism constitutes a clinical diagnosis of Hashimoto's thyroiditis.

10. When is it useful to measure levels of serum thyroglobulin?
Levels of thyroglobulin may be used as an indicator of the presence of functional thyroid tissue. As such they are a sensitive and specific marker for tumor recurrence in patients with a history of thyroid cancer. However, all functional normal thyroid tissue must first be eradicated for this test to be useful; in other words, patients must first undergo thyroidectomy followed by ablation with radioactive iodine. Such therapies, of course, are routine in patients with thyroid cancer.

11. Under what circumstances is it useful to measure levels of calcitonin?
Calcitonin is a product of the C cells in the thyroid gland. Medullary carcinoma of the thyroid (MCT) represents neoplastic growth of C cells. Thus measurements of calcitonin levels are used to follow patients with MCT and to identify family members at risk of MCT. Basal measurements of calcitonin can be used for this assessment if the levels are elevated. However, a more sensitive test measures levels of calcitonin in response to stimulation by pentagastrin, alone or combined with calcium. Indeed, screening for the presence of C-cell disease in a patient with MCT or a family member must include a pentagastrin or calcium-pentagastrin test as well as a screen for pheochromocytoma and elevated calcium. The frequency and duration of such screening tests are debatable, but they probably should be performed on a yearly basis until age 35–45 years in first-degree members of a family with MCT. Of course, even families in which only one member has sporadic MCT should undergo evaluations initially and periodically to detect other potentially affected members. However, if two or more family members are known to have MCT or multiple endocrine neoplasia syndrome 2 (MEN-2), then screening of all family members becomes even more important.

12. What are the major methods used to image the thyroid gland?
Various imaging studies are useful in identifying abnormalities of the thyroid gland, including isotopic methods, such as the technetium scan and radioactive iodine scan and uptake, as well as nonisotopic methods, primarily ultrasound, computed tomography (CT), and magnetic resonance imaging (MRI). In general, imaging studies based on accumulation of isotope by the thyroid gland should be carried out in the absence of thyroid hormonal supplementation and, if possible, antithyroidal medications (e.g., propylthiouracil or methimazole). In addition, the administration of iodinated contrast may interfere with such imaging studies for weeks after exposure to the contrast agent.

13. What role does technetium scanning play in evaluation of the thyroid gland?
Technetium is trapped but not organified by the thyroid gland. Imaging of technetium distribution allows visualization of the gland with contrast enhancement of any "hot" or "cold" areas. It is very useful in assessing the functional status of palpable thyroid nodules. This distinction is useful in determining the malignant potential of a thyroid nodule, because a cold nodule is much more likely to be malignant than a warm or hot nodule. In hyperthyroid individuals, technetium scanning allows distinction among various causes of hyperthyroidism. Graves' disease, otherwise known as diffuse toxic goiter, is characterized by an overactive thyroid gland in which technetium is distributed homogeneously, whereas toxic multinodular goiter (MNG) is associated with heterogeneous distribution of technetium.

14. How does measurement of radioactive iodine uptake contribute to the assessment of thyroid disorders?
The measurement of radioactive iodine (^{131}I or ^{123}I) uptake is useful in distinguishing hyperthyroid conditions such as Graves' disease (in which uptake is usually enhanced) from forms of

thyroiditis in which hyperthyroidism is associated with decreased iodine uptake. The table below indicates conditions in which radioactive iodine uptake is elevated or reduced. Measurements of radioactive iodine uptake are also used to calculate the required dose of radioactive iodine therapy for treatment of Graves' disease. A normal radioactive iodine uptake is about 8–30%, depending on the iodine content in the diet.

Increased uptake	Decreased uptake
Graves' disease	Subacute thyroiditis
Toxic MNG	Painless thyroiditis
Toxic autonomous nodule	Thyrotoxicosis factitia
TSH pituitary adenoma	Struma ovarii
Trophoblastic tumor	

15. What are the contributions of ultrasonography, MRI, and CT in imaging of the thyroid gland?

Ultrasonography is used most often to help to evaluate a palpable thyroid nodule (i.e., to distinguish solid from cystic lesions). It reveals nodules as small as 2 mm and often discloses multinodularity in glands otherwise presumed to have a single nodule. It is also useful in guiding a needle biopsy of a nodule and in the periodic monitoring of the size of a nodule.

MRI and CT scanning of the thyroid are useful in identifying recurrent or metastatic lesions of thyroid cancer. They also may be useful in assessment of a substernal goiter and are helpful for assessing changes in lymph nodes or residual thyroid masses over time. At present, MRI and CT seem to be comparable in this regard. We prefer MRI, however, because we believe that it provides better resolution of small structures in the neck and because we are concerned that CT will be performed with contrast material, despite orders to the contrary. Contrast material may impair the ability to use radioactive isotope scanning and therapy for weeks or months.

BIBLIOGRAPHY

1. Beckers C, Corvette C, Thalasso M: Evaluation of serum thyroxine by radioimmunoassay. J Nucl Med 14:317, 1973.
2. Cavaleri R: The effects of nonthyroid disease and drugs on thyroid function tests. Med Clin North Am 75:27, 1991.
3. Cavaleri R: Thyroid radioiodine uptake: Indications and interpretation. The Endocrinologist 2:341, 1992.
4. Clark F, Horn DB: Assessment of thyroid function by combined use of serum protein bound iodine and resin uptake of 131-I triiodothyronine. J Clin Endocrinol Metab 25:39, 1965.
5. Gorman CA: Thyroid function testing: A new era. Mayo Clin Proc 63:1026, 1988.
6. Gow SM, Kellett HA, Seth J, et al: Limitations of new thryoid function tests in pregnancy. Clin Chim Acta 152:32, 1985.
7. Hay ID, Klee GG: Thyroid dysfunction. Endocrinol Metab Clin North Am 17:473, 1988.
8. Klee GG, Hay ID: Assessment of sensitive thyrotropin assays for expanded role in thyroid function testing: Proposed criteria for analytic performance and clinical utility. J Clin Endocrinol Metab 64:461, 1987.
9. Ladenson PW: Diseases of the thyroid gland. Endocrinol Metab Clin North Am 14:145, 1985.
10. Smith BR, McLachlin SM, Furmaniak J: Autoantibodies to the thyrotropin receptor. Endocr Rev 9:106, 1988.
11. Van Herle AJ: Serum thyroglobulin measurement in the diagnosis and management of thyroid disease. Thyroid Today 4:1, 1981.
12. Weetman AP, MacGregor AM: Autoimmune thyroid disease: Development in our understanding, Endocr Rev 5:309, 1984.
13. Zarkarija M, MacKenzie JM: The spectrum and significance of autoantibodies reacting with the thyrotropin receptor. Endocrinol Metab Clin North Am 16:343, 1987.

29. HYPERTHYROIDISM

William L. Lasswell, Jr., M.D., Ph.D., and Kenneth D. Burman, M.D.

1. Which thyroid disorders are most commonly associated with hyperthyroidism?

It is important to distinguish between primary and secondary forms of hyperthyroidism. Primary hyperthyroidism is due to overactivity of the thyroid gland and comprises the great majority of cases. Secondary hyperthyroidism is a much less common problem that on rare occasions may result from a pituitary tumor that secretes thyroid-stimulating hormone (TSH) or overmedication with thyroid hormone supplements. Three forms of primary hyperthyroidism account for the great majority of cases: Graves' disease, toxic multinodular goiter, and the solitary toxic nodule.

2. What constitutes a diagnosis of primary hyperthyroidism?

Because primary hyperthyroidism is due to oversecretion of thyroid hormones, the serum levels of thyroxine (T_4) and/or triiodothyronine (T_3) are elevated. In addition, suppression of the pituitary gland results in an undetectable level of serum TSH. Usually the overactive thyroid gland accumulates an elevated amount of radioactive iodine, which is measured as 24-hour radioactive iodine uptake (RAIU). An increase in the RAIU and abnormal thyroid function tests are common to most types of primary hyperthyroidism. Therefore, other methods, such as the thyroid scan, often are needed to distinguish among the conditions. In the case of Graves' disease, the distribution of tracer is homogeneous throughout the gland, whereas distribution is heterogeneous in multinodular goiter and almost completely restricted to the nodule in patients with a solitary toxic nodule.

Thyroid scans are performed with technetium or radioactive iodine. There are no major clinical differences between the two agents. Usually, ^{123}I is used for scans and ^{131}I for RAIU studies. [123]I is more expensive and administratively difficult to use because of its short half-life of 6 hours, whereas ^{131}I gives significantly more radiation exposure but has a half-life of about 7 days. No isotope should be given to a women who is or may be pregnant.

3. What is Graves' disease?

Graves' disease is an autoimmune disorder characterized by production of antibodies to the TSH receptor. These antibodies have various effects. Hyperthyroidism results when thyroid-stimulating immunoglobulins (TSI) act as agonists at the TSH receptor, stimulating synthesis of thyroid hormone and enlargement of the thyroid gland. Some cases of Graves' disease represent part of a more extensive autoimmune process associated with such conditions as pernicious anemia, vitiligo, diabetes mellitus, autoimmune adrenal insufficiency, and systemic lupus erythematosus.

Graves' disease, along with Hashimoto's disease, is classified as an autoimmune thyroid disease. The antibody profiles and clinical manifestations of the two disorders overlap considerably. As a result, many believe that the two diseases represent part of a spectrum of autoimmune thyroid diseases based on a similar process.

4. What are the manifestations of Graves' disease?

Patients with Graves' disease usually present with symptoms typical of thyrotoxicosis. Frequent complaints include rapid heart rate, palpitations, nervousness, and tremor. Patients sometimes complain of sleep disturbances, weight loss, inability to concentrate, and profound fatigue when performing any sort of demanding physical activity. Physical findings include tachycardia, a hand tremor that is fine and usually bilateral, and warm, sometimes velvety skin. The thyroid gland is diffusely enlarged in nearly all patients, often with an audible bruit.

5. Are any physical findings in hyperthyroid individuals unique to Graves' disease?

Graves' disease is unique among hyperthyroid disorders because of certain concomitant autoimmune phenomena, including ophthalmopathy, acropachy, and pretibial myxedema.

Graves' ophthalmopathy, which occurs as a result of autoimmune-mediated inflammation in the ocular and retroorbital area, may be manifest as proptosis, often accompanied by disordered movement of the extraocular muscles. The precise pathogenesis is unknown, but it likely represents either a proliferation of retroocular fibroblasts with cytokine production and resultant cellular synthesis of proteins or primary involvement of the extraocular muscles with antibodies binding to specific proteins. Autoimmune ophthalmopathy may occur before, during, or after the onset of hyperthyroidism but usually manifests within 1 year of disease onset. Pretibial myxedema also probably represents an inflammatory reaction that is autoimmune-mediated. The result is the accumulation of glycosaminoglycans and other constituents within the dermis of the skin, typically, but not always, on the anterior surface of the lower legs. Skin lesions of pretibial myxedema are typically nontender and elevated with a rough surface. The process causing acropachy, or clubbing, is thought to be similar to the process that causes pretibial myxedema.

6. What are the options for treatment of Graves' disease?
Options for definitive treatment of Graves' disease include medical therapy, radioactive iodine therapy, and surgery. The choice of therapy depends on variables such as age, patient preference, underlying medical conditions, and complicating features (e.g., thyroid nodules). Evidence suggests that cold, or inactive, thyroid nodules in a patient with Graves' disease have a higher likelihood of being malignant. As a result, some clinicians recommend surgery in such cases, although this is controversial.

7. Do radioactive iodine and surgery play important roles in the treatment of hyperthyroidism?
The most commonly used therapy for Graves' disease is radioactive iodine. This therapy can be given on an outpatient basis, usually about 8–12 mCi. The desired result is hypothyroidism due to complete destruction of the gland, which usually occurs within 2–3 months. It is important to monitor thyroid function tests and to provide supplemental L-thyroxine once the gland is completely destroyed and hypothyroidism ensues. Radioactive iodine is usually well tolerated, but exacerbation of signs or symptoms of thyrotoxicosis may occur within 1–2 weeks after therapy. In addition, radioactive iodine has the potential to precipitate thyroid storm by releasing thyroid hormone from radiation-damaged thyrocytes. This risk, which is highest in elderly and debilitated individuals, may be addressed by prior therapy with antithyroidal medications, such as propylthiouracil (PTU) or methimazole (MMI). PTU and MMI must be discontinued for several days before administration of radioactive iodine. Surgery for Graves' disease is usually not indicated but may be appropriate in the presence of a thyroid nodule that is suspicious for carcinoma.

8. What are some of the features of antithyroidal medications?
Hyperthyroidism of most types, including Graves' disease, can be treated effectively with the thionamide antithyroidal drugs (ATDs). Approximately 20–50% of patients achieve remission on these medications. The ATDs approved for use in the United States are PTU and MMI. Both drugs inhibit synthesis of thyroid hormone. In addition, PTU inhibits peripheral conversion of T_4 to T_3. PTU has a shorter serum half-life and should be given in multiple daily doses, whereas MMI may be used once daily. Serious side effects are rare, although granulocytopenia, skin rash, and liver toxicity are possible. In an effort to reduce such complications, it is important to monitor liver function tests periodically and to warn the patient to consult a physician for new-onset skin rash or sign of infection. Furthermore, we believe that a complete blood count (CBC) with differential should be obtained every 2–4 weeks during administration of antithyroidal drugs. A gradual decline in white blood cells may herald the onset of granulocytopenia.

9. What is multinodular goiter?
Multinodular goiter (MNG) is most commonly seen in elderly patients. The cause of MNG is unknown, but the natural history is such that hyperthyroidism may eventually occur. Thyrotoxicosis associated with MNG is treated by the same methods as those used for Graves' disease. However, long-term remissions cannot be induced by antithyroidal drugs in toxic MNG.

Moreover, higher doses of ^{131}I are required to treat patients with toxic MNG, which seems to be more resistant to the effects of antithyroidal drugs and ^{131}I therapy.

10. How does therapy with propranolol and corticosteroids contribute to the treatment of hyperthyroidism?

Propranolol has proved to be a valuable asset in the treatment of hyperthyroidism. It reduces not only the tachycardia and tremor but also the peripheral conversion of T_4 to T_3. Because of its rapid onset, propranolol is useful as an adjunct to radioactive iodine therapy and also as a means of preparing a thyrotoxic patient for urgent or emergent surgery. Any beta blocker may be used, although only propranolol inhibits conversion of T_4 to T_3. We prefer a long-acting, cardioselective agent such as atenolol. Beta blockers do not inhibit synthesis of thyroid hormone and on rare occasions patients may get worse with these medications. Corticosteroids also are useful in inhibiting the peripheral conversion of T_4 to T_3

11. What other medications are useful in treating hyperthyroidism?

Although the medications discussed above are usually chosen for treatment of hyperthyroidism, other medications are sometimes useful, including ipodate and iodine. Ipodate is an iodine-containing contrast agent that has a dual effect. It directly inhibits synthesis of thyroid hormone and also releases iodine, which acutely inhibits further organification of iodine by the thyroid gland (Wolff-Chaikoff effect). The therapeutic effects of iodine solutions are based on the same mechanism. Both agents act rapidly, causing dramatic reductions of thyroid hormone levels in 2–3 days and often normalizing levels within 7–14 days. These agents, however, must be administered concurrently with ATDs, which inhibit synthesis of thyroid hormone, because the thyroid gland typically escapes the inhibitory effects of iodine and worsens the hyperthyroidism. Such iodine-induced thyrotoxicosis is extremely difficult to treat.

12. What is subacute thyroiditis?

Subacute thyroiditis is an inflammation of the thyroid gland that often occurs in association with infections of the upper respiratory tract. Patients typically present with a tender, enlarged gland. In the natural history of the disorder, an initial phase of hyperthyroidism due to release of thyroid hormone from damaged thyrocytes is followed by a hypothyroid phase and then by a return to euthyroidism and restoration of normal glandular function. Not every patient manifests each phase. The disease usually runs its course in 2–3 months. Symptomatic therapy for the hyperthyroid and hypothyroid phases is appropriate.

13. What is postpartum thyroiditis?

Postpartum thyroiditis is a disorder frequently seen in women (perhaps 5–10%) after delivery. The cause is unknown. Its course is similar to subacute thyroiditis in that three distinct phases may occur: an initial hyperthyroid phase followed first by hypothyroidism and later by euthyroidism. The disorder usually resolves within 1 year or less after delivery. However, as in the case of subacute thyroiditis, recurrent episodes may result in permanent hypothyroidism. Postpartum thyroiditis is common, occurring in about 5–10% of women in the postpartum period. It may manifest as depression and must be differentiated from postpartum depression. Many other signs and symptoms erroneously attributed to having and caring for an infant in fact may be related to abnormalities in thyroid function.

BIBLIOGRAPHY

1. Bierwaltes WH: The treatment of hyperthyroidism with iodine-131. Semin Nucl Med 8:95, 1978.
2. Burch HB, Wartofsky L: Life-threatening thyrotoxicosis. Endocrinol Metab Clin North Am 22:263, 1993.
3. Char DH: Thyroid Eye Disease, 2nd ed. New York, Churchill Livingstone, 1990.
4. Cooper DS: Antithyroid drugs. N Engl J Med 311:1353, 1984.
5. Greer MA: Treating Graves' disease. Endocrinologist 4:69, 1994.
6. Kay TWH, d'Emden MC, Andrews JT, Martin FIR: Treatment of nontoxic multinodular goiter with radioactive iodine. Am J Med 84:19, 1988.

7. Mazzaferri EL, de los Santos ET, Rofagha-Keyhani: Solitary thyroid nodule: Diagnosis and management. Med Clin North Am 72:1177, 1988.
8. Rojeski MT, Gharib H: Nodular thyroid disease: Evaluation and management. N Engl J Med 313:428, 1985.
9. Solomon DH: Treatment of Graves' hyperthyroidism. In Ingbar SH, Braverman LE (eds): The Thyroid, 5th ed. Philadelphia, J.B. Lippincott, 1986.
10. Teuscher J, Peter HJ, Gerber H, et al: Pathogenesis of nodular goiter and its implications for surgical management. Surgery 103:87, 1988.
11. Wartofsky L: Guidelines for the treatment of hyperthyroidism, Am Fam Physician 30:199, 1984.

30. HYPOTHYROIDISM

Bryan R. Haugen, M.D., and E. Chester Ridgway, M.D.

1. How common is hypothyroidism?

Hypothyroidism is relatively common, with a prevalence of 2–3% in the general population. The mean age at diagnosis is the mid-50's. Hypothyroidism is much more common in women with a female-to-male ratio of 10:1. Postpartum hypothyroidism, a transient hypothyroid phase after pregnancy, is found in 5–10% of women.

2. What is subclinical hypothyroidism?

Subclinical hypothyroidism is a mild and much more common form of hypothyroidism, often with few or no symptoms. As many as 10–20% of women over 50 years old have subclinical hypothyroidism. Hypercholesterolemia and subtle cardiac abnormalities have been associated. Biochemically, the levels of thyroxine (T_4) or free T4 are normal, whereas the level of thyroid-stimulating hormone (TSH) is mildly elevated. When patients are treated with thyroxine they have an improved sense of well-being (compared with placebo), and the cardiac and lipid abnormalities resolve. Therefore, treatment is generally recommended. Thyroid antibodies, an indicator of autoimmune thyroid disease, may help to predict which patients will progress to clinical hypothyroidism; testing is recommended for patients with a minimally elevated TSH.

3. What causes hypothyroidism?

Many disorders can cause hypothyroidism. The two most common causes are chronic lymphocytic thyroiditis (Hashimoto's disease), an autoimmune form of thyroid destruction, and radioiodine-induced hypothyroidism after treatment of Graves' disease (autoimmune hyperthyroidism). Postpartum thyroiditis occurs in approximately 10% of women, two-thirds of whom experience a transient hypothyroid phase (6–12 months) requiring treatment.

Other less common causes of hypothyroidism include subacute thyroiditis, external irradiation to the neck, medications (antithyroid drugs, amiodarone, interferon), infiltrative diseases, central (pituitary/hypothalamic) hypothyroidism, congenital defects, and endemic (iodine-deficient) goiter, which is fairly common outside of the U.S.

4. What symptoms are associated with hypothyroidism?

Hypothyroidism commonly presents with nonspecific symptoms such as fatigue, cold intolerance, depression, weight gain, weakness, joint aches, constipation, dry skin, hair loss, and menstrual irregularities.

5. What findings on physical examination are consistent with hypothyroidism?

Physical examination may be normal with mild or subclinical hypothyroidism and should not deter further work-up if clinical suspicions are high. Common signs of moderate-to-severe hypothyroidism include hypertension, bradycardia, coarse hair, periorbital swelling, yellow skin, (due to elevated levels of beta carotene), carpal tunnel syndrome, and delayed relaxation of the deep tendon reflexes. The thyroid may be enlarged, normal, or small in size, but thyroid consistency is usually firm.

Unusual presentations of hypothyroidism include megacolon, cardiomegaly, and congestive heart failure (CHF). Severe CHF in one patient scheduled for cardiac transplant resolved with thyroid hormone replacement alone.

6. What laboratory tests may be abnormal during hypothyroidism?

Laboratory clues to hypothyroidism include normochromic, normocytic anemia (menstruating women may also have iron deficiency anemia due to excess bleeding from irregular menses), hyponatremia, hypercholesterolemia, and elevated levels of creatine phosphokinase (CPK).

7. What tests best confirm the diagnosis of hypothyroidism in the outpatient setting?

Many thyroid function tests are available to the clinician, including assessments of TSH, T_4, T_3, resin uptake, free T_4, free T_3, and reverse T_3. In the outpatient setting only one test is usually necessary: assessment of TSH. TSH, which is synthesized and secreted from the anterior pituitary gland, is the most sensitive indicator of thyroid function in the nonstressed state. Basically, if the TSH is normal (normal range 0.5–5 mIU/ml), the patient is euthyroid; if the TSH is elevated (greater than 5 mIU/ml), the patient has primary gland failure.

Care must be taken in interpreting total T_4 levels (occasionally done on health-screening panels). Many conditions unrelated to thyroid disease cause low or elevated levels of total T_4, because more than 99% of T_4 is protein-bound and total T_4 levels depend on the amount of thyroid-binding proteins, which may vary greatly. Total T_4 levels must always be compared with the T_3 resin uptake (T3RU), which reflects the amount of thyroid hormone-binding protein.

8. What tests best confirm hypothyroidism in the inpatient setting?

Interpretation of the thyroid function test in the acutely ill inpatient is more difficult when hypothyroidism is suspected. Acute nonthyroidal illness may cause suppression of the T_4 and T_3 levels, and TSH may be elevated in the recovery phase. Medications such as dopamine and glucocorticods may suppress the TSH. Severe illness may even cause low levels of free T_4. When hypothyroidism is suspected in the stressed, hospitalized patient, a combination of clinical signs (inappropriate bradycardia, puffy facies, dry skin, delayed relaxation of the deep tendon reflexes) and laboratory tests (TSH and free T_4 levels) are necessary to exclude or confirm the diagnosis of hypothyroidism. If these tests are equivocal, a reverse T_3 level that is normal or elevated in nonthyroidal illness and low in hypothyroidism may prove helpful. Inpatient TSH testing also may be confounded by normal diurnal variations in TSH. TSH levels in a euthyroid person may exceed the normal range at night, when patients are frequently admitted. A morning test may help to clarify the significance of a mildly elevated TSH.

9. Which thyroid hormone preparation should I use?

Since 1891 when sheep thyroid extract was first used to treat myxedema, many preparations have been developed and are still available. The best replacement regimen at this time is levothyroxine (LT_4). Brand-name levothyroxine (Synthroid, Levothroid, Levoxine) is preferred over the generic preparations, because cost is a minor issue (generic costs $4/month, whereas brand names cost about $7–10/month) and because generic LT_4 may vary 15–20% in bioavailability. Other thyroid hormone preparations include triiodothyronine (LT_3), which is reserved for special cases because of its potency and short half-life, and desiccated thyroid and thyroglobulin, which give unpredictable concentrations of serum thyroid hormone because of varied content and bioavailability.

10. What is the best dose of levothyroxine for replacement in a hypothyroid patient?

Otherwise healthy, young patients may be started on full replacement doses of LT_4 (1.6 µg/kg). Elderly patients and patients with known or suspected cardiac disease should be started on low doses of LT_4 (25 µg/day), which are increased gradually by 25 µg/day every 2–3 months until the TSH is normal.

11 How should the clinician approach surgery in the hypothyroid patient?

There are two broad categories to consider: emergent/cardiac surgery and elective surgery. Hypothyroidism is associated with minor postoperative complications—gastrointestinal (prolonged constipation, ileus) as well as neuropsychiatric (confusion, psychosis); in addition, the incidence of fever with infections is lower. However rates of mortality and major complications (blood loss, arrythmias, impaired would healing) are similar to the rates in euthyroid patients.

Current recommendations are to proceed with emergent surgery in the hypothyroid patient and to monitor for potential postoperative complications during replacing therapy with LT4. Patients with ischemic coronary artery disease requiring surgery should proceed without LT_4 replacement, because T_4 increases myocardial oxygen demand and may precipitate worsening cardiac symptoms if given before surgery. Postoperatively the patient should receive replacement therapy with LT_4 at a slow rate and be followed for CHF (increased in hypothyroid patients undergoing cardiac surgery).

Patients scheduled for elective surgery should wait until TSH is normalized because of the postoperative complications associated with hypothyroidism.

12. How does myxedema differ from hypothyroidism?

Myxedema is a severe form of prolonged hypothyroidism. Complications include hypoventilation, cardiac failure, fluid and electrolyte abnormalities, and coma. Myxedema coma is frequently precipitated by an intercurrent systemic illness, surgery, or narcotic/hypnotic drugs. Patients with myxedema coma should receive replacement therapy with 300–500 μg of intravenous LT_4 followed by 50–100 μg each day. Because conversion of T_4 to T_3 (active hormone) is decreased with severe illness, patients with profound cardiac failure that requires pressors or patients unresponsive to 1–2 days of LT_4 therapy should be given LT_3 at 12.5 μg intravenously every 6 hours.

BIBLIOGRAPHY

1. Roti E, Minelli R, Gardini E, Braverman LE: The use and misuse of thyroid hormone. Endocr Rev 14:401–423, 1993.
2. Mandel SJ, Brent GA, Larsen PR: Levothyroxine therapy in patients with thyroid disease. Ann Intern Med 119:492–502, 1993.
3. Rosenthal MJ, Hunt WC, Garry PJ, Goodwin JS: Thyroid failure in the elderly: Microsomal antibodies as discriminant for therapy. JAMA 258:209–213, 1987.
4. Cooper DS, Halpern R, Wood LC, et al: L-thyroxine therapy in subclinical hypothyroidism. Ann Intern Med 101:18–24, 1984.
5. Elder J, McLelland A, O'Reilly SJ, et al: The relationship between serum cholesterol and serum thyrotropin, thyroxine, and tri-iodothyronine concentrations in suspected hypothyroidism. Ann Clin Biochem 27:110–113, 1990.
6. Ladenson PW: Recognition and management of cardiovascular disease related to thyroid dysfunction. Am J Med 88:638–641, 1990.
7. Patel R, Hughes RW: An unusual case of myxedema megacolon with features of ischemic and pseudomembranous colitis. Mayo Clin Proc 67:369–372, 1992.
8. Arem R, Patsch W: Lipoprotein and apolipoprotein levels in subclinical hypothyroidism. Arch Intern Med 150:2097–2100, 1990.
9. Ladenson PW, Levin AA, Ridgeway EC, Daniels GH: Complications of surgery in hypothyroid patients. Am J Med 77:261–266, 1984.
10. Hay ID, Duick DS, Vliestra RE, et al: Thyroxine therapy in hypothyroid patients undergoing coronary revascularization: A retrospective analysis. Ann Intern Med 95:456–457, 1981.

31. THYROIDITIS

Robert C. Smallridge, M.D., COL, MC

1. Give the differential diagnosis for thyroiditis.
 1. Acute (suppurative)
 2. Subacute (granulomatous)
 3. Autoimmune
     Chronic lymphocytic (Hashimoto's disease)
     Atrophic (primary myxedema)
     Juvenile
     Postpartum
 4. Painless (nonpostpartum)
 5. Riedel's struma

2. What causes acute thyroiditis?
This rare disease is infectious and usually bacterial; at times, however, fungal, tuberculous, parasitic, or syphilitic infections have been reported. *Pneumocytis carinii* has been observed in patients with acquired immunodeficiency syndrome (AIDS). Treatment involves drainage and antibiotics.

3. Describe the four stages of subacute thyroiditis (see figure).
 Stage I: Patients have a painful (uni- or bilateral) thyroid and may have systemic symptoms. Inflammatory destruction of thyroid follicles causes release of excessive thyroxine (T_4) and triiodothyronine (T_3) into the blood, and thyrotoxicosis may ensue.
 Stage II: A transitory period (1–2 weeks) of euthyroidism occurs after the T_4 is cleared from the body.
 Stage III: With severe disease, patients may become hypothyroid until the thyroid gland repairs itself.
 Stage IV: A euthyroid state returns.

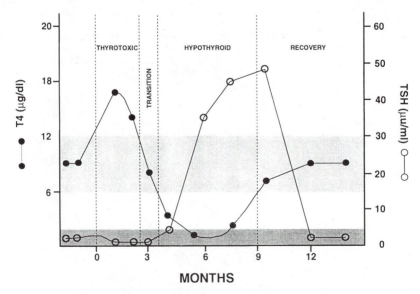

Thyroid function during subacute thyroiditis.

4. What is the natural history of subacute thyroiditis?

Subacute thyroiditis is probably viral in origin. Although patients almost always recover clinically, serum thyroglobulin levels remain elevated and intrathyroidal iodine content is low for many months. Patients are also more susceptible to iodine-induced hypothyroidism at a later time. Such findings suggest persistent subclinical abnormalities after an episode of subacute thyroiditis.

5. What is the most common cause of thyroiditis?

Autoimmune thyroid disease is most common. It is recognized by the presence of microsomal antibodies (thyroid peroxidase) and, less frequently, thyroglobulin antibodies in serum.

6. Give the clinical characteristics of autoimmune thyroid disease.

Chronic lymphocytic thyroiditis usually presents as a euthyroid goiter that progresses to hypothyroidism in middle-aged and older persons, especially women. Atrophic thyroiditis is characterized by a very small thyroid gland in a hypothyroid patient. Some evidence suggests that thyroid growth inhibitory antibodies may account for the lack of a goiter. Two-thirds of adolescents with goiter have autoimmune (juvenile) thyroiditis.

7. Does postpartum thyroiditis follow a different clinical course from that of other types of autoimmune thyroiditis?

Yes. Postpartum disease develops in women between the third and ninth month after delivery. It typically follows the stages seen in patients with subacute thyroiditis.

8. How common is postpartum thyroiditis?

After delivery 5–10% of women develop bicohemical evidence of thyroid dysfunction. About one-third of affected women develop symptoms (usually hypothyroidism) and benefit from 6–12 months of therapy with L-thyroxine.

9. What are the differences between subacute and postpartum thyroiditis?

Patients with subacute thyroiditis have thyroid pain, an elevated sedimentation rate, and a transient rise in thyroid antibodies. Most are positive for the HLA-B35 antigen, and histologic examination shows giant cells and granulomas in the thyroid. In postpartum disease there is no pain, the sedimentation rate is normal, and thyroid antibodies are positive both before and after the episode. The prevalence of HLA-DR3 and HLA-DR5 antigens is increased, and histologic examination shows lymphocytic infiltration of the thyroid gland.

10. Why do women develop postpartum thyroiditis?

It is thought that women who develop postpartum thyroiditis have underlying asymptomatic autoimmune thyroiditis. During pregnancy the maternal immune system is partially suppressed, with a dramatic rebound rise in thyroid antibodies after delivery. Although microsomal antibodies are not believed to be cytotoxic, they are currently the most reliable marker of susceptibility to postpartum disease.

11. Does thyroid function in patients with postpartum thyroiditis return to normal, as it does in subacute thyroiditis?

Not always. Approximately 20% of women become permanently hypothyroid, and an equal number have persistent mild abnormalities.

12. Do any factors identify women at increased risk of developing postpartum thyroiditis?

Women with a higher microsomal antibody titer are, in general, more likely to develop thyroiditis. Recently it has been shown that approximately 25% of women with type I diabetes mellitus develop thyroiditis after delivery. For high-risk patients, screening for thyroid antibodies and careful monitoring of thyroid function are indicated.

13. What is painless thyroiditis?

Both men and women may present with thyrotoxic symptoms that are transient. As with subacute thyroiditis, they often experience subsequent hypothyroidism. Unlike subacute disease, this disorder is painless. It has been given a variety of names, including hyperthyroiditis, silent thyroiditis, transient painless thyroiditis with hyperthyroidism, and lymphocytic thyroiditis with spontaneously resolving hyperthyroidism. Of interest, this disease was first described in the 1970s and reached its peak incidence in the early 1980s. It seems to occur less often now.

14. What is the etiology of painless thyroiditis?

Some investigators believe that it is a variant of subacute thyroiditis, because a small percentage of patients with biopsy-proved subacute disease have had no pain. Others believe that painless thyroiditis is a variant of Hashimoto's disease, because the histology of the two is similar.

15. What is destruction-induced thyroiditis?

Destruction-induced thyroiditis refers to the three disorders (subacute, postpartum, and painless thyroiditis) in which an inflammatory infiltrate destroys thyroid follicles and excessive amounts of T_4 and T_3 are released into the circulation.

16. When a patient presents with hyperthyroid symptoms, an elevated level of T_4 and a suppressed level of TSH, what is the next test that should be ordered?

A 24-hour radioactive iodine uptake (RAIU) should be performed. When the thyroid is overactive (as in Graves' or toxic nodular disease), the RAIU is elevated. In destruction-induced thyroiditis the RAIU is low, as a result of both suppression of TSH by the acutely increased level of serum T_4 and the diminished ability of damaged thyroid follicles to trap and organify iodine.

17. What is the appropriate therapy for patients with any of the destructive thyroiditides?

In the thyrotoxic stage, beta blockers relieve adrenergic symptoms. All forms of antithyroid therapy (drugs, radioactive iodine ablation, and surgery) are absolutely contraindicated. Thyroid hormone promptly relieves hypothyroid symptoms and should be continued for 6–12 months, depending on the severity of disease. Many patients need no therapy.

18. What is Riedel's struma?

Riedel's struma is a rare disorder in which the thyroid becomes densely fibrotic and hard. Local fibrosis of adjacent tissues may produce obstructive symptoms that require surgery. In some cases, fibrosis of other tissues (fibrosing retroperitonitis, sclerosing cholangitis) may occur.

BIBLIOGRAPHY

1. Amino N, Mori H, Iwatani Y, et al: High prevalence of transient postpartum thyrotoxicosis and hypothyroidism. N Engl J Med 306:849, 1982.
2. Fein HG, Metz S, Nikolai TF, et al: HLA antigens in thyroiditis: Differences between silent and postpartum lymphocytic forms, and comparison with subacute and goitrous autoimmune thyroiditis. In Walfish PG, Wall JR, Volpe R (eds): Autoimmunity and the Thyroid. New York, Academic Press, 1985.
3. Gerstein HC: Incidence of postpartum thyroid dysfunction in patients with Type I diabetes mellitus. Ann Intern Med 118:419, 1993.
4. Guttler R, Singer PA: *Pneumocystis carinii* thyroiditis. Arch Intern Med 153:393, 1993.
5. Hamburger JI: The various presentations of thyroiditis. Ann Intern Med 104:219, 1986.
6. Hay ID: Thyroiditis: A clinical update. Mayo Clin Proc 60:836, 1985.
7. Hayslip CC, Fein HG, O'Donnell VM, et al: The value of serum antimicrosomal antibody testing in screening for symptomatic postpartum thyroid dysfunction. Am J Obstet Gynecol 159:203, 1988.
8. Lamberton P, Jackson IMD: Thyroiditis. In Becker KL (ed): Principles and Practice of Endocrinology and Metabolism. Philadelphia, J.B. Lippincott, 1990.
9. Nikolai TF, Coombs GJ, McKenzie AK: Lymphocytic thyroiditis with spontaneously resolving hyperthyrodism and subacute thyroiditis: Long-term follow-up. Arch Intern Med 141:1455, 1981.

10. Othman S, Phillips DIW, Parkes AB, et al: A long-term follow-up of postpartum thyroiditis. Clin Endocrinol 32:559, 1990.
11. Roti E, Minelli R, Gardini E, et al: Iodine-induced hypothyroidism in euthyroid subjects with a previous episode of subacute thyroiditis. J Clin Endocrinol Metab 70:1581, 1990.
12. Smallridge RC, De Keyser FM, Van Herle AJ, et al: Thyroid iodine content and serum thyroglobulin: Cues to the natural history of destruction-induced thyroiditis. J Clin Endocrinol Metab 62:1213, 1986.
13. Solomon BL, Fein HG, Smallridge RC: Usefulness of antimicrosomal antibody titers in the diagnosis and treatment of postpartum thyroiditis. J Fam Pract 36:177, 1993.
14. Woolf PD: Transient painless thyroiditis with hyperthyroidism: A variant of lymphocytic thyroiditis? Endocr Rev 1:411, 1980.

32. THYROID NODULES AND GOITER

William J. Georgitis, M.D., COL, MC

PATHOGENESIS

1. The five cases represented in the figure on the facing page are hyperthyroid, as indicated by the undetectable levels of thyroid-stimulating hormone (TSH). Match the appropriate diagnosis and pathogenic mechanism to the appropriate case. (Answers appear at the end of the chapter.)

Case No.	Diagnosis	Pathogenesis
__1__	_____	_____
__2__	_____	_____
__3__	_____	_____
__4__	_____	_____
__5__	_____	_____

Possible diagnoses:

DTG	=	Diffuse toxic goiter
TMNG	=	Toxic multinodular goiter
SAT	=	Subacute thyroiditis
LT/SRH	=	Lymphocytic thyroiditis with spontaneously resolving hyperthyroidism (painless thyroiditis)
STN	=	Solitary toxic nodule
FH	=	Factitious hyperthyroidism

Pathogenesis:

A. Surreptitious ingestion of thyroid hormone
B. Autoimmune production of thyroid-stimulating IgG immunoglobulin
C. Inflammatory thyroiditis, probably of viral origin
D. Excessive production of thyroid hormone by an autonomous follicular adenoma
E. Excessive production of thyroid hormone by multiple autonomous follicular adenomas
F. Lymphocytic thyroiditis with low-uptake form of hyperthyroidism

2. What is the pathogenesis of diffuse nontoxic goiter?

No one knows for sure. The traditional concept holds that TSH-dependent enlargement of the thyroid compensates for diminished efficiency of thyroid hormone production due to environmental goitrogens, deficiency or excess of iodine, or inherited biosynthetic defects. Goiter regression with iodine supplementation or thyroxine suppression of TSH supports this mechanism, but elevated levels of TSH have never been convincingly demonstrated in cross-sectional studies of populations with simple goiter. An alternative pathogenesis may involve factors other than TSH that are capable of inducing thyroid growth without stimulating hyperfunction, much like certain immunoglobulins found in diffuse toxic goiter.

3. What is the natural history of diffuse nontoxic goiter?

Simple goiter over time becomes multinodular and demonstrates a tendency toward autonomous function, defined as TSH-independent production and secretion of thyroid hormone. In this setting, a load of iodine may result in thyrotoxicosis (Jod-Basedow hyperthyroidism). Epidemics of this disorder were described in iodine-deficient areas of the world after the initiation of iodine supplementation programs.

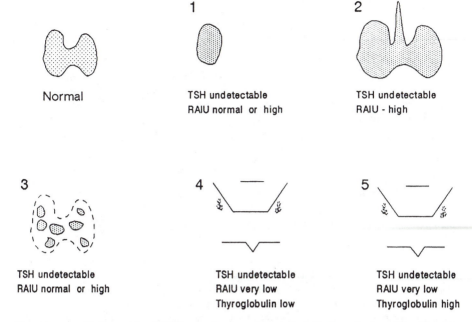

1

TSH undetectable
RAIU normal or high

2

TSH undetectable
RAIU - high

Normal

3

TSH undetectable
RAIU normal or high

4

TSH undetectable
RAIU very low
Thyroglobulin low

5

TSH undetectable
RAIU very low
Thyroglobulin high

Thyroid scans and iodine uptakes (RAIU) are no longer routinely included in the evaluation of thyroid nodules and goiter. However, coupled with measurements of serum thyroid hormones, thyroglobulin, and thyrotropin, nuclear medicine tests clearly define the pathophysiology of most thyroid disorders. These cases illustrate concepts relevant to diagnosis and management. Cost-effective or optimal approaches for specific thyroid conditions are discussed in articles listed at the end of the chapter.

4. How does lithium cause goiter?

Lithium, like iodine, blocks the release of thyroid hormone. Rising levels of TSH cause thyroid enlargement. In patients with chronic lymphocytic thyroiditis or prior radioiodine treatment, lithium may precipitate overt hypothyroidism.

CLINICAL MANIFESTATIONS

5. What diagnosis should be suspected if patient no. 1 from question 1 reports the sudden painful enlargement of her thyroid nodule?

Hemorrhagic degeneration with cyst formation should be suspected. Expansion of the nodule stretches visceral pain fibers in the thyroid capsule. The resulting deep aching pain may be referred to the jaw or ear. Although both the hyperthyroidism and the nodule may resolve, persistence of the nodule may require percutaneous needle aspiration or surgery.

6. How can patients nos. 2, 5, and 6 from question 1, all with forms of hyperthyroidism associated with low uptake of iodine, be differentiated?

LT/SRH and SAT present quite differently. A prodromal illness characterized by myalgias and fever coupled with either upper respiratory or gastrointestinal symptoms generally precedes the onset of neck pain in SAT. The erythrocyte sedimentation rate is usually markedly elevated.

In contrast, LT/SRH does not cause neck pain, although a painful variant has been described. This disorder lacks constitutional symptoms and is prone to appear in the postpartum period. Sedimentation rates are normal. Positive titers of antithyroid microsomal antibody favor LT/SRH but are undetectable often enough to be of little differential value.

A patient surreptitiously ingesting excessive thyroid hormone should not have a goiter, and levels of serum thyroglobulin are low in contrast to the normal or high levels in patients with hyperthyroidism due to thyroiditis.

7. How are most thyroid cancers discovered?

Most thyroid cancers are discovered by chance in asymptomatic patients. A lump in the neck may be noted first by the patient, by an examining physician, or during imaging studies to investigate structures adjacent to the thyroid. Thyroid nodules are common, with a lifetime occurrence approaching 6% and an autopsy prevalence of 50%. The frequency of thyroid cancer in surgical series before the widespread use of fine-needle aspiration averaged about 10%.

EVALUATION

8. List a differential diagnosis for nodules of the thyroid.

Adenoma	Cyst	Metastatic cancer/
Carcinoma	Thyroiditis	lymphoma/sarcoma
Parathyroid cyst		Thyroid hemiagenesis

9. Can the nature of a thyroid nodule be suspected on the basis of history or physical examination?

Although most patients with thyroid nodules have no symptoms or signs, certain features are worth noting on examination. Symptoms attributable to a neck mass, such as hoarseness, dysphagia, dyspnea, or on rare occasions, hemoptysis from tracheal invasion suggest malignancy. Most patients with thyroid cancer have normal thyroid function. Therefore, thyroid nodules in hyperthyroid or hypothyroid patients are more likely to be benign. Recent painless growth rather than the sudden appearance of thyroid pain, as seen with SAT or cystic degeneration of a nodule, typifies thyroid cancer. Family history is usually not helpful except in medullary thyroid cancers associated with the multiple endocrine neoplasia syndromes, which are inherited in an autosomal dominant pattern. Nodules fixed to adjacent neck structures or accompanied by enlarged cervical lymph nodes are likely to be cancerous.

10. If a nodule is cancer, what kind is it likely to be?

Thyroid Cancer Classified in Descending Order of Frequency	
Papillary	50–70%
Follicular	10–15%
Medullary	1–2%
Anaplastic	Rare
Primary thyroid lymphoma	Rare
Metastatic to thyroid	Rarely detected in vivo

11. Is examination of thyroid cyst fluid helpful in making a diagnosis?

First, the amount and gross appearance of cyst fluid is worth recording. After aspiration, about one-third of cysts reaccumulate fluid. If the volume of fluid obtained on sequential aspirations does not decline surgical removal of the cyst should be considered.

Simple thyroid cysts have yellow, burgundy, or chocolate-colored fluid and are generally benign, whereas complex cysts may be malignant. Cytology of cyst fluid is almost always nonspecific, showing histiocytes and crenated erythrocytes. Fine-needle biopsy directed at any solid component palpable after the fluid has been drained may help to define the benign or malignant nature of the lesion.

Crystal-clear watery fluid is indicative of a parathyroid cyst. Because hyperparathyroidism is associated with about one-half of parathyroid cysts, the level of serum calcium should be checked.

12. What is the risk of cancer in patients with multinodular goiter and Hashimoto's disease?
Although autopsy series indicate that up to 75% of thyroid nodules are multiple and that malignancy is rare, any thyroid nodule can be cancerous. Contrary to old axioms, a nodule in the presence of multinodular goiter or lymphocytic thyroiditis has the same risk of cancer as the solitary nodule.

13. What is the role of fine-needle aspiration biopsy in the evaluation of a thyroid nodule?
Fine-needle aspiration is a safe, outpatient procedure with an accuracy of 90–95% in adequate specimens interpreted by experienced cytopathologists. The majority of biopsies return with benign diagnoses, including adenomatous hyperplasia (benign multinodular goiter), colloid adenoma, or autoimmune thyroiditis. Surgery is thus avoided. A reading of papillary thyroid cancer helps the surgeon to plan the operation of choice. Follicular neoplasms are more vexing, because aspiration biopsy cannot differentiate adenoma from carcinoma, and even frozen sections of intraoperative specimens do not distinguish malignancy reliably. Finally, fine-needle aspiration is inadequate in about 15% of patients. An inadequate result deserves further investigation. In summary, the information obtained from fine-needle biopsy of the thyroid nodule helps to direct proper management; therefore, all palpable thyroid nodules should be biopsied.

14. What is the difference between a "cold," "warm," and "hot" thyroid nodule on thyroid scan?
The cold nodule displays diminished radiolabeling compared with surrounding normal thyroid tissue. The majority of cold nodules are benign, but virtually all thyroid cancers are poor at concentrating iodine compared with normal thyroid tissue. The hot nodule avidly absorbs tracer, whereas uptake by the remainder of the thyroid is suppressed, as demonstrated by patient no. 1 in question 1. Solitary toxic nodules (STN) are usually larger than 3 cm in diameter and most frequently occur in patients over the age of 40 years. Patients with STN tend not to appear hypermetabolic like patients with diffuse toxic goiter and often present a profile of T_3 toxicosis, with suppressed TSH, normal T_4 and elevated T_3. Toxic adenomas are never cancerous. In contrasts, the warm nodule may be malignant. The personality spectrum of warm nodules is characterized by indecision. Some warm nodules are really cold nodules that appear warm because they are invested by normal thyroid tissue. Others are autonomous nodules like the STN but fail to secrete sufficient thyroid hormone to suppress uptake of TSH and tracer by extranodular thyroid tissue. Repeat scanning after treatment with thyroxine helps to resolve the nature of the nodule. Autonomous nodules may be observed, whereas all others deserve fine-needle biopsy to exclude thyroid cancer.

MANAGEMENT

15. What surgeon devised the incision for conventional transverse cervical thyroidectomy?
Swiss surgeon Theodor Kocher (1841–1917) devised the incision. But a word of caution—he was an innovator. If you call for a "Kocher" in the operating room, you may receive a forceps, a wrist operation, or a right subcostal incision designed to approach the gallbladder instead of the thyroid!

16. Which treatment was first used for diffuse toxic goiter—radioactive iodine or antithyroid medications?
Both were used initially in the early 1940s. Thiourea, the first goitrogenic substance to be used, had undesirable toxicities and soon was replaced by methimazole and propylthiouracil. Of the fission products developed during World War II, [130]I was used before ^{131}I, which became widely available in 1946.

17. What thyroid conditions are treated with radioactive iodine?

Radioiodine treatment is effective in diffuse toxic goiter and toxic nodular goiter of both the solitary and multinodular varieties. Compressive symptoms from benign multinodular goiters in patients judged to be poor surgical risks can be relieved by radioactive iodine, although the goiter shrinks on average less than 30%. Finally, radioactive iodine as an adjunctive therapy for differentiated forms of thyroid cancer decreases rates of recurrence.

18. When is suppressive therapy with thyroxine useful?

When a patient describes recent thyroid enlargement and is found to be hypothyroid with an elevated level of TSH, thyroxine treatment may cause goiter regression. However, recent investigations in euthyroid patients with thyroid nodules question the efficacy of thyroxine suppression. Nonetheless, incontrovertible data in patients with irradiation-associated thyroid disease initially treated by simple lobectomy indicate that suppression of thyroxine decreases the incidence of subsequent thyroid nodules in the remaining lobe.

* * * *

Answers: 1, STN, D; 2, DTG, B; 3, TMNG, E; 4, FH, A; 5, SAT, C or LT/SRH, F

BIBLIOGRAPHY

1. Braverman LE, Utiger RD (eds): Werner and Ingbar's The Thyroid: A Fundamental and Clinical Text. Philadelphia, J. B. Lippincott, 1991.
2. Gharib H: A strategy for the solitary thyroid nodule. Hosp Pract 27:53–60, 1992.
3. Massaferri EL: Management of a solitary thyroid nodule. N Engl J Med 328:553–559, 1993.
4. Mortensen JD. Gross and microscopic findings in clinically normal thyroid glands. J Clin Endocrinol Metab 15:1270–1280, 1955.
5. Ridgeay EC. Clinician's evaluation of a solitary thyroid nodule. J Clin Endocrinol Metab 74:231–235, 1992.
6. Rojeski MT: Nodular thyroid disease. N Engl J Med 313:428–436, 1985.
7. Ross DS: Evaluation of the thyroid nodule. J Nucl Med 32:2181–2192, 1991.
8. Sakiyama R: Thyroiditis: A clinical review. Am Fam Physician 48:615–621, 1993.
9. Smallridge RC: Metabolic and anatomic thyroid emergencies: A review. Crit Care Med 20:276–291, 1992.
10. Wool MS: Thyroid nodules. The place of fine-needle aspiration biopsy in management. Postgrad Med 94:111–122, 1993.

33. THYROID CANCER

Arnold A. Asp, M.D.

1. What are the most common types of thyroid cancer?

The thyroid consists predominantly of follicular epithelial cells, which incorporate iodine into thyroid hormone to be stored in follicles, and of smaller numbers of parafollicular cells, which produce calcitonin. Malignant transformation of either type of cell may occur, but the parafollicular malignancy (medullary carcinoma of the thyroid) is much less common than cancers derived from follicular epithelial cells. Malignancies originating from follicular epithelial cells are designated according to their microscopic appearance and include papillary, follicular, and anaplastic carcinomas.

Papillary carcinoma and its variants comprise approximately 60–80% of thyroid cancers, whereas follicular carcinoma makes up approximately 15–30% of primary thyroid malignancies. These two forms are frequently referred to as the differentiated thyroid carcinomas. Medullary carcinoma of the thyroid (MCT) comprises 2–10% of thyroid carcinomas, whereas anaplastic forms of thyroid carcinoma make up 1–10%.

2. What are the differentiated forms of thyroid carcinoma?

Malignant transformation of the iodine-concentrating cells of the thyroid follicle results in two main forms of differentiated thyroid carcinoma: papillary and follicular carcinoma. The two malignancies are histologically distinct. Papillary carcinoma is generally an unencapsulated tumor marked by enlarged cells with dense cytoplasm and overlapping nuclei that have granular, powdery, chromatin, nucleoli, and pseudonuclear inclusion bodies (often called as "Orphan Annie eyes"), all arranged in papillary fronds. Follicular carcinoma is generally characterized by atypical-appearing thyroid cells with dense, uniform, overlapping nuclei and a disorganized microfollicular architecture. Follicular carcinoma cannot be differentiated reliably from benign follicular adenomas on cytomorphologic criteria alone; follicular cancer must demonstrate invasion of the tumor capsule or blood vessels. Tumors that contain histologic elements of both types of carcinoma are classified as mixed papillary-follicular cancer and are considered to be variants of papillary carcinoma.

Papillary and follicular carcinoma also behave as clinically distinct entities. Most endocrinologists consider follicular carcinoma to be the more aggressive of the differentiated cancers, with a higher rate of metastases, more frequent recurrence after therapy, and an exaggerated mortality rate compared with the relatively indolent papillary carcinoma. This view is not universal. Some authors believe that the sharp dichotomy between the clinical courses of papillary and follicular cancer is artificial and attribute the apparent aggressiveness of follicular carcinoma to its occurrence in an elderly population; they argue that when cases are controlled for age, outcomes of patients with either form of differentiated carcinoma are comparable.

3. What is the clinical course of papillary carcinoma?

Papillary carcinoma usually presents as a painless nodule within the thyroid gland or cervical lymphatics. The disease may occur at any age but has a peak incidence during the fourth decade. Women are more commonly affected than men and comprise 62–81% of patients in most series. The primary tumor is rarely encapsulated (4–22% in most series) but is less aggressive if a capsule is present. Papillary carcinoma is more commonly multifocal within the thyroid than is follicular carcinoma; 20–80% of glands have multiple lesions at resection. Extrathyroidal invasion through the capsule of the thyroid occurs in 5–16% of cases.

Papillary carcinoma frequently metastasizes to regional cervical and high mediastinal lymphatics. At the time of surgery 35–43% of patients have enlarged regional lymph nodes that harbor cancer. If lymph nodes are systematically "picked" and examined for microscopic foci, the prevalence of cervical metastases increases to 90%. Unlike other neoplasms, the presence of papillary carcinoma in regional lymph nodes does not increase mortality; it does, however, increase the likelihood of recurrence after therapy. Up to 20% of recurrent lesions cannot subsequently be eradicated. Although lymphatic metastases are common, only 3–7% of patients with papillary carcinoma manifest distant metastatic lesions during initial therapy. Distant metastases involve the lung (76% of distant foci), bone (23% of distant foci), and brain (15% of distant foci).

Compared with other malignancies, papillary carcinoma is relatively indolent. Cancer-related death occurs in only 4–12% of patients during 20-year follow-up. Prognostic factors at the time of diagnosis that augur a poor outcome include male sex, age > 40 years, extrathyroidal invasion, distant metastases, and large primary tumor (> 1.5 cm diameter).

4. What is the clinical course of follicular carcinoma?

Follicular carcinoma usually presents as an asymptomatic nodule within the thyroid, but unlike papillary carcinoma, it may present as an isolated metastatic pulmonary or osseous focus without a palpable thyroid lesion. Very rarely metastatic foci of follicular carcinoma retain hormonal synthetic capability and overproduce thyroid hormones, causing thyrotoxicosis. Follicular carcinoma may occur at any age, but has a later peak incidence (fifth decade) than papillary carcinoma. Women outnumber men, comprising approximately 60% of cases. Follicular carcinoma occurs more commonly in areas of iodine deficiency; incidence of the malignancy has decreased as iodine supplementation has increased. The tumor is nearly always encapsulated, and the degree of vascular or capsular invasiveness (minimal to extensive) is indicative of malignant potential. Follicular carcinoma is usually unifocal (<10% multifocal).

Hematogenous metastasis occurs in follicular carcinoma; for this reason cervical and mediastinal lymphatic involvement is less common than in papillary carcinoma (only 6–13% of patients during initial surgery.) In contrast to cases of papillary carcinoma, the presence of cervical metastases indicates advanced disease. Distant metastases to the lung, bone, and central nervous system (in descending order of occurrence) are discovered more commonly in follicular than in papillary carcinoma, occurring in 12–33% of cases. Death due to follicular carcinoma occurs in 13–59% of patients followed for 20 years. Prognostic factors at the time of initial therapy that portend a poor outcome include age greater than 50 years, male sex (in some settings), marked degree of vascular invasion, and distant metastases.

5. Do any other factors predict the course of differentiated carcinoma?

Differentiated carcinoma is discovered in 5–10% of the surgical resections performed for the treatment of Graves' disease. In some series of patients with Graves' disease, up to 45% of palpable nodules contain papillary carcinoma. Such data have led to speculation that the thyroid-stimulating immunoglobulins responsible for thyrotoxicosis may potentiate the growth of neoplastic cells and predispose to aggressive forms of differentiated carcinoma.

Chronic lymphocytic thyroiditis is found concomitantly with papillary carcinoma in 5–10% of cases. Local recurrence and metastatic disease are less common in such cases and may indicate a favorable effect of Hashimoto's disease.

Distant metastatic disease, as mentioned above, occurs more commonly in follicular carcinoma than in papillary cancer. Regardless of the primary type of cancer, the prognosis associated with distant metastases is dismal. Overall, 50–66% of patients with pulmonary, osseous, or central nervous system lesions die within 5 years. On rare occasions pulmonary metastases may be compatible with 10–20-year survival in younger patients. Metastases to the bone are associated with brief survival, despite aggressive therapy.

6. How are the differentiated carcinomas treated?

No other subject in the field of endocrinology inflames passions or sparks controversy more than the therapy of differentiated thyroid carcinoma. Meetings of specialists are all to often subjected to the sad spectacle of fisticuffs between members as the merits of therapy are debated; balding men in bowties circle one another, fists and arms gamely pumping the air, while female counterparts shriek biostatistics peppered with vernacular epithets and common finger gestures seldom encountered outside the confines of the roller-derby rink. Simply stated, therapy of differentiated thyroid carcinoma is based on the surgical removal of the primary tumor and eradication of all metastatic disease with radioactive iodine (^{131}I). Lifelong suppression of thyroid-stimulating hormone (TSH) with exogenous thyroid hormone subsequently reduces the risk of recurrence.

7. What type of surgery is preferred?

Opinions about the extent of initial surgical resection have been tempered by the possible complications of thyroid surgery; recurrent laryngeal nerve damage with resultant hoarseness and/or iatrogenic hypoparathyroidism occur in 1–5% of thyroid resections. Fear of complications, coupled with the relatively low mortality rate associated with differentiated thyroid carcinoma, has prompted some surgeons to remove only the thyroid lobe in which cancer is apparent at the time of exploration. Most surgeons, however, are cognizant of the frequency of clinically inapparent multicentric lesions, the increased recurrence rates in patients treated with simple lobectomy, and the low rate of postsurgical complications; thus they have rejected simple lobectomy and instead prefer near-total thyroidectomy, which entails the removal of the thyroid lobe containing the tumor, the isthmus, and the majority of the contralateral thyroid lobe. The posterior capsule of the contralateral lobe is left undisturbed in an attempt to preserve the underlying parathyroid glands and the recurrent laryngeal nerve. With this procedure, the surgeon is able to remove the primary tumor and the bulk of normal thyroid tissue that may harbor microscopic malignancy.

Cervical and high mediastinal lymph nodes that appear to harbor metastatic disease are harvested at the time of surgery. Radical neck dissections do not reduce mortality or rate of recurrence and should be avoided, unless there is direct extensions of the tumor throughout the neck. In the event that a single, small (<1.5 cm) papillary carcinoma is discovered, lobectomy and isthmusectomy may be curative.

8. How does ^{131}I therapy benefit the patient?

Most (but not all) differentiated thyroid malignancies retain the ability to trap inorganic iodine when stimulated by TSH. When ^{131}I is concentrated within normal or malignant thyroid tissue, beta-irradiation results in cellular damage or death. If a metastatic lesion is capable of concentrating radioiodine, it becomes visible with a gamma camera; if it absorbs enough ^{131}I to impart 8,000 rad of irradiation, the tumor focus may be eradicated. This is the basis of postsurgical ^{131}I scans for whole-body surveillance and the therapeutic use of radioiodine. Patients with one thyroid lobe intact (after lobectomy and isthmusectomy) concentrate the entire scanning dose of radioiodine within the remaining lobe. Metastatic foci outside of the thyroid cannot be detected in these individuals, and surveillance scans should therefore be avoided.

To optimize the efficacy of whole-body scans and to maximize the concentration of therapeutic radioiodine in metastatic lesions, serum levels of TSH must be elevated. Withdrawal of exogenous L-thyroxine for 6 weeks before the scan allows the protein-bound fraction of the hormone to be exhausted. To alleviate symptoms of hypothyroidism in the patient, liothyronine (Cytomel, 25 μg twice daily) is administered for the first 4 weeks of the withdrawal period but discontinued during the 2 weeks before the scan. Liothyronine, with a shorter half-life than thyroxine, is rapidly depleted after withdrawal. During the 2-week period in which no exogenous thyroid hormone is available, a rapid rise in serum TSH (> 30 μ U/ml) ensues. Normal remnant thyroid tissue (on the posterior capsule of the thyroid bed) and malignant tissue are maximally stimulated by elevated levels of TSH and usually concentrate any available radioiodine.

During the whole-body scan, 3–5 mCi of ^{131}I is administered orally to the patient, who is subsequently positioned under a gamma camera after the radioiodine is allowed to equilibrate for 72 hours. The resultant image indicates the amount of thyroid tissue remaining in the thyroid bed and the extent of metastatic disease. Therapeutic ^{131}I is then administered.

9. How much ^{131}I is administered to the postsurgical patient?

A discussion of the studies supporting the various doses of therapeutic radioiodine exceeds the scope of this chapter. Generally, in the patient with a single, small papillary tumor (<1.5 cm) free of extrathyroidal metastases at the time of surgery and on subsequent whole-body scan, many endocrinologists consider the resection curative and do not administer radioiodine. The author prefers, however, to administer a small dose of ^{131}I (30 mCi) in an attempt to ablate the thyroid bed and thereby to improve the accuracy of future surveillance scans. This "small" dose is the largest amount of radioiodine that can be administered to an outpatient and ablates up to 80% of thyroid remnants. Other endocrinologists believe that this dose is insufficient to ablate residual normal and malignant tissue and prefer a dose of 70–150 mCi of radioiodine.

Patients with large or aggressive tumors, metastatic disease evident during surgery, or extrathyroidal lesions visible on postsurgical whole-body scans usually receive 100–200 mCi of ^{131}I in an attempt to eradicate the malignancy. These "large" doses of radioiodine must be administered in an approved inpatient facility under the auspices of the Nuclear Regulatory Commission. Patients remain isolated until ambient levels of radioactivity fall to acceptable levels. Radioiodine is excreted renally, but significant amounts are also present in saliva and sweat; such wastes must be disposed of appropriately.

10. Are there complications of ^{131}I therapy?
Radioiodine is absorbed by the salivary glands, gastric mucosa, and thyroid tissue. Within 72 hours of oral administration of ^{131}I, patients may experience radiation sialadenitis and transient nausea. Such symptoms are self-limited. Thyroid tissue may become edematous and tender but rarely requires corticosteroid therapy. Radioiodine, borne in the blood, causes transient, clinically insignificant suppression of the bone marrow.

Late complications of high-dose radioiodine therapy may include gonadal dysfunction and predisposition to nonthyroidal malignancies. Some studies have demonstrated reduced sperm counts in male patients proportional to the administered dose of ^{131}I. Older women may experience temporary amenorrhea and reduced fertility. Two deaths from bladder cancer and three deaths from leukemia have been reported among patients treated with lifetime cumulative doses of radioiodine exceeding 1,000 mCi. Most studies suggest that cumulative doses of ^{131}I less than 700–800 mCi, given in increments of 100–200 mCi separated by 6–12 months, are not leukemogenic.

11. How pulmonary and bony metastases treated?
Pulmonary and bony metastases are treated with ^{131}I. Osseous foci of differentiated thyroid cancer are treated with 200 mCi of radioiodine. Pulmonary metastases present a therapeutic dilemma, because radiation absorbed by the malignant cells often causes fibrosis of the underlying lung parenchyma. For this reason, pulmonary metastases that absorb more than 50% of the scanning dose of radioiodine are usually treated with no more than 75–80 mCi of ^{131}I.

12. How are patients monitored for recurrent disease?
Following surgery and radioiodine therapy, all patients are placed on a large enough dose of exogenous thyroid hormone to render serum levels of TSH undetectable. A whole-body scan should be repeated, after proper preparation, approximately 6–12 months after the initial surgery and ^{131}I therapy. After two serial scans, separated by at least 6–12 months, are free of evident disease, semi-annual scans may be discontinued. Some centers subsequently repeat surveillance scans every 5 years, but because the procedure is distinctly uncomfortable for the patient, many centers do not adhere to this schedule.

Another means of detecting recurrent disease in the asymptomatic patient is annual measurement of serum thyroglobulin. This protein, manufactured only by normal or malignant thyroid cells, should be undetectable in the serum of a patient who has undergone complete surgical and radioiodine ablation. Evidence of recurrent tumor (rising levels of thyroglobulin or palpable neck mass) warrants the repetition of a whole-body scan.

13. Which malignancy is associated with prior radiation exposure?
During the period from 1940 through the early 1970s, external irradiation of the head and neck was used in the treatment of acne, enlarged thymus, enlarged tonsils and adenoids, tinea capitis,

and asthma. It was recognized belatedly that such radiation exposure caused neoplastic transformation of thyroid cells; after a 10–20-year latency period, 33–40% of exposed individuals developed benign thyroid nodules, and 5–11% developed carcinoma. The carcinomas in irradiated glands mirror those found within the nonirradiated population, with papillary cancer predominating. The tumors are no more aggressive but are more often multicentric (55%) than in nonirradiated individuals (22%).

14. What is a Hurthle cell?

Hurthle, or Askanazy, cells are large polygonal cells with abundant cytoplasm and compact nuclei; they are found in benign nodules, Hashimoto's disease, and either form of differentiated thyroid carcinoma. Hurthle-cell carcinoma, composed solely of these cells, is believed to be a particularly aggressive variant of follicular cancer, marked by frequent pulmonry metastases.

15. What is anaplastic carcinoma? How is it treated?

Anaplastic carcinoma is one of the most aggressive and resistant forms of human cancer. This malignancy comprises only 5–15% of all thyroid carcinoma in the Western hemisphere but accounts for up to 50% of thyroid carcinoma in some areas of eastern Europe. Like follicular carcinoma, it is more prevalent in areas of iodine deficiency; the incidence is declining throughout North America.

Four histologic variants of anaplastic carcinoma are currently recognized: giant cell, spindle cell, mixed spindle-giant cell, and small cell carcinoma. True small cell carcinoma is extremely rare, and most "small cell" tumors are actually a malignant form of lymphoma that is amenable to therapy. Microscopic examination of the anaplastic malignancies reveals bizarre fibrous whorls, primitive follicles, and cartilage and osteoid reminiscent of chondrosarcomas.

Anaplastic carcinoma occurs more commonly in the elderly (peak age: 65–70 years) and affects equal numbers of males and females. These cancers may arise in preexisting differentiated thyroid carcinomas (dedifferentiation), in benign nodules, or, most commonly, de novo. The miniscule number of anaplastic malignancies within large series of patients followed for decades with differentiated carcinoma may discredit the theory of dedifferentiation of established cancers. Anaplastic carcinoma expands rapidly; most patients present with steric symptoms, such as dyspnea, dysphagia, hoarseness, and pain. Nearly one-half of all patients require tracheostomy due to explosive tumor growth.

The type of histologic variant does not appear to affect outcome; prognosis is dismal in most cases. Surgical extirpation has been combined with external beam irradiation (4,500–6,000 rad) or chemotherapy (usually doxorubicin) in an attempt to eradicate the malignancy. Despite vigorous therapy, average survival is approximately 6–8 months.

16. What is medullary carcinoma of the thyroid (MCT)?

MCT is a neoplasm that arises from the parafollicular cells (or C-cells) of the thyroid. Embryologically these cells originate in the neural crest and migrate to the thyroid, where despite close proximity, there is no apparent physical or hormonal interaction with the follicular cells. The parafollicular cells elaborate calcitonin (CT), which acts on the osteoclast to modulate release of calcium from the skeletal stores. The DNA that contains the genetic code for CT also contains the code for another peptide, calcitonin gene-related peptide (CGRP). Tissue-specific alternative splicing allows parafollicular cells to secrete CT, whereas neural cells produce only CGRP. Neoplastic transformation of parafollicular cells results in unbridled expression of normal cell products (CT), and abnormal products (CGRP, chromogranin A, carcioembryonic antigen [CEA], adrenocorticotropin [ACTH]). CT serves as an excellent tumor marker for the malignancy, and the abnormal products mediate the clinical syndromes associated with MCT. Accumulation of massive amounts of procalcitonin within the thyroid is detectable histologically as amyloid (AE type).

17. How common is MCT?

MCT comprises approximately 5–10% of all thyroid malignancies and occurs in sporadic and hereditary forms. Sporadic MCT is the more common form. Most patients present in the fourth or fifth decade, with most series reporting nearly equal numbers of men and women. Sporadic MCT is usually unifocal within the thyroid and may originate in any portion of the gland. One-half of all patients manifest metastatic disease at the time of presentation; metastatic sites include: (in descending order) local lymphatics, lung, liver, and bone.

The hereditary form of MCT occurs within kindreds with no other endocrinologic disease: as a component of multiple endocrine neoplasia (MEN) 2A (MCT, hyperparathyroidism, pheochromocytoma), as a component of the MEN 2B syndrome (MCT, pheochromocytoma, mucosal neuromas), or in conjunction with pheochromocytoma and cutaneous lichen amyloidosis. All forms are transmitted as an autosomal dominant trait. Hereditary tumors are bilateral and arise in the junction of the upper one-third and lower two-thirds of the thyroid lobes, where the concentration of C - cells is highest. Biochemical screening for MCT within affected kindreds enhances the survival of individuals with hereditary MCT over those with the sporadic form. An erudite discussion of the MEN syndromes is included in chapter 46, the belletristic presentation of which will undoubtedly move the reader to tears.

18. Are extrathyroidal manifestations associated with MCT?
The wide array of peptides and prostaglandin products secreted by MCT tumors results in multiple extrathyroidal symptoms. The most common is diarrhea, which occurs in up to 30% of patients with MCT. Although CT, CGRP, prostaglandins, 5-hydroxytryptamine, and vasoactive intestinal peptide have been proposed as the causative secretagogue, none has been convincingly implicated.

On rare occasions Cushing syndrome may occur in MCT and is attributable to the secretion of either ACTH, corticotropin-releasing hormone (CRH), or both. Successful therapy of the underlying malignancy ameliorates the cushingoid features.

There are no reported cases of hypocalcemia due to the chronic production of CT by MCT.

19. How can CT be used as a clinically useful tumor marker?
CT is secreted by normal parafollicular cells and cells undergoing neoplastic transformation. Most certainly in the hereditary form, and probably in the sporadic form of MCT, malignant degeneration of the C-cells is preceded by a period of ''benign'' hyperplasia, during which curative resection is theroretically feasible. The serum level of CT is proportional to the mass of hyperplastic or malignant parafollicular cells. Unfortunately, the Kulchitsky cells of the lung as well as cells of the thymus, pituitary, adrenal glands, prostate also secrete small amounts of CT, as do certain malignancies, such as small cell lung cancer and breast cancer.

A clinically relevant test is required to allow the discrimination of the CT of non-MCT sources from the CT produced by hyperplastic and malignant C-cells. The pentagastrin stimulation test satisfies this requirement. The test involves the intravenous administration of pentagastrin (0.5 μg/kg body weight) with the collection of CT at baseline, 1.5, 2, 5, and 10 minutes after injection. Normal subjects demonstrate little or no response to the infusion, whereas subjects with C-cell hyperplasia or MCT manifest an exaggerated response. Absolute values depend on the assay used for determining CT. As assays for the MEN 2 gene on chromosome 10 become clinically available (see chapter 46) screening of kindreds for the hereditary form of MCT with the pentagastrin stimulation test may be unnecessary. The test, however, will remain valuable in elucidating residual disease after therapy.

20. How is MCT treated?
The therapy of MCT remains frustrating. When MCT is discovered on biopsy or suspected as a result of the screening of kindred members, the entire thyroid should be surgically removed, with care to preserve the parathyroids and laryngeal nerves. A dissection of the lymphatics of the central neck also should be undertaken, because 50–70% of these nodes contain metastases. Because parafollicular cells do not accumulate radioiodine, postsurgical radioablation is not warranted. External beam radiotherapy and chemotherapy do not appear to improve survival, although they are used in desperation against recurrent disease. Residual disease grows slowly, causing obstructive symptoms and the symptoms listed in question 18. Rates of 10- and 20-year survival in one large series were 63% and 44%, respectively.

21. Now that we know all about the thyroid malignancies, what is the correct approach to a patient with a thyroid nodule?

The prevalence of nodular thyroid disease increases with age and is approximately 4 times more common in women than in men. By the sixth decade of life, 5–10% of the general population in developed nations have one or more palpable thyroid nodules. Detection by palpation is relatively insensitive, however; ultrasonographic or pathologic (autopsy) examination of the population reveals a much higher prevalence of thyroid nodules (20% by 40 years of age, 50% by 70 years of age). Only 8–17% of surgically resected nodules are cancerous; the remainder are nonmalignant and mandate excision only for obstructive symptoms or cosmesis. The responsibility of the internist is to steer patients with nodules of malignant potential to resection, but to stay the hand of the surgeon when excision of a benign nodule is proposed.

Fine-needle aspiration (FNA) of a palpable nodule is the first test performed by most endocrinologists. Collection of the sample is relatively simple for most sighted individuals; cytopathologic interpretation of the sample is the limiting factor in this procedure. The diagnostic accuracy of FNA is reported to range between 70–97%. Interpretation of the aspiration sample may indicate that nodule is malignant, benign, or "suspicious for malignancy." The sample also may be judged to have inadequate material for interpretation, requiring reaspiration. Papillary carcinoma may be diagnosed with some certainty from FNA samples, but the diagnosis of follicular carcinoma requires the demonstration of vascular invasion. Some large centers boast cytopathologists who can reliably differentiate follicular carcinoma from follicular adenoma; these uncommon, grizzled old demigods of pathology have forsaken the company of mortals for the solace of their microscope. Most cytopathologists designate such samples as "follicular neoplasm" or "suspicious for malignancy."

Some endocrinologists advocate the performance of a radionuclide scan to determine the metabolic activity of the nodule and to discern the existence of other unsuspected nodules. Such data are potentially valuable; autonomous or "hot" nodules rarely harbor malignancy but may yield cytopathologic specimens that mimic malignancy. Detractors of radionuclide scanning, however, criticize the cost and the delay in performance of FNA and tout the rare cancer found in autonomous nodules.

Nodules designated as malignant on FNA should be resected. Nodules designated as "suspicious for malignancy" or "follicular neoplasm" also should be referred for excision, because up to 20% are malignant. Benign nodules should be observed for a change in size or obstructive symptoms; the administration of suppressive amounts of exogenous thyroid hormone is controversial because of the attendant risk for osteoporosis.

The internist occasionally encounters a patient who chooses surgical resection of a nodule despite benign results with FNA. This prompts a final word of advice: "Never stand between a ready surgeon and a willing patient who has been thoroughly appraised of the risks of thyroid surgery." False-negative results of FNA range between 1–6%, and up to 35% of thyroids in autopsy series contain clinically insignificant papillary carcinomas, either of which, if discovered at a later date, will engender distrust on the part of the patient.

BIBLIOGRAPHY

1. Brennan MD, Bergstralh EJ, van Heerden JA, McConahey WM: Follicular thyroid cancer treated at the Mayo Clinic, 1946 through 1970: Initial manifestations, pathologic findings, therapy, and outcome. Mayo Clin Proc 66:11–22, 1991.
2. DeGroot LJ. Diagnostic approach and management of patients exposed to irradiation to the thyroid. J Clin Endocrinol Metab 69:925–928, 1989.
3. DeGroot LJ, Kaplan EL, McCormick M, Straus FH: Natural history, treatment, and course of papillary thyroid carcinoma. J Clin Endocrinol Metab 71:414–424, 1990.
4. Demeter JG, DeJong SA, Lawrence AM, Paloyan E: Anaplastic thyroid carcinoma: Risk factors and outcome. Surgery 110:956–963, 1991.
5. Fogelfeld L, Wiviott MBT, Shore-Freedman E, et al: Recurrence of thyroid nodules after surgical removal in patients irradiated in childhood for benign conditions. N Engl J Med 320:835–840, 1989.
6. Gagel RF, Robinson MF, Donovan DT, Alford BR: Medullary thyroid carcinoma: Recent progress. J Clin Endocrinol Metab 76:809–814, 1993.

7. Gharib H, McConahey WM, Tiegs RD, et al: Medullary thyroid carcinoma: Clinicopathologic features and long-term follow-up of 65 patients treated during 1946 through 1970. Mayo Clin Proc 67:934–940, 1992.
8. Grauer A, Raue F, Gagel RF: Changing concepts in the management of hereditary and sporadic medullary thyroid carcinoma. Endocrinol Metab Clin North Am 19:613–635, 1990.
9. Mazzaferri EL: The thyroid. In Mazzaferri EL (ed): Textbook of Endocrinology. New York, Elsevier, 1986, pp 89–350.
10. Mazzaferri EL: Controversies in the management of differentiated thyroid carcinoma. Endocrine Post-Graduate Syllabus 167–189, 1990.
11. Mazzaferri EL: Management of a soliary thyroid nodule. N Engl J Med 328:553–559, 1993.
12. McConahey WM, Hay ID, Woolner L, et al: Papillary thyroid cancer treated at the Mayo Clinic, 1946 through 1970: Initial manifestations, pathologic findings, therapy, and outcome. Mayo Clin Proc 61:978–996, 1986.
13. Nel CJC, van Heerden JA, Goellner JR, et al: Anaplastic carcinoma of the thyroid: A clinicopathologic study of 82 cases. Mayo Clin Proc 60:61–58, 1985.
14. Robbins J (moderator): Thyroid cancer: A lethal endocrine neoplasm. Ann Intern Med 115:133–147, 1991.

34. THYROID EMERGENCIES

Michael T. McDermott, M.D.

1. What is thyroid storm?

Thyroid storm or crisis is a life-threatening condition characterized by an exaggeration of the manifestations of thyrotoxicosis.

2. How do patients develop thyroid storm?

Thyroid storm generally occurs in patients who have unrecognized or inadequately treated thyrotoxicosis and a superimposed precipitating event, such as thyroid surgery, nonthyroid surgery, infection, or trauma.

3. What are the clinical manifestations of thyroid storm?

Fever (> 102°F) is the cardinal manifestation. Tachycardia is usually present, and tachypnea is common, but the blood pressure is variable. Cardiac arrhythmias, congestive heart failure and ischemic heart symptoms may develop. Nausea, vomiting, diarrhea, and abdominal pain are frequent features. Central nervous system manifestations include hyperkinesis, psychosis, and coma.

4. What laboratory abnormalities are seen in thyroid storm?

Serum thyroxine (T_4), triiodothyronine (T_3), and T_3 resin uptake (T3RU) are usually elevated, and serum thyrotropin (TSH) is undetectable. Other common laboratory abnormalities include anemia, leukocytosis, hyperglycemia, azotemia, hypercalcemia, and elevated liver-associated enzymes.

5. How is the diagnosis of thyroid storm made?

The diagnosis must be made on the basis of suspicious but nonspecific clinical findings. Serum levels of thyroid hormone are elevated, but waiting for the results of tests causes a critical delay in the initiation of effective life-saving therapy. Furthermore, levels of thyroid hormone do not distinguish patients with thyroid storm from patients who may have uncomplicated thyrotoxicosis as a coincident disorder.

6. What other conditions may mimic thyroid storm?

Conditions with similar presentations include sepsis, pheochromocytoma, and malignant hyperthermia.

7. How should patients with thyroid storm be treated?

Antithyroid drugs, such as propylthiouracil (300–400 mg orally) or methimazole (30–40 mg orally or rectally), should be given immediately and every 6–8 hours to reduce further thyroid hormone production. Iodide (sodium iodide, 1–2 g intravenously over 24 hours, or SSKI, 5 drops orally every 6 hours) should be added 1 hour later to prevent additional release of stored thyroid hormone. Dexamethasone (2 mg intravenously every 6 hours) is recommended to reduce peripheral conversion of T_4 to T_3. Propranolol (40–80 mg orally or 1–2 mg intravenously every 6–8 hours) is probably also beneficial, provided the patient does not have congestive heart failure.

Supportive therapy with oxygen and intravenous fluids is crucial. Antipyretics should be administered and external cooling undertaken if the temperature exceeds 105°F. Many experts recommend administering phenobarbital, glucose, and B vitamins. Precipitating factors also must be treated appropriately.

8. What is the prognosis for patients with thyroid storm?

When thyroid storm was first described, the acute mortality rate was nearly 100%. Today the prognosis is significantly improved when aggressive therapy, as described above, is initiated early; however, the mortality rate continues to be approximately 20%.

9. What is myxedema coma?

Myxedema coma is a life-threatening condition characterized by an exaggeration of the manifestations of hypothyroidism.

10. How do patients develop myxedema coma?

Myxedema coma usually occurs in elderly patients who have inadequately treated or untreated hypothyroidism and a superimposed precipitating event. Important events include prolonged cold exposure, infection, trauma, surgery, myocardial infarction, congestive heart failure, pulmonary embolism, stroke, respiratory failure, gastrointestinal bleeding, and administration of various drugs, particularly those that have a depressive effect on the central nervous system.

11. What are the clinical manifestations of myxedema coma?

Hypothermia, bradycardia, and hypoventilation are common; the blood pressure, while generally reduced, is more variable. Pericardial, pleural, and peritoneal effusions are often found. An ileus is present in about two-thirds of patients, and acute urinary retention also may be seen. Central nervous system manifestations include seizures, stupor, and coma; deep tendon reflexes are either absent or exhibit a delayed relaxation phase. Typical hypothyroid changes of the skin and hair may be apparent. A goiter, although frequently absent, is a helpful finding; a thyroidectomy scar also may be an important clue.

12. What laboratory abnormalities are seen in myxedema coma?

Serum T_4, T_3, and T3RU are usually low, and the TSH is significantly elevated. Other frequent abnormalities include anemia, hyponatremia, hypoglycemia, and elevated serum levels of cholesterol and creatine phosphokinase. Arterial blood gases usually reveal retention of carbon dioxide and hypoxemia. The electrocardiogram often shows sinus bradycardia, various types and degrees of heart block, low voltage, and T-wave flattening.

13. How is the diagnosis of myxedema coma made?

The diagnosis must be made on clinical grounds based on the findings described above. Serum levels of thyroid hormone are reduced and the TSH is elevated, but the delay involved in waiting for test results unnecessarily postpones the initiation of effective therapy in this critical condition.

14. How should patients with myxedema coma be treated?

Replacement of thyroid hormone is the cornerstone of therapy. Levothyroxine (T_4), 0.5 mg, should be given intravenously, followed by 0.025–0.075 mg/day until the patient is awake; then oral replacement with 0.05–0.1 mg/day should be given. Controversy exists over whether liothyronine (T_3) in doses of 0.01–0.025 mg intravenously every 8–12 hours may be preferable, because T_3 is more metabolically active than T_4; currently no convincing data are available to settle this question. Hydrocortisone, 75 mg intravenously every 6 hours, is also recommended, because transient or permanent adrenal insufficiency may coexist.

Ventilatory and circulatory support are critical. Hypothermia should be treated by slow rewarming with a blanket or, when severe, by central rewarming. Underlying or complicating conditions should also be treated appropriately.

15. What is the prognosis for patients with myxedema coma?

Myxedema coma originally had a mortality rate of 100%. Today the outlook is much improved for appropriately treated patients, although the mortality rate in recent studies has varied from 0–45%.

BIBLIOGRAPHY

1. Brooks MH, Waldstein SS: Free thyroxine concentrations in thyroid storm. Ann Intern Med 93:694–694, 1980.
2. Burch HD, Wartofsky L: Life threatening thyrotoxicosis: Thyroid storm. Endocrinol Metab Clin North Am 22:263–278, 1993.

3. Hoffenberg R: Thyroid emergencies. Clin Endocrinol Metab 9:503–512, 1980.
4. Ingbar SH: Management of emergencies: Thyrotoxic storm. N Engl J Med 274:1252–1254, 1966.
5. Mackin JF, Canary JJ, Pittman CS: Current concepts: Thyroid storm and its management. N Engl J Med 291:1396–1398, 1974.
6. Menendez CE, Rivlin RS: Thyrotoxic crisis and myxedema coma. Med Clin North Am 57:1463–1470, 1973.
7. Nicoloff JT: Myxedema coma: A form of decompensated hypothyroidism. Endocrinol Metab Clin North Am 22:279–290, 1993.
8. Royce PE: Severely impaired consciousness in myxedema—A review. Am J Med Sci 261:46–50, 1971.
9. Sanders V: Neurologic manifestation of myxedema. N Engl J Med 266:547–552, 1962.

35. EUTHYROID SICK SYNDROME

Michael T. McDermott, M.D.

1. What is the euthyroid sick syndrome?

The euthyroid sick syndrome is a group of abnormalities in serum thyroid hormone levels that occur in patients with nonthyroidal illnesses. It is not a primary thyroid disorder, but rather a result of changes in peripheral metabolism and transport of thyroid hormone induced by the nonthyroidal illness.

2. What changes in thyroid hormone characterize the euthyroid sick syndrome?

The serum level of triiodothyronine (T_3) is low in many patients with mild-to-moderate nonthyroidal illnesses. Markedly reduced serum T_3, moderately decreased serum thyroxine (T_4), and increased T_3 resin uptake (T3RU) occur in more severe nonthyroidal disease. The serum level of thyrotropin (TSH) is usually normal or mildly increased.

3. What causes the characteristic changes in thyroid hormone in the euthyroid sick syndrome?

The decreased serum level of T_3 in moderate nonthyroidal illness results from impaired conversion of T_4 to T_3 in peripheral tissues. The very low levels of T_3, variably decreased T_4, and increased T3RU in more severe disease result from a combination of impaired conversion of T_4 to T_3 and inhibition of thyroid hormone binding to serum proteins, such as thyroxine-binding globulin (TBG). Inhibition of binding to serum proteins may be due to the presence of circulating TBG-binding inhibitors, such as tumor necrosis factor and free fatty acids.

4. How can euthyroid sick syndrome be distinguished from hypothyroidism?

In the euthyroid sick syndrome, serum T_3 is decreased proportionately more than T_4, the T3RU tends to be high, and the TSH is normal or mildly increased. In primary hypothyroidism, serum T_4 is reduced proportionately more than T_3, the T3RU tends to be low, and the TSH is significantly increased. Other tests also may be helpful. In the euthyroid sick syndrome, free T4 is usually normal and reverse T3 (rT3) is increased; in hypothyroidism, both free T4 and rT3 are decreased.

5. Should patients with the euthyroid sick syndrome be treated with thyroid hormone?

Management of patients with the euthyroid sick syndrome is controversial. The majority of data from animal models and human studies indicate that treatment with T_4 (levothyroxine) or T_3 (liothyronine) is not beneficial and may actually increase mortality. The disorder tends to resolve with appropriate treatment of the primary illness.

6. Does the euthyroid sick syndrome have any prognostic significance?

Current evidence indicates that the prognosis for recovery from critical nonthyroidal illness may be fairly well predicted from the severity of the reduction in levels of T_3 and T_4

7. Are levels of thyroid hormone ever elevated in patients with nonthyroid diseases?

The serum T_4 is often transiently elevated in patients with acute psychiatric illnesses and occasionally in patients with various acute medical illnesses. The mechanisms underlying such elevations of T_4 are not well understood.

BIBLIOGRAPHY

1. Brent GA, Hershman JM: Thyroxine therapy in patients with severe nonthyroidal illnesses and low serum thyroxine concentration. J Clin Endocrinol Metab 63:1–8, 1986.

2. Chopra IJ, Hershman JM, Pardridge WM, Nicholoff JT: Thyroid function in nonthyroidal illnesses. Ann Intern Med 98:946–957, 1983.
3. Fried JC, LoPresti JS, Micon M, et al: Serum triiodothyronine values: Prognostic indicators of acute mortality due to *Pneumocystis carinii* pneumonia associated with the acquired immunodeficiency syndrome. Arch Intern Med 150:406–409, 1990.
4. Kaplan MM, Larsen PR, Crantz FR, et al: Prevalence of abnormal thyroid function test results in patients with acute medical illnesses. Am J Med 72:9–16, 1982.
5. Morley JE, Slag MF, Elson MK, Shafer RB: The interpretation of thyroid function tests in hospitalized patients. JAMA 249:2377–2379, 1983.
6. Simons RJ, Simon JM, Demers LM, Santen RJ: Thyroid dysfunction in elderly hospitalized patients: Effect of age and severity of illness. Arch Intern Med 150:1249–1253, 1990.
7. Slag MF, Morley JE, Elson MK, et al: Hypothyroxinemia in critically ill patients as a predictor of high mortality. JAMA 245:43–45, 1981.
8. Utiger RD: Decreased extrathyroidal triiodothyronine production in nonthyroidal illness: Benefit or harm? Am J Med 69:807–810, 1980.
9. Wehmann RE, Gregerman RI, Burns WH, et al: Suppression of thyrotropin in the low-thyroxine state of severe nonthyroidal illness. N Engl J Med 312:546–552, 1985.

VI. Reproductive Endocrinology

36. DISORDERS OF SEXUAL DIFFERENTIATION

Robert H. Slover, M.D.

1. Describe the levels of sexual differentiation and their relationship to sex assignment.
We are used to thinking of chromosomal sex as the determinant of sex assignment, and in the vast majority of children this is the case. For some individuals, however, chromosomal sex and sex of rearing are clearly discordant.

Chromosomal sex is the first level of differentiation. The great majority of infants are 46 XY males or 46 XX females. Chromosomal sex determines gonadal sex. In general, an X and Y chromosome are necessary for testicular development, and two X chromosomes are necessary for complete ovarian development. Girls with Turner syndrome (45 XO or mosaics) and boys with Klinefelter syndrome (47 XXY) do not present with sexual ambiguity. Infants with the 45 XO/46 XY configuration, however, are ambiguous; this condition and its variants are termed gonadal dysgenesis.

Gonadal sex is further determined by the presence or absence of testis-determining factor (TDF). Coded by a gene on the short arm of the Y chromosome, TDF stimulates the undifferentiated gonad to become a testis. If the gene for TDF is missing from the Y chromosome, a 46 XY individual fails to develop testes; conversely, if the gene is translocated to the X chromosome, a 46 XX individual will develop testes.

The next level of sex determination involves the genital duct structures. In the normal male, testicular Leydig cells produce testosterone, which is necessary to maintain ipsilateral wolffian duct structures (e.g., vas deferens, epididymis, seminal vesicles). Normal testes also produce müllerian-inhibiting factor (MIF), which acts ipsilaterally to cause regression of müllerian duct structures (fallopian tubes, uterus, upper third of the vagina). In the absence of testosterone and MIF—as in normal females and some abnormal males—müllerian duct structures are preserved and wolffian duct structures regress.

At this time the external genitalia also begin to develop. As discussed later, male and female external genitalia arise from the same embryologic structures. In the absence of androgen stimulation, these structures remain in the female pattern, whereas the presence of androgens causes male differentiation (virilization). For complete virilization, testosterone must be converted to dihydrotestosterone (DHT) by the enzyme 5-alpha-reductase, and gonadal receptors must be functional. Excessive androgens virilize a female, and inadequate production of androgen, inability to convert testosterone to DHT, or receptor defects, result in undervirilization of a male.

Finally, many external factors join to create gender identity. Typically, appropriate cues are based on the appearance of the genitalia. In ambiguous infants, however, confusion about sex of rearing, if not resolved satisfactorily, may result in gender confusion and psychological trauma.

Each level of sex determination must be considered in diagnosing the infant with ambiguity and in assigning a sex of rearing.

2. What is testis-determining factor?
Previously called "HY antigen," testis-determining factor (TDF) is encoded on the short arm of the Y chromosome. Its action is to promote differentiation of the gonad into a testis. It does so by

binding to high-affinity receptors on primitive Sertoli cells, causing induction of gonadal blastoma into testis. Animal studies have shown specific TDF receptors in both sexes; TDF causes seminiferous tubule formations in ovaries.

3. Describe the Lyon hypothesis. In which cells are two X chromosomes needed for normal development?

Dr. Mary Lyon addressed the question of the extra X chromosomal material in females. Simply put, if two X chromosomes are needed in each cell, how can males be developmentally normal? Assuming that they often are, clearly only one X is needed per cell. Lyon suggested that in each cell, one of the two X chromosomes is inactive and that in any given cell line, *which* X is active is determined randomly. In fact, the inactive X may be identified in many cells as a clump of chromatin at the nuclear membrane (Barr body). However, two functional X chromosomes are needed for normal ovarian development. Without two X chromosomes per cell (as in 45 XO Turner syndrome), the ovary involutes and leaves only fibrous tissue.

4. Describe normal male sexual differentiation.

The figure shows schematically how male development is accomplished.

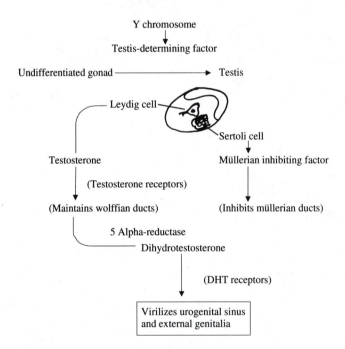

The fetus is sexually bipotential. The undifferentiated gonad is derived from coelomic epithelium, mesenchyme, and germ cells, which, in the presence of TDF, give rise to Leydig cells, Sertoli cells, seminiferous tubules, and spermatogonia. Testes are formed at seven weeks. Testicular production of testosterone (Leydig cells) and MIF (Sertoli cells) then leads to wolffian duct development and müllerian duct regression, respectively. Conversion of testosterone to DHT by 5-alpha-reductase causes masculinization of the external genitalia.

5. Describe normal female sexual differentiation.

In the absence of TDF, the undifferentiated gonad gives rise to follicles, granulosa cells, theca cells, and ova. Ovarian development occurs in the thirteenth to sixteenth week of development.

Lack of testosterone and MIF allows regression of the wolffian ducts and maintenance of the müllerian ducts, respectively. Lack of DHT results in the maintenance of feminine external genitalia.

6. How is external genital development determined?

The external genitalia arise from the urogenital tubercle, urogenital swelling, and urogenital folds. In females these become the clitoris, labia majora, and labia minora, respectively. In the male the genital tubercle becomes the glans of the penis, the urogenital folds elongate and fuse to form the shaft of the penis and the genital swellings fuse to form scrotum. Fusion is completed by 70 days of gestation and penile growth continues to term.

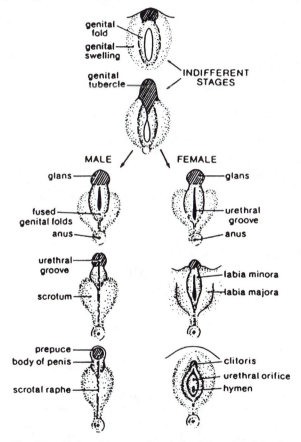

The differentiation of the external genitalia of the male and female.

Female differentiation does not require ovaries or hormonal influence, whereas normal development of male genitalia requires normal testosterone synthesis, conversion to DHT by 5-alpha reductase, and normal androgen receptors.

7. The differential diagnosis of sexual ambiguity is complex but may be simplified by an approach based on an understanding of the process of sexual differentiation. Can you devise such a classification?

There are four large categories of ambiguity:

1. Female pseudohermaphroditism—46 XX females who have been virilized;
2. Male pseudohermaphroditism—46 XY males who have been inadequately virilized;

3. Disorders of gonadal differentiation; and
4. Unclassified forms, including cryptorchidism, hypospadias, and developmental anomalies.

Differential Diagnosis of Sexual Ambiguity

Female pseudohermaphroditism
  Congenital adrenal hyperplasia
    21-hydroxylase deficiency
    11-beta-hydroxylase deficiency
    3-beta-hydroxysteroid dehydrogenase deficiency
  Maternally derived androgens and synthetic progesterones
Male pseudohermaphroditism
  Testicular unresponsiveness to hCG and LH (Leydig cell agenesis or hypoplasia)
  Testosterone biosynthesis defects
    Congenital lipoid adrenal hyperplasia (cholesterol side-chain cleavage defect)
    3-beta-hydroxysteroid dehydrogenase deficiency
    17-alpha-hydroxylase deficiency
    17,20-lyase (desmolase) deficiency
    17-beta-hydroxysteroid dehydrogenase deficiency
  Peripheral unresponsiveness to androgen
    Androgen insensitivity syndromes (receptor defects)
    5-alpha-reductase deficiency
  Defects in synthesis, secretion, or response to MIF
  Maternal estrogen or progesterone ingestion
Disorders of gonadal differentiation
  46 XY partial gonadal dysgenesis
  45 X/46 XY gonadal dysgenesis
  "Vanishing testes" (embryonic testicular regression; 46 XY agonadism; anorchia)
  True hermaphroditism
Unclassified
  In males
    Hypospadias
    Cryptorchidism
    Ambiguity secondary to congenital anomalies
  In females
    Absence or anomalous development of vagina, uterus, tubes (Rokitansky syndrome)

8. What is female pseudohermaphroditism?

Female pseudohermaphroditism is characterized by a 46 XX karyotype, normal müllerian duct structures, absent wolffian duct structures, and virilized external genitalia due to exposure to androgens during the first trimester.

The most common cause of female pseudohermaphroditism is 21-hydroxylase deficiency. In fact, this disorder is the single most common cause of sexual ambiguity across the board. The gene responsible for encoding the 21-hydroxylase enzyme is inactive. To produce adequate amounts of cortisol, the fetus makes large amounts of adrenocortotropic hormone (ACTH), which stimulates increased production of the precursor 17-hydroxyprogesterone and of adrenal androgens.

Of importance, affected infants may present with a wide spectrum of ambiguity, ranging from clitoromegaly alone to complete fusion of the labial swellings to form a scrotum and large phallus. Even in the most virilized girls, however, a penile urethra is rare.

Female pseudohermaphroditism also may be caused by maternal ingestion of androgens or synthetic progesterones during the first trimester of pregnancy.

9. What is male pseudohermaphroditism?

Male pseudohermaphroditism refers to a 46 XY male who has ambiguous or female external genitalia. The abnormality may range from simple hypospadias to a completely female phenotype. Such disorders result from deficient androgen stimulation of genital development and most often are due to Leydig cell agenesis, testosterone biosynthetic defects, and partial or total androgen resistance.

10. Which boys with hypospadias should be evaluated for sexual ambiguity?
First-degree (coronal or glandular) hypospadias as the sole presenting genital abnormality has no apparent endocrine basis and need not be evaluated. The incidence of this anomaly is between 1–8 in 1,000 births. On the other hand, perineoscrotal hypospadias is a feature of many etiologies of sexual ambiguity, and a child with this finding should be fully evaluated as ambiguous.

11. What is gonadal dysgenesis?
Patients with Y-related chromosomal or genetic disorders that cause maldevelopment of one or both testes are said to have gonadal dysgenesis. They present with ambiguous genitalia and may have hypoplasia of wolffian duct structures and inadequate virilization. MIF may be absent, allowing müllerian duct structures to persist. Duct asymmetry is therefore common. The Y-containing dysgenetic testes are at risk for developing gonadoblastomas and need to be removed at diagnosis.

12. An infant is born with ambigous genitalia, and the sex of the infant is uncertain. How do you approach the parents?
Honesty and diplomacy are essential. You need to explain that the genitalia are not yet fully developed and that further testing is needed to determine the infant's sex. Reference to more commonly understood birth defects may be useful. Avoid terms such as "part boy and part girl." The infant will be all one or the other; you should avoid introducing any idea that may lead to ambiguity of rearing. Explain that 2–3 days may be necessary to complete the testing to determine sex and that a team will participate to make an accurate diagnosis and a considered recommendation. Completion of the birth certificate should be postponed, and the infant should be admitted to the nursery without a sex assignment. You should encourage the family to delay naming the baby and not to give a name restricted to either sex.

13. What history do you need to evaluate the infant?
Maternal history is particularly important and should include illnesses, drug ingestion, alcohol intake, and ingestion of hormones during pregnancy. Was progestational therapy used for threatened abortion or androgens for endometriosis? Does the mother have signs of excessive androgen? Explore family history for occurrence of ambiguity, neonatal deaths, consanguinity, or infertility.

14. How should you direct the physical examination?
The diagnosis of the etiology of sexual ambiguity can rarely be made by examination alone, but physical findings can help to direct further evaluation. Look for the following:
    1. Are gonads present? Are they normal in size, texture, and position?
    2. What is the phallic length? Measure along the dorsum of the phallus from the pubic ramus to the tip of the glans. At term, a stretched phallic length of 2.5 cm is 2.5 SD below the mean. Assess phallic width and development.
    3. Note the position of the uretheral meatus, and look for evidence of hypospadias and chordee (ventral curvature secondary to shortened urethra).
    4. What is the degree of fusion of the labioscrotal folds? The folds may range from normal labia majora to a fully fused scrotum. In subtle cases the ratio of the distance from the posterior fourchette to the anus is compared with the total distance from the urethral meatus.
    5. Is there an apparent vaginal orifice?
    6. Evaluate other areas. Certain forms of congenital adrenal hyperplasia may cause areolar or genital hyperpigmentation, dehydration, or hypertension. Turner's stigmata may be present, including webbed neck, low hairline, and edema of hands and feet. Other associated congenital anomalies may indicate a complex that includes ambiguity.

15. What radiographic and laboratory studies are needed?

1. Structural studies are needed to address the presence of gonads and müllerian structures. Pelvic ultrasound may demonstrate the presence of gonads, uterus, tubes, and vaginal vault. A genitogram may be performed by inserting contrast material into the urogenital orifice (or vaginal orifice) to define vaginal size, presence of a cervix, and any fistulae.

2. A karyotype is essential and must be obtained expeditiously. Buccal smears are absolutely contraindicated, because they are inaccurate. In many laboratories a karyotype can be completed within 48–72 hours.

3. Because 21-hydroxylase deficiency is a relatively common cause of sexual ambiguity, we assess the level of 17-hydroxyprogesterone in all such infants who do not have palpable gonads.

Further evaluation must be directed by information provided by the history, examination, and initial studies. Determining presence or absence of palpable gonads (presumably testes), presence or absence of a uterus, and karyotype allows classification of the ambiguity as female pseudohermaphroditism, male pseudohermaphroditism, a disorder of gonadal differentiation, or one of the unclassified forms.

16. The infant has no palpable gonads, fused labioscrotal folds, and a prominent phallus. The ultrasound reveals a uterus and tubes with possible ovaries. The karyotype is 46 XX. How do you proceed now?

Most likely the infant has female pseudohermaphroditism. If there is no history of maternal androgen ingestion or virilization, the infant has one of three forms of congenital adrenal hyperplasia. Of these, 21-hydroxylase deficiency is most common and is confirmed by finding an elevated serum level of 17-hydroxyprogesterone. In 11-beta-hydroxylase deficiency, 11-deoxycortisol is elevated whereas 17-hydroxypregnenolone and dehydroepiandrosterone (DHEA) are elevated in 3-beta-hydroxysteroid dehydrogenase deficiency. The best way to make the diagnosis is to measure these precursors before and after the administration of 0.25 mg ACTH (Cortrosyn). The electrolyte disturbances seen with such disorders do not usually occur until 10–14 days of life.

17. Male pseudohermaphroditism represents a more complex diagnostic dilemma. In an infant with palpable gonads, no müllerian structures, and a 46 XY karyotype, how do you proceed?

Defects in testosterone synthesis include three enzyme blocks of the adrenal pathway (cholesterol side-chain cleavage defect, 3-beta-hydroxysteroid dehydrogenase deficiency, and 17-alpha-hydroxylase deficiency). Enzyme blocks are diagnosed with ACTH stimulation testing and measurement of precursors. Cholesterol side-chain cleavage defects have no measurable precursors but show high levels of ACTH and low cortisol response. Patients with 17-alpha-hydroxylase deficiency have elevated levels of progesterone, desoxycorticosterone and corticosterone with associated hypertension. Infants with 3-beta hydroxysteroid dehydrogenase deficiency have elevated levels of 17-hydroxypregnenolone and DHEA.

The two remaining defects in testosterone synthesis involve deficiencies of testicular rather than adrenal enzymes: 17,20-lyase and 17-beta-hydroxysteroid dehydrogenase. Thus, they are not associated with elevations of ACTH or electrolyte disturbances. Both deficiencies are diagnosed by measuring the precursor response to administration of hCG. Infants with 17,20-lyase deficiency have elevated levels of 17-hydroxypregnenolone and 17-hydroxyprogesterone, whereas infants with 17-beta-hydroxysteroid dehydrogenase deficiency have elevated levels of DHEA and androstenedione.

Infants with Leydig cell hypoplasia have low levels of testosterone after hCG stimulation, but normal adrenal function. Testicular biopsy reveals normal seminiferous tubules but absent or few Leydig cells.

Stimulation with hCG also allows measurement of the testosterone-to-dihydrotestosterone ratio. If the ratio is elevated, 5-alpha-reductase deficiency should be suspected and may be confirmed by cultures of genital skin fibroblasts.

Finally, normal testosterone levels with no abnormalities in ACTH and hCG testing lead to the diagnosis of partial androgen insensitivity or receptor defects. The diagnosis is made by demonstrating abnormal androgen binding in cultures of genital skin fibroblasts in a research laboratory.

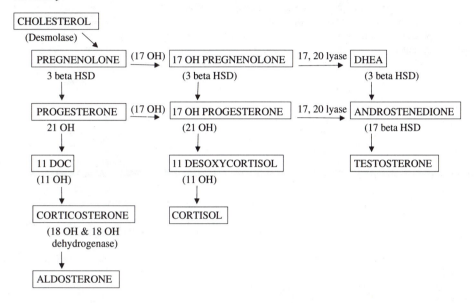

Testosterone synthesis pathway.

18. What is complete androgen insensitivity?

Strictly speaking, complete androgen insensitivity (testicular feminization) rarely presents as ambiguity in the newborn period of early childhood. Unless the testes have descended and are palpable in the labia majora, affected infants appear as phenotypically normal females.

The androgen receptor, encoded on the X chromosome, binds testosterone and more avidly, dihydrotestosterone. Androgen insensitivity results from abnormalities of the androgen receptor. Complete androgen resistance occurs with a frequency of 1 in 20,000 to 1 in 64,000 males and is the third most common cause of primary amenorrhea (after Turner syndrome and congenital absence of the vagina). Affected children grow as normal females until puberty. They feminize with normal breast development, because high levels of testosterone are aromatized to estrogen, but have no pubic and axillary hair and no menses. Because they produce MIF, they lack müllerian duct structures. Wolffian duct structures are also rudimentary or absent because they lack normal testosterone receptors. Gender identity is clearly female; patients come to medical attention because of primary amenorrhea.

The intraabdominal testes are at risk for malignancy, particularly after the onset of puberty. Timing of gonadectomy is debated. Because the risk of malignancy is low until puberty, some prefer to leave the gonads intact until spontaneous pubertal development; on the other hand, because carcinoma in situ has been found in prepubertal patients, others recommend early removal. If the testes are removed before puberty, low-dose estrogen therapy is necessary for normal pubertal progression. Because the upper section of the vagina is müllerian in origin, affected girls may have shortened vaginas and need plastic surgical repair.

19. Describe the clinical picture in children with 5-alpha-reductase deficiency.

Deficiency of 5-alpha-reductase impairs the conversion of testosterone to DHT, leading to incomplete virilization and differentiation of the external genitalia. The disorder is particularly well documented in a large kindred in the Dominican Republic, in whom it is inherited as an autosomal recessive condition.

Male infants with 5-alpha-reductase deficiency are born with sexual ambiguity. External genitalia range from a penis with simple hypospadias to a blind vaginal pouch and a clitorislike phallus. The most common presentation is a urogenital sinus with a blind vaginal pouch. During puberty, affected boys undergo virilization; affected females are normal.

Traditionally, infants with 5-alpha-reductase deficiency were raised as females until puberty, then continued life as males and, in some cases, achieved fertility. Recently, however, the condition has been recognized early in life, and affected males now are raised from infancy as boys.

20. What is a "true hermaphrodite"?

"True hermaphroditism," a disorder of gonadal differentiation, refers to individuals with both ovarian and testicular elements. Affected children may have bilateral ovotestes, an ovary or testis on one side with an ovotestis on the other, or an ovary on one side and a testis on the other. Because the effects of MIF and testosterone on duct structures are ipsilateral and localized, internal duct development is often asymmetrical. Thus a fallopian tube and unicornuate uterus, with absent or vestigial male duct structures, may develop on the side without testicular elements, whereas epididymis, vas deferens, and seminal vesicles without müllerian structures may develop on the side with testicular elements. The genitalia may be male, female, or ambiguous, depending on functioning testicular tissue.

21. Why is a multidisciplinary team needed in approaching an infant with sexual ambiguity?

Sexual ambiguity is a complex issue in numerous ways. Accurate diagnosis is essential and may take a fair amount of time. Sex of assignment must be based not only on underlying diagnosis and karyotype but also on potential for adult sexual function, fertility, and psychological health. For these reasons, input from several specialties, including endocrinology, genetics, neonatalogy, psychology, and urology, is important. All members of the team must communicate adequately with each other, and parents must receive a single message. Poor communication initially may lead to serious psychological problems later.

22. Once the etiology of sexual ambiquity has been determined in an infant, what factors should be considered assigning a sex of rearing?

Arriving at a precise diagnosis provides the treating team an understanding of potential risks and benefits of either sex assignment. For example, in a poorly virilized male, the difference in outcome among children with defects in testosterone synthesis, complete androgen insensitivity, and 5-alpha-reductase deficiency is enormous. A child with defective synthesis of testosterone may be raised male or female, depending on other factors; a child with complete androgen insensitivity should be raised female; and a boy with 5-alpha reductase deficiency usually is raised male. Yet children affected by any of the three conditions all have normal 46 XY karyotypes.

Three factors must be considered: (1) what is the potential for an unambiguous genital appearance? (2) what is the potential for normal sexual function? (3) is there a potential for fertility? Phallic size, urethral position, vaginal anatomy, and presence or absence of müllerian or wolffian duct structures, as well as gonadal characteristics and karyotype, must be considered.

Virilized females (female pseudohermaphrodites) should be assigned a female sex. They have normal ovaries as well as müllerian structures and, with surgical correction and steroid replacement, can have normal sexual function and achieve fertility.

Male pseudohermaphrodites are usually infertile; sex assignment is based on phallic size. Because a stretched penile length of 2.5 cm at term is 2.5 SD below the mean, an infant with a phallus smaller than 2.5 cm usually is assigned a female sex of rearing. Deficiency of 5-alpha-reductase is an obvious exception. If male sex assignment is contemplated, a trial of depot testosterone (50 mg every 3–4 weeks) for 1–3 months indicates whether phallic growth is possible.

In patients with gonadal dysgenesis and Y chromosomal material, gonadectomy is necessary and fertility is not possible. Internal duct structure is also frequently deranged. Small phallic size usually leads to a female sex assignment.

True hermaphrodites who have a unilateral ovary and müllerian structures may have spontaneous puberty and normal fertility and are raised as females. External genital size and structure may allow male assignment, but more commonly external genitalia are poorly virilized, and affected infants are assigned a female sex.

BIBLIOGRAPHY

1. Goodall J: Helping a child to understand her own testicular feminization. Lancet 337:33, 1991.
2. Jasso N, Boussin L, Knebelmann B, et al: Anti-mullerian hormone and intersex states. Trends Endocrinol Metab 2:227, 1991.
3. Kaplan S: Clinical Pediatric Endocrinology, Philadelphia, W.B. Saunders, 1990.
4. McGillivray BC: The newborn with ambiguous genitalia. Semin Perinatol 16:365, 1992.
5. Meyers-Seifer CH, Charest NJ: Diagnosis and management of patients with ambiguous genitalia. Semin Perinatol 16:332, 1992.
6. Pagona R: Diagnostic approach to the newborn with ambiguous genitalia. Pediatr Clin North Am 34:1019, 1987.
7. Penny R: Ambiguous genitalia. Am J Dis Child 144:753, 1990.
8. Thigpen AE, Davis DL, Gautier T, et al: Brief report: The molecular basis of steroid 5 alpha-reductase deficiency in a large Dominican kindred. N Engl J Med 327:1216, 1992.

37. DISORDERS OF PUBERTY

Robert H. Slover, MD

1. What physiologic events initiate puberty?

Maturation of the hypothalamic-pituitary axis initiates puberty. The hypothalamus begins to secrete gonadotropin-releasing hormone (GNRH) in pulses during sleep and eventually during waking hours as well. GNRH pulses stimulate the pituitary gland to secrete pulses of luteinizing hormone (LH) and follicle-stimulating hormone (FSH). LH and FSH, in turn, stimulate the gonads to enlarge and to secrete sex steroids that circulate and promote the development of secondary sex characteristics.

2. What is the normal pattern of puberty in males?

In the United states, normal puberty usually occurs between 9 and 14 years of age in boys (Fig. 1). In both sexes, puberty requires maturation of gonadal function and increased secretion of adrenal androgen (adrenarche). Puberty begins in 98% of boys with testicular enlargement, followed within 6 months by pubic hair and within 12–18 months by phallic enlargement. The growth spurt is a late pubertal event in boys, beginning with phallic enlargement and peaking in the final stage of genital growth.

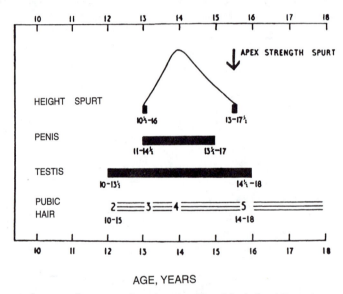

Sequence of events at puberty in males. (From Marshall and Tanner.)

3. Describe the normal pattern of female pubertal development.

As with males, female pubertal development depends on gonadal maturation and adrenarche. Breast development, linear growth, vaginal maturation, and changes in body habitus are mediated by ovarian estrogen, whereas development of pubic and axillary hair, acne, and body odor are androgen-dependent. Girls normally begin puberty between ages 18 and 13 years. In 85% of girls, the initial pubertal event is appearance of breast buds; 15% begin by developing pubic hair. The growth spurt, in contrast to boys, occurs early in girls, beginning with the onset of breast budding.

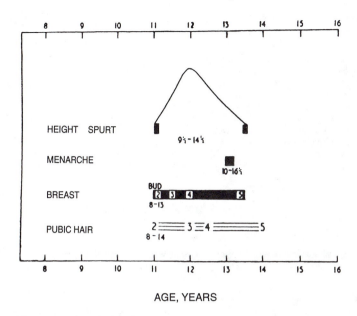

AGE, YEARS

The sequence of events at puberty in females. An average is represented in relation to the scale of ages. (From Marshall and Tanner.)

Menarche usually occurs 18–24 months from the onset of breast development (mean age:12.8 years; range:10–16 years).

4. How is pubertal development measured?

Sexual maturity is determined by examination and described by a scale devised by John Tanner in 1969. The Tanner stages are outlined below. Because of the distinct actions of adrenal androgens and gonadal steroids, it is important to distinguish between breast and pubic hair development in girls and between genital and pubic hair development in boys. In all cases, Tanner stage I is prepubertal.

Pubertal Development in Girls and Boys

	GIRLS		
STAGE	BREAST DEVELOPMENT CHARACTERISTICS	STAGE	PUBIC HAIR DEVELOPMENT CHARACTERISTICS
I	Prepubertal; elevation of the papilla only	I	Prepubertal; no pubic hair
II	Breast buds are noted or palpable; enlargement of the areola	II	Sparse growth of long, straight or slightly curly, minimally pigmented hair, mainly of the labia
III	Further enlargement of the breast and areola, with no separation of their contours	III	Considerably darker and coarser hair spreading over the mons pubis
IV	Projection of areola and papilla to form a secondary mound above the level of the breast	IV	Thick, adult-type hair that does not yet spread to the medial surface of the thighs.
V	Adult contour breast with projection of papilla only	V	Hair adult in type and distributed in the classic inverse triangle

BOYS

STAGE	GENITAL DEVELOPMENT CHARACTERISTICS	STAGE	PUBIC HAIR DEVELOPMENT CHARACTERISTICS
I	Prepubertal; testicular length < 2.5 cm	I	Prepubertal; no pubic hair
II	Testes >2.5 cm in the longest diameter and scrotum thinning and reddening	II	Sparse growth of slightly pigmented, slightly curly pubic hair, mainly at the base of the penis
III	Growth of the penis in width and length and further growth of the testes	III	Thicker, curlier hair, spread to the mons pubis
IV	Penis further enlarged; testes larger, with darker scrotal skin color	IV	Adult-type hair that does not yet spread to the medial thighs
V	Genitalia adult in size and shape	V	Adult-type hair spread to the medial thighs

Data from Marshall WE, Tanner JM: Variations in the pattern of pubertal changes in girls. Arch Dis Child 44:291–303, 1969; and Marshall WE, Tanner JM: Variations in the pattern of pubertal changes in boys. Arch Dis Child 45:13–23, 1970.

In addition to the physical examination, the tools to assess pubertal development include determination of bone age, growth velocity and pattern, and specific endocrine studies.

5. What constitutes precocity in boys and girls?

If the lower limit of normal is defined as two standard deviations from the mean, a boy entering puberty before the age of 9 years or a girl entering puberty before the age of 8 years should be considered precocious. In practice, however, even 8-year-old girls or 9-year-old boys may be worrisome; frequently children coming to medical attention at these ages entered puberty at an even younger age and in fact are precocious. In addition, the tempo of puberty may be more rapid than normal, suggesting an unusual underlying event; therefore, one may evaluate pubertal development in girls under age 9 years and boys under age 10 years.

6. In which sex is precocity more prevalent? Why?

Precocious puberty predominantly affects girls, with a female-to-male ratio of 4:1. In fact, the prevalence of organic etiologies (central nervous system lesions, gonadal tumors, and specific underlying diseases) is similar in both sexes. The disparity in overall prevalence of precocity is explained by the large numbers of precocious girls with central idiopathic precocity, a condition that is unusual in boys. At least 80% of all precocious puberty in girls is central idiopathic in nature.

7. Two common benign conditions in girls are often confused with precocious puberty. The first is premature thelarche. How is it diagnosed and treated?

Premature thelarche (breast development) is a benign, self-limited condition of girls, usually in the preschool years. It is not associated with true precocity, because there are no other estrogen effects. Breasts may reach midpubertal (Tanner stage III) maturity. Premature thelarche may result from increased sensitivity of breast tissue to the normal low prepubertal levels of estradiol.

A careful history should exclude exogenous intake of estrogen and additional signs of precocity, such as vaginal maturity, growth spurt, and androgen production. Physical examination must exclude genital maturity, pubic and axillary hair, accelerated growth, nipple and areolar maturation, and thyroid disorders. Bone age films should not show advanced skeletal maturity, and levels of gonadotropins and estradiol should be in the prepubertal range. GNRH stimulation may provoke an FSH-predominant response as opposed to the typical LH-predominant response in true central precocity.

Premature thelarche requires only observation and periodic reexamination. Because thelarche is usually the first event of puberty for girls, affected children should be monitored to ensure that they do not progress into true puberty.

8. The second benign condition is premature adrenarche. How is it diagnosed and treated?
Premature adrenarche (adrenal maturation) is also a benign, self-limited condition in which adrenal production of dehydroepiandrosterone sulfate (DHEA-S) reaches pubertal levels at an earlier age than usual. As a result, the patient develops pubic and axillary hair, body odor, and perhaps mild acne. This condition usually develops after age 6 years in boys or girls and may be associated with a slight acceleration of growth and a slight advance in bone age.

The rest of pubertal development, including breast development and vaginal maturity in girls, and genital and testicular enlargement in boys, is not affected; true puberty proceeds at a normal pace.

Evaluation is directed at exclusion of androgen-producing tumors and should include assessment of levels of DHEA-S, androstenedione, and testosterone as well as bone age. Careful examination should exclude other findings of true precocity. Specifically, girls show no evidence of estrogen production, and in boys genitalia remain immature.

No therapy is required, but periodic reexamination, observation, and reassurance are important.

9. How is the diagnosis of true precocity made?
In simple terms, the diagnosis of true precocity requires the appearance of the physical signs of puberty before the age of 8 years in girls and the age of 9 years in boys. The disorders that cause precocity are either GnRH-dependent (central) or GnRH-independent (peripheral). The first mechanism involves activation of the GnRH pulse-generator, increase in gonadotropins, and resultant increase in production of sex steroids. The second form does not involve GnRH and gonadotropins.

The first question to be asked is whether the child in fact is precocious. No matter which mechanism is involved the answer is yes if:

1. Both growth velocity and bone age are markedly increased.

2. Levels of sex steroids are elevated. (Levels may be difficult to measure, however, early in the course of pubertal development.)

3. Girls show evidence of both androgen and estrogen events (such as breast development and pubic hair) or menses.

4. Boys show bilateral testicular enlargement with virilization.

History may include behavioral changes, menses or vaginal discharge, growth spurt, erections, acne, and pubic or axillary hair. Physical examination should emphasize Tanner stage, height, and growth rate. A bone age film is essential. Baseline gonadotropins may not be elevated early in puberty, because they are episodically released, most often during sleep. Levels of sex steroids also may be fairly low.

10. What are the diagnostic possibilities in the child with true precocious puberty?
Causes of Isosexual Precocious Puberty
    Central (GnRH-dependent)
      Idiopathic true precocious puberty*
      CNS tumors (hamartomas,* hypothalamic tumors)
      CNS disorders (meningitis, encephalitis, hydrocephalus, trauma,
        abscesses, cysts, granulomas)
      Profound hypothyroidism
    Peripheral (GnRH-independent)
      Males
        hCG-secreting tumors (CNS, liver)
        Androgen excess
          Congenital adrenal hyperplasia (21-hydroxylase deficiency,
            11-hydroxylase deficiency)
          Adrenal tumors
          Leydig cell testicular tumor
          Familial gonadotropin-independent Leydig cell maturation (testotoxicosis)

Females
   Follicular cysts*
   Ovarian tumor
   Adrenal tumor
   Exogenous estrogen
   McCune-Albright syndrome (polyostotic fibrous dysplasia)
Causes of Contrasexual Precocious Puberty (rare)
Feminization in males
   Adrenal tumor (feminizing)
   Increased peripheral steroid-to-estrogen conversion
Virilization in females
   Congenital adrenal hyperplasia (21-hydroxylase deficiency*,
      11-hydroxylase deficiency, 3-beta-hydroxydehydrogenase deficiency)
   Adrenal tumors (virilizing)
   Ovarian tumors (virilizing)

* More common. CNS = central nervous system; hCG = human chorionic gonadotropin.

11. After the general diagnosis of precocity is made, how does one proceed to a specific diagnosis?
It may be impossible to distinguish GnRH-dependent from GnRH-independent precocity on examination. Although the possible etiologies of peripheral precocious puberty are more numerous (see below), central precocity accounts for the overwhelming majority of cases.

Measurement of sex steroid and gonadotropin levels and determination of the response to GnRH are important in elucidating the cause of precocity. A child with GnRH-dependent (central) precocity may have pubertal levels of gonadotropin and sex steroids and a pubertal response to GnRH. If levels of sex steroids are elevated but levels of gonadotropin are low and the response to GnRH is prepubertal, the etiology is likely to be peripheral or GnRH-independent.

In children with central precocity, magnetic resonance imaging (MRI) of the brain with contrast is needed to rule out an expanding lesion or hamartoma. In children with peripheral precocity, scanning is necessary to determine a gonadal or adrenal source of sex steroids. If LH is elevated in a boy, a human chorionic gonadotropin (hCG)-secreting tumor should be suspected.

Differential Diagnosis of Precocious Puberty

BOYS	GIRLS
Central precocious puberty	Central precocious puberty
Serum gonadotropins pubertal; pubertal GnRH test	Serum gonadotropins pubertal; pubertal GnRH test
Pubertal value of testosterone	Pubertal value of estradiol
Normal pubertal testicular enlargement	Ovarian and uterine enlargement
Peripheral precocious puberty	Peripheral precocious puberty
Gonadotropin secreting tumor	Feminizing adrenal tumor
High hCG or LH; no rise in LH response to GnRH	Low serum gonadotropins; prepubertal GnRH response
Pubertal or higher serum testosterone	High serum estradiol and DHAS
Slight to moderate uniform testicular enlargement	Ovaries prepubertal
Leydig cell tumor	Granulosa cell tumor
Low serum gonadotropins; GnRH response suppressed	Low serum gonadotropins; GnRH response suppressed
Very high serum testosterone	Very high estradiol
Irregular, asymmetric enlargement of testes	Ovarian enlargement on physical, ultrasound, CT, or MRI

Table continued on following page.

Differential Diagnosis of Precocious Puberty (Continued)

BOYS	GIRLS
Familial testotoxicosis	Follicular cyst
Low serum gonadotropins; GnRH response suppressed	Low serum gonadotropins; prepubertal LH response to GnRH but FSH may rise above normal
Pubertal or higher serum testosterone	
Testes larger than 2.5 cm but smaller than expected for pubertal stage	Estradiol low to high depending on stage of cyst
	Cysts may be visible on sonogram

From Wheeler M, Styne D: Diagnosis and management of precocious puberty. Pediatr Clin North Am 37:1255, 1990, with permission.

12. How is central idiopathic precocious puberty treated?

Children (usually girls) with central idiopathic precocious puberty face the immediate problems of psychosocial trauma, inappropriately early behavioral changes, and embarrassment. They also are at risk for short adult stature, because they have rapid skeletal maturation and bone closure. Affected youngsters are exceptionally tall as they mature but become short adults. Until a decade ago, such children could be treated only with progestational agents that stopped menses and some aspects of pubertal maturation but did not alter linear growth.

Current therapy relies on GnRH agonists. Such agents, investigated since the early 1980s, only recently gained approval from the Food and Drug Administration (FDA) and became commercially available. Their mechanism of action is to bind to the GnRH receptors at the pituitary level, blocking the normal pulsatile message of GnRH and "turning off" the process of puberty. GnRH agonists are effective in decreasing the secretion of gonadotropin and sex steroids, rates of linear growth and skeletal maturation, and development of secondary sex characteristics. They are given commonly in monthly depot parenteral form and have no serious side effects. Therapy is continued until the child reaches normal pubertal age and has a reasonable height prediction.

13. What is the association of hypothyroidism with precocity?

Precocious puberty has been described in girls with severe acquired hypothyroidism. Although affected children exhibit secondary sex characteristics of precocity, growth is delayed—and perhaps bone ages—because of the hypothyroidism. Additional indications include large follicular cysts and elevated levels of TSH and prolactin. The mechanism for this association is not known, but elevated levels of TSH may cross-react with ovarian gonadotropin receptors to stimulate ovarian enlargement and secretion of estrogen.

Patients are easily diagnosed with studies of thyroid function and treated with thyroxine. Only after thyroid replacement is established is it possible to determine whether the patient has concurrent central precocity that requires therapy with GnRH analogs.

14. What is McCune-Albright syndrome? How is it treated?

McCune-Albright syndrome is a triad consisting of irregular (Coast-of-Maine) café-au-lait lesions, polyostotic fibrous dysplasia, and GnRH-independent precocious puberty. It affects both sexes but is seen infrequently in boys. In girls, breast development and vaginal bleeding occur with sporadic increases in estradiol and ovarian cysts. GnRH testing elicits a prepubertal response, and gonadotropins are low; with time, however, increased estradiol may mature the hypothalamus, thus leading to true central GnRH-dependent precocity.

The syndrome is often associated with other endocrine dysfunction, including hyperthyroidism, adrenal hyperplasia, Cushing's syndrome, gigantism, and hyperparathyroidism.

Metabolic abnormalities demonstrate hyperfunction of hormone-secreting tissues and have in common cells that respond to extracellular signals through the activation of the adenylate cyclase system and cyclic adenosine monophosphate (c-AMP) but not through trophic hormones. In specific, recent investigations have demonstrated alterations in G (guanine nucleotide-binding) proteins necessary to signal transduction in hormone synthesis.

Therapy is controversial and experimental. Some girls have been treated with oral medroxyprogesterone. More recently, testolactone, an aromatase inhibitor, has been used to block synthesis of estradiol and estrone from testosterone and androstenedione. If true GnRH-dependent precocity intervenes, a GnRH agonist is useful.

15. Describe testotoxicosis.

Familial testotoxicosis is an autosomal dominant, gonadotropin-independent form of male precocity. Boys with this condition begin to develop true precocity with testicular and phallic enlargement and growth acceleration by the age of 4 years. Serum gonadotropins are low, and GnRH studies show a prepubertal response, but the serum testosterone level is high. By mid-adolescence to adulthood GnRH stimulation demonstrates a more typical LH-predominant pubertal response.

Treatment options include medroxyprogesterone (inhibition of testosterone synthesis), ketoconazole (inhibition of adrenal and gonadal synthesis), or a combination of testolactone and spironolactone (aromatic inhibition plus androgen receptor blockade).

16. How does non–salt-wasting congenital adrenal hyperplasia present in boys?

The most common adrenogenital syndrome is deficiency of 21-hydroxylase. Girls present with virilization in utero, resulting in a degree of sexual ambiguity. They are discovered at birth and should be diagnosed within the first days of life by the finding of greatly elevated levels of 17-hydroxyprogesterone. In the more common salt-losing form of this disease, boys present with vomiting, shock, and electrolyte disturbances at 7–10 days of age. A small subset of affected boys, however, do not waste salt; they present with precocity consisting of pubic hair, acne, body odor, deepening of the voice, penile but not testicular enlargement, acceleration of linear growth, and skeletal maturation in early or late childhood. A similar presentation occurs in boys with the much less common 11-hydroxylase deficiency, which also may cause hypertension.

Treatment is directed at reducing androgen levels by replacing corticosteroids that reduce secretion of adrenocorticotropic hormone (ACTH).

17. What is adolescent gynecomastia?

At least 75% of boys experience transient gynecomastia with areolar enlargement and palpable and often tender breast buds. Gynecomastia typically occurs at Tanner stage II or III and is transient; it may be unilateral or bilateral and may be symmetric. In boys with gynecomastia that lasts longer than 2 years, surgical removal may be required. Testosterone therapy may accentuate the condition because of aromatase activity and conversion to estradiol. Dihydrotestosterone has been used experimentally with reportedly good results, but it is not commercially available. Clearly, in obese boys, weight reduction is of value not only in reducing adipose tissue but also in reduction of glandular tissue. Pathologic gynecomastia occurs in boys with Klinefelter syndrome or partial androgen insensitivity.

18. At what age does failure to enter puberty necessitate investigation?

Boys are brought to medical attention for pubertal delay more frequently than girls, in part, perhaps because of social bias. Three percent of children are statistically delayed in pubertal development. Serious evaluation is warranted in girls with no breast development by age 13 years or no menses by age 15 years. Boys should be evaluated if they have not reached a testicular length of 2.5 cm by age 14 years. The majority of children are constitutionally delayed and, given time, will enter puberty spontaneously.

19. What should the history and physical examination include in an adolescent with pubertal delay?

Growth velocity and pattern are important; children with constitutional delay typically have been short throughout childhood, whereas adolescents with hypogonadotropic hypogonadism have normal childhood growth but lack the normal pubertal growth spurt. Questions about the timing of puberty may reveal partial development but failure of normal progression, suggestive of partial hypogonadotropic hypogonadism. Underlying illness, drug therapy, and psychosocial issues are influential.

On physical examination, body proportions should be determined. Eunuchoidal proportions occur early in patients with Klinefelter syndrome and late in those with hypogonadotropic hypogonadism. Pubic hair may represent only adrenal androgen function. Testicular length of greater than 2.5 cm indicates gonadotropin stimulation. Estrogen effect is evaluated by breast development and vaginal maturity. In addition, visual field and olfaction should be evaluated (80% of boys with Kallmann syndrome have reduced or absent sense of smell). The stigmata of gonadal dysgenesis include high arched palate, low hairline, widely spaced nipples, ptosis, pterygium colli, shortened fourth metacarpals, cardiac murmurs, cubitus valgus, and pigmented nevi. Signs of hypothyroidism and Cushing's syndrome must also be evaluated.

20. What laboratory tests help in the diagnosis of pubertal delay?
Initial evaluation should include screening for underlying disorders with complete blood count, urinalysis, erythrocyte sedimentation rate, chemistries, and thyroid function studies; bone age and levels of somatomedin-C should be assessed if growth velocity is subnormal. Screening for levels of LH and FSH is very important. Levels that are high for the child's stage of sexual maturity indicate hypergonadotropic hypogonadism (primary gonadal failure). Low values, however, do not distinguish between constitutional delay and hypogonadotropic hypogonadism. However, patients with low levels of gonadotropins and a bone age of more than 13 years are likely to have underlying pathology, whereas patients with low levels of gonadotropins and bone age of 11 years or under are much more likely to have a good prognosis for normal pubertal development. Patients who progress through normal puberty have a progressive rise in LH and FSH over 6–12 months.

The GnRH test is difficult to interpret in prepubertal or peripubertal children. Whereas GnRH testing may suggest the diagnosis if there is a clear rise in levels of LH, the overlap in response among prepubertal, hypogonadotropic, and early pubertal children is significant. Use of a GnRH agonist may help in this conundrum by causing a rise in LH (over 12.5 IU/L at 3 hours) and FSH (over 6.0 IU/L at 8–12 hours) in children with constitutional delay as opposed to a reduced response in boys with hypogonadotropic hypogonadism. The agonist also stimulates production of testosterone in most boys with constitutional delay. Alternatively, the GnRH test may be repeated after time to establish a pattern.

Testicular responsiveness (or even presence of a testis) may be evaluated by giving hCG and measuring the testosterone response. Additional tests, if clinically indicated, include assessment of prolactin and karyotype. Structural studies may include MRI, skull films, formal visual field testing, and pelvic ultrasound.

21. How does constitutional delay affect puberty?
Constitutional delay of growth is frequently diagnosed in childhood as a common cause of short stature, more often in boys than in girls. However, some delayed children from genetically taller families may grow within normal parameters and may not present for medical attention until puberty is delayed. Characteristic features include the following:

1. Puberty is not delayed beyond 16 years in boys or 18 years in girls.
2. Onset of puberty correlates with bone age appropriate for puberty (e.g., 11 years in girls and 12 years in boys).
3. The physiologic decline in growth velocity is exaggerated before puberty.
4. When puberty begins, linear growth and pubertal changes proceed normally.
5. The prolonged prepubertal growth period, followed by normal pubertal progression and growth spurt, result in achievement of expected genetic height.

It is challenging to differentiate between constitutional delay and hormonal disorders of pubertal development, such as gonadotropin deficiency, in the prepubertal period. Time and careful observation are important tools.

22. Other than the constitutional delay, what causes delay in pubertal development?
It seems useful to classify pubertal delay in adolescence by the initial levels of gonadotropin. Primary gonadal failure results in hypergonadotropic hypogonadism as gonadotropins rise to stimulate unresponsive gonads. Hypogonadotropic hypogonadism, on the other hand, is a disorder of the hypothalamic-pituitary axis, which fails to produce gonadotropins.

A subset of girls who begin puberty at a normal age fail to progress to menarche. The majority of such girls have müllerian duct abnormalities but normal levels of gonadotropin. In addition, 46XY phenotypic females with androgen insensitivity (testicular feminization) have primary amenorrhea but elevated levels of gonadotropins.

Causes of Delayed Adolescence in the Phenotypic Male and Female

Hypergonadotropic Conditions
    Variants of ovarian and testicular dysgenesis
    Gonadal toxins (antimetabolite and/or radiation treatment)
    Enzyme defects (17-alpha-hydroxylase deficiency in the genetic male or female and 17-ketosteroid
       reductase deficiency in the genetic male)
    Androgen insensitivity (testicular feminization)
    Other miscellaneous disorders
Hypogonadotropic Conditions
    Multiple tropic hormone deficiency
    Isolated growth hormone deficiency
    Isolated gonadotropin deficiency
    Miscellaneous syndrome complexes (e.g., Prader-Willi syndrome)
    Systemic conditions, nutritional and psychogenic disorders, increased energy expenditure
    Other endocrine causes, hypothyroidism, glucocorticoid excess, hyperprolactinemia
    Constitutional delay in growth and development
Eugonadotropic Conditions: Delayed Menarche
    Gonadal dysgenesis variants with residually functioning ovarian tissue
    Polycystic ovarian disease
    Hyperprolactinemia

From Rosenfeld R: Diagnosis and management of delayed puberty. J Clin Endocrinol Metab 70:559, 1990, with permission.

23. The family of a boy with constitutional delay of puberty asks what can be done for their son, who is 14 years old, infantile, and miserable at school. What might you suggest?
Most boys with constitutional delay of puberty, especially if it is mild, are able to wait and accept reassurance. For others, however, psychological issues become overwhelming, and they need help in maturing. In the past several years, studies have shown that physiologic doses of testosterone do not compromise final adult height. A 6-month course of low-dose depot testosterone increases growth rate in 75% of boys and advances puberty. A dose of 50–100 mg intramuscularly every 3–4 weeks seems effective and safe. Such small doses have a remarkable effect on secondary sex characteristics such as voice, acne, phallic length, and, to a lesser degree, sexual hair.

24. Do body habitus and lifestyle influence the timing of puberty and final height?
In the early 1980s a number of reports suggested that extremely active and thin girls had a high incidence of primary amenorrhea and delay of puberty. Gymnasts, runners, and ballet dancers, among others, were evaluated. A high incidence of primary amenorrhea, secondary amenorrhea, and dysmenorrhea was found among this group of athletes and appears to be related to fat-lean ratio as well as to exercise. Indeed, when forced by injury to discontinue activity, such athletes gained weight and quickly progressed to menarche.

A recent study evaluated the effect of intensive physical training during puberty on final height in girls. Predicted height decreased significantly with time in gymnasts but not in swimmers. The author concluded that heavy training in gymnastics starting before and lasting through puberty, may reduce final adult height.

25. What is Turner syndrome? How is it treated?
Any consideration of pubertal delay in girls must include the possibility of Turner syndrome. The minimal diagnostic criterion for Turner syndrome is an abnormal karyotype in at least one tissue of the body in which a portion or all of an X chromosome is missing. Turner syndrome has an

incidence of approximately 1:2500 live female births. In the absence of a second functional X chromosome, oocyte degeneration is accelerated, leaving fibrotic streaks in place of normal ovaries. Because of primary gonadal failure, gonadotropins rise and are elevated at birth and again at the normal time of puberty.

Between 5–15% of girls with Turner syndrome undergo spontaneous puberty; the remainder require hormonal replacement. The timing of estrogen replacement is critical; it is frequently delayed to allow maximal prepubertal growth, especially if growth hormone is used. In mid-adolescence, estrogen is replaced, often as unopposed estradiol or conjugated estrogen for a year, followed by cycling with estrogen and progestins.

Clinical Findings Commonly Described in Patients with Turner Syndrome

PRIMARY DEFECTS	SECONDARY FEATURES	INCIDENCE (%)
Physical features		
Skeletal growth disturbances	Short stature	100
	Short neck	40
	Abnormal upper to low segment ratio	97
	Cubitus valgus	47
	Short metacarpals	37
	Madelung deformity	7.5
	Scoliosis	12.5
	Genu valgum	35
	Characteristic facies with micrognathia	60
	High arched palate	36
Lymphatic obstruction	Webbed neck	25
	Low posterior hairline	42
	Rotated ears	common
	Edema of hands/feet	22
	Severe nail dysplasia	13
	Characteristic dermatoglyphics	35
Unknown factors	Strabismus	17.5
	Ptosis	11
	Multiple pigmented nevi	26
Physiologic features		
Skeletal growth disturbances	Growth failure	100
	Otitis media	73
Germ cell chromosomal defects	Gonadal failure	96
	Infertility	99.9
	Gonadoblastoma	4.0
Unknown factors— embryogenic	Cardiovascular anomalies	55
	Hypertension	7
	Renal and renovascular anomalies	39
Unknown factors—metabolic	Hashimoto's thyroiditis	34
	Hypothyroidism	10
	Alopecia	2
	Vitiligo	2
	Gastrointestinal disorders	2.5
	Carbohydrate intolerance	40

From Hall J, Gilchrist D: Turner syndrome and its variants. Ped Clin North Am 37:1421, 1990, with permission.

26. Why do boys with Klinefelter syndrome have pubertal delay?

Klinefelter syndrome, or seminiferous tubular dysgenesis, is the most common cause of testicular failure. It results from at least one extra X chromosome; thus the most common karyotype is 47 XXY. The incidence is 1:1000 male births. Eunuchoid proportions are present from early childhood. Other features include gynecomastia, tall stature, small testes, elevated gonadotropins, and sometimes retardation. Seminiferous tubular dysgenesis is universal in patients with Klinefelter syndrome, but Leydig cell function (testosterone production) is variable; thus they may have either delay in pubertal onset or failure to progress normally through puberty. In most patients, testosterone replacement is necessary.

Features which May Be of Value in the Clinical Detection of Klinefelter Syndrome

FEATURES	CHILD	ADULT
Psychosocial	Delay in language development; placid; poorly organized motor function	Increased psychopathology; disturbed body image
Testes	May be small in size (decreased germ cell mass)	Small size with halinization; incomplete virilization or fibrosis; gynecomastia
Phallus	May be small in size; may have hypospadias	Small size secondary to inadequate testosterone production
Body habitus	Long legs with decreased upper to lower segment ratio; slim build with decreased weight for height; hypoplasia of the middle phalanges of the fifth fingers; limitation of pronation and supination of forearms	Eunuchoid habitus; increased truncal adiposity and decreased muscle mass

From Rosenfeld R: Diagnosis and management of delayed puberty. J Clin Endocrinol Metab 70:559, 1990, with permission.

27. What is Kallmann syndrome?
Kallmann syndrome is one of a class of disorders called idiopathic hypogonadotropic hypogonadism or idiopathic hypothalamic hypogonadism (IHH). It occurs as frequently as 1:10,000 boys and 1:50,000 girls. The classic form is characterized by hypogonadotropic hypogonadism with hyposmia or anosmia and associated with hypoplasia or aplasia of other structures of the rhinencephalon (e.g., cleft lip/cleft palate, congenital deafness, and color blindness). Undescended testes and gynecomastia are common.

In boys with Kallmann syndrome (or any of the IHH disorders), testosterone therapy affects puberty and normal growth; in fact the delay in puberty increases final adult height. For affected individuals to achieve fertility, however, therapy with both gonadotropins (hCG and human menopausal gonadotropin [hMG]), and pulsatile GnRH has been used with good results.

28. How is long-term testosterone therapy given?
In boys with primary hypogonadism or hypogonadotropic hypogonadism for whom fertility is not an immediate issue, long-term testosterone therapy is required. While the patient is growing, careful attention must be paid to velocity and bone age.

Most commonly, depot testosterone esters (enanthate or cypionate) are used in 25–50 mg doses every 3–4 weeks for the first 1–2 years of therapy. By the second or third year the dose is raised to 50–100 mg intramuscularly every 3–4 weeks. The adult maintenance level is 200–300 mg intramuscularly every 3–4 weeks.

Oral testosterone undecanoate, given 2–3 times/day, has been used in Europe with fairly poor response; 17-alpha-alkylated testosterone products are orally active but potentially hepatotoxic. Testosterone patches are not yet satisfactory or commercially available.

The most common side effect of testosterone therapy in males is gynecomastia due to aromatization of the testosterone to estradiol. Acne, oily skin, 2–3% weight gain, and 10–15% decline in HDL cholesterol are also seen. The goal of therapy is to achieve pubertal and sexual growth with testosterone levels in the normal range 6–8 days after each injection.

29. Can a girl be treated on a short-term basis for delay of puberty?
Treatment of delayed puberty in girls is more controversial and less frequent. After a thorough initial evaluation, however, some endocrinologists use low doses of conjugated estrogen (Premarin, 0.3 mg) or ethinyl estradiol (5–10 µg) daily for 3–4 months. Therapy is then stopped, and physical changes are evaluated. Withdrawal bleeding is unusual after one course of estrogen

therapy but may occur with subsequent courses. In older girls with significant pubertal development but lack of menses, a single course of medroxyprogesterone (Provera) is often given to stimulate withdrawal bleeding and to reassure both patient and physician.

30. Can long-term estrogen therapy be safely given?

Oral estrogen therapy is successful and should be given at the lowest dose that provides effect. Long-term, unopposed estrogen therapy should be avoided, even in girls without a uterus.

Typically we initiate replacement therapy with estrogen alone, either as ethinyl estradiol (5–10 µg) or as Premarin (0.15–0.3 mg) daily for 12–18 months. At that point, we add progesterone cyclically to produce menses, either by using a combination of estrogen for 25 days and adding Provera (5–10 mg) for the last 12 days or by using oral contraceptives.

During the years of growth, bone maturation and height must be carefully monitored, although low-dose estrogen is not likely to compromise final adult height.

BIBLIOGRAPHY

1. Comite F et al: Cyclical ovarian function resistant to treatment with an analogue of luteinizing hormone releasing hormone in McCune-Albright syndrome. N Engl J Med 311:1032, 1984.
2. Evans SJ: The athletic adolescent with amenorrhea. Pediatr Ann 13:605, 1984.
3. Frisch R, Wyshak G, Vincent L: Delayed menarche and amenorrhea in ballet dancers. N Engl J Med 303:17, 1980.
4. Hall J, Gilchrist D: Turner syndrome and its variants. Pediatr Clin North Am 37:1421, 1990.
5. Ibanez L, et al: Natural history of premature pubarche and auxological study. J Clin Endocrinol Metab 74:254, 1992.
6. Kaplan S (ed): Clinical Pediatric Endocrinology. Philadelphia, W. B. Saunders, 1990.
7. Kaplan S, Grumbach M: Pathophysiology and treatment of sexual precocity. J Clin Endocrinol Metab 71:785, 1990.
8. Kulin H, Rester E: Managing the patient with a delay in pubertal development. Endocrinologist 2:231, 1992.
9. Levine M: The McCune-Albright syndrome: The whys and wherefores of abnormal signal transduction. N Engl J Med 325:1738, 1991.
10. Pescovitz O: Precocious puberty. Pediatr Rev 11:229, 1990.
11. Rosenfeld R: Diagnosis and management of delayed puberty. J Clin Endocrinol Metab 70:559, 1990.
12. Theinz G, et al: Evidence for a reduction of growth potential in adolescent female gymnasts. J Pediatr 122:306, 1993.
13. Wheeler M, Styne D: Diagnosis and management of precocious puberty. Pediatr Clin North Am 37:1255, 1990.
14. Zachmann M: Therapeutic indications for delayed puberty and hypogonadism in adolescent boys. Horm Res 35:141, 1991.

38. MALE HYPOGONADISM

Allan R. Glass, M.D.

1. What is male hypogonadism?

Male hypogonadism refers to the clinical and/or laboratory syndrome that results from a failure of the testis to work properly. The normal testis has two functions: synthesis and secretion of testosterone (from the Leydig cells) and production of sperm (from the seminiferous tubules). Deficiency of both functions is termed male hypogonadism. In addition, a decrease in sperm output without deficient production of testosterone is not uncommon and results in male infertility; some view infertility as a form of male hypogonadism. Conversely, a decrease in production of testosterone without a decline in production of sperm is possible but highly unusual; this disorder is generally viewed as a variant of male hypogonadism. In rare instances, the peripheral tissues are unable to respond to normal production of testosterone. Such situations are usually congenital (e.g., testicular feminization) and may fall under the general category of male hypogonadism.

2. How is production of testosterone normally regulated?

Luteinizing hormone (LH) secreted from the anterior pituitary stimulates production of testosterone by Leydig cells. After secretion from the testis into the bloodstream, testosterone gives negative feedback to the hypothalamic-pituitary unit and thus inhibits output of LH. This classic endocrine feedback loop serves to maintain serum testosterone at a predetermined level; if serum testosterone falls below the set point, the pituitary is stimulated to secrete LH, which in turn stimulates testicular output of testosterone until serum levels return to the set point. Conversely, if serum testosterone rises above the set point, decreased output of LH results in decreased testicular output of testosterone until serum levels have declined to the set point.

3. How is production of sperm normally regulated?

The regulation of sperm production appears to be more complicated and certainly is less clearly understood than regulation of testosterone levels. The Sertoli cells within the seminiferous tubules seem to play an important coordinating role. Follicle-stimulating hormone (FSH) secreted by the pituitary gland is thought to stimulate spermatogenesis, probably by acting through the Sertoli cell. Concurrently, FSH also stimulates the release of a polypeptide hormone, termed inhibin, from the Sertoli cells into the circulation. Circulating inhibin appears to inhibit the output of FSH from the pituitary gland, thus completing a feedback loop. In theory, if spermatogenesis declines, production of inhibin also should decline; thus the negative feedback effect on the pituitary would be reduced. This decline in inhibin should lead to increased output of FSH, which then presumably stimulates spermatogenesis. However, not all aspects of this feedback loop (FSH-inhibin-spermatogenesis) have been verified experimentally. In addition to the FSH-inhibin feedback loop, spermatogenesis also seems to depend on intratesticular production of testosterone (see question 2).

4. Define primary hypogonadism and secondary hypogonadism.

Failure of testicular function may result from a defect either in the testis or at the hypothalamic-pituitary level. Testicular disorders leading to hypogonadism are termed primary hypogonadism whereas disorders of hypothalamic-pituitary function leading to hypogonadism are termed secondary hypogonadism.

5. What are the causes of primary hypogonadism?

Currently the most common cause of primary hypogonadism is testicular dysfunction resulting from cancer chemotherapy. Particularly potent are the alkylating agents; their effects are usually much more devastating on production of sperm than on production of testosterone. Another common cause is Klinefelter's syndrome, a congenital disorder associated with an abnormal chromosomal complement (two X chromosomes and 1 Y chromosome instead of the single X and single Y found in normal males). It is often associated with gynecomastia and azoospermia (sperm count of zero); production of testosterone is usually reduced by about 50%. In addition, genetic defects may lead to loss of one of the enzymes required for testosterone synthesis; such rare congenital disorders often result in ambiguous genitalia. Testicular trauma, exposure to x-rays, and infections, such as postpubertal mumps orchitis, also may lead to primary hypogonadism. Certain systemic disorders—either congenital, such as myotonic dystrophy, or acquired, such as renal failure—are also associated with primary hypogonadism. A considerable number of cases of primary hypogonadism are idiopathic.

6. Is normal aging associated with primary hypogonadism?
A number of cross-sectional studies have noted that older men seem to have reduced levels of serum testosterone compared with younger men. Whether this decline reflects hypogonadism that is an intrinsic part of the aging process or the various chronic diseases that develop as one ages has not been established conclusively.

7. What are the causes of secondary hypogonadism?
Pituitary adenomas may cause secondary hypogonadism, usually by interfering with the output of LH and FSH. Perhaps the most common type of pituitary adenoma that results in hypogonadism is prolactinoma; the overproduction of prolactin seems to have various deleterious effects on gonadal function in addition to those expected from any space-occupying lesion in the pituitary. However, pituitary adenomas that produce growth hormone (acromegaly) or adrenocorticotropic hormone (Cushing's disease), among others, also may lead to hypogonadism, as well as pituitary tumors with no obvious hormonal output. Hypothalamic-pituitary dysfunction after surgery or trauma and infiltrative diseases, such as hemochromatosis, may cause hypogonadism. Congenital disorders in which output of LH and FSH is impaired, such as Kallmann's syndrome (associated with anosmia), also lead to secondary hypogonadism.

8. What clinical symptoms are seen in male hypogonadism?
Loss of the sperm-producing function of the testis leads to infertility, usually defined as failure of a normal female partner to conceive after 12 months of unprotected intercourse. Loss of the testosterone-producing function of the testis may lead to loss of libido and erectile dysfunction as well as diminution of secondary sexual characteristics, such as facial and pubic hair. Decreased production of testosterone also may lead to more generalized symptoms, such as decreased muscle strength, malaise, and fatigue. In boys who develop hypogonadism before sexual maturation, delay or absence of the onset of puberty is typical.

9. What physical findings are observed in male hypogonadism?
Reduction in testis size is seen in virtually all cases of male hypogonadism, except those of recent onset. Because most of the testis volume is composed of seminiferous tubules, the decline in testis size usually correlates roughly to the decline in production of sperm. Decrease in production of testosterone may lead to reduction in body hair, arrest of temporal balding pattern, and small prostate size. Gynecomastia, which usually reflects a decrease in androgen/estrogen ratio, is also common, particularly in primary hypogonadism. Onset of hypogonadism before the epiphyses of the long bones fuse may lead to prolonged longitudinal growth of the extremities and development of eunuchoidal proportions, in which the ratio of the upper body segment (pubis to vertex) to the lower body segment (pubis to floor) is less than 0.9. Impaired production of testosterone during fetal development may lead to ambiguous external genitalia.

10. What laboratory tests are useful in confirming a suspected diagnosis of male hypogonadism?

The main functions of the testis, production of sperm and production of testosterone, are readily assessed by semen analysis and measurement of serum testosterone, respectively. Because sperm density is highly variable from day to day in any individual, accurate assessment usually involves several semen analyses. Serum testosterone in a given individual also varies considerably from moment to moment and from morning to night; again, several specimens may be needed to establish an accurate measurement. In addition, most testosterone in serum is bound to plasma proteins, particularly sex hormone-binding globulin (SHBG); thus, in patients in whom levels of plasma protein may be disrupted, measurement of the physiologically active free testosterone may prove informative.

11. Can laboratory tests help in distinguishing primary hypogonadism from secondary hypogonadism?

As noted previously, the testis is normally regulated by a series of negative feedback loops. LH from the pituitary stimulates production of testosterone by the testis, and serum testotserone then inhibits output of LH. FSH from the pituitary stimulates spermatogenesis, which then inhibits FSH via inhibin. Consequently, primary hypogonadism resulting from a testicular disorder leads to a decline in production of testosterone and sperm, with a consequent decrease in the negative feedback effects on the pituitary and thus a corresponding increase in serum levels of LH and FSH. Conversely, in secondary hypogonadism due to a hypothalamic-pituitary defect, serum LH and FSH may be subnormal. Normal levels of serum LH and FSH also are seen with secondary hypogonadism; in such cases, the bioactivity of the hormones may be reduced.

12. What other diagnostic tests are useful in defining the cause of male hypogonadism?

Additional diagnostic testing should be based on clinical suspicion and results of preliminary testing. For example, in cases of secondary hypogonadism, measurement of serum prolactin and pituitary radiography (preferably magnetic resonance imaging [MRI]) are often useful. Visual field testing and measurement of other pituitary hormones also may be appropriate to assess possible hormone overproduction by a tumor or tumor-related hypopituitarism. Likewise, the initial findings in primary hypogonadism may suggest additional tests. For example, small testes, gynecomastia, azoospermia, modestly reduced serum testosterone, and high levels of serum LH and FSH in a young man may lead to chromosome analysis to confirm a presumptive diagnosis of Klinefelter's syndrome. Measurement of serum estradiol levels may be helpful when feminization is prominent clinically, as with secondary hypogonadism related to production of estrogen by testicular or adrenal tumors. Testis biopsy rarely provides information that is useful in establishing a specific diagnosis or in assisting with prognosis or treatment.

13. How is hypogonadism treated?

Deficiency of testosterone is easily treated with testosterone replacement therapy. At the present time, the most effective means of treatment is periodic intramuscular injection of testosterone esters, such as testosterone enanthate or cypionate. Generally, these medications are given in a dosage of 200 mg every 2 weeks or 100 mg every week. Less frequent injections may lead to a period of inadequate testosterone replacement between injections. Some older men with testosterone deficiency are unconcerned about sexual function and may not desire testosterone replacement, although it should be recalled that testosterone has beneficial effects on bone and hematopoiesis apart from its more commonly recognized effects on libido and potency. Currently available oral formulations of testosterone are generally rather ineffective and potentially dangerous. Newer, more convenient methods of testosterone replacement are under development, including transdermal patches and several forms of long-acting preparations of depot testosterone. Because of its potential for abuse by athletes and others, testosterone is presently designated a schedule III drug.

14. Is testosterone treatment dangerous?

Testosterone administration is generally quite safe; as with any drug, however, there is always the potential for adverse effects. Gynecomastia and acne may occur in the first few months after initiating testosterone treatment; these may resolve with continued treatment, although temporary dose reduction may be helpful. Abnormalities in liver function are quite uncommon with currently used injectable preparations but are much more frequent with oral formulations. In older men, effects of testosterone on the prostate must be considered, including the possibility of precipitating urinary retention due to testosterone-induced enlargement of the prostate. In addition, because of the potential for testosterone stimulation of occult prostate carcinoma, it is advisable to monitor prostate-specific antigen (PSA) in older men receiving testosterone replacement. A testosterone-induced increase in hematocrit is common, although clinically significant polycythemia is quite rare. Testosterone treatment may also precipitate sleep apnea; marked increases in hematocrit may be a clue to this side effect. In boys who have not yet gone through puberty, the rapid increase in serum testosterone after initial treatment may lead to considerable psychological difficulties; initiating treatment with smaller doses may be helpful. Testosterone treatment may also have an adverse effect on lipid profiles.

15. How does one treat the deficiency of sperm production?
In men with primary hypogonadism, as manifested by elevated levels of serum FSH, there seems to be no effective treatment for increasing sperm count. If one plans to use a medication that is known to cause hypogonadism (e.g., cancer chemotherapeutic agents), it may be desirable to cryopreserve semen specimens before treatment, provided that treatment is not unduly delayed. The outlook is much less pessimistic with secondary hypogonadism, particularly if the condition developed after puberty. Treatment with gonadotropins (human chorionic gonadotropin with or without added FSH) may be successful in restoring production of sperm as well as testosterone. The pretreatment size of the testis is often a clue to prognosis: larger testis size is associated with a better outcome. Production of testosterone and sperm in men with secondary hypogonadism also may be restored with pulsatile administration of gonadotropin-releasing hormone (GNRH) via a portable infusion pump, provided that the pituitary retains the capability to make gonadotropins. Treatment with gonadotropins or GNRH tends to be both costly and prolonged.

16. Does prolactin-related hypogonadism require a special approach?
Yes. The mechanism by which hyperprolactinemia, usually from a pituitary adenoma, causes hypogonadism is not clearly defined. However, prolactin seems to have an inhibitory effect on the action of testosterone in addition to other effects on its production. Thus, patients with high levels of serum prolactin and low levels of serum testosterone often do not respond clinically to testosterone replacement therapy (as outlined above) unless serum concentrations of prolactin are lowered. The most effective way to lower serum concentrations of prolactin in such circumstances is usually treatment with dopamine agonists, such as bromocriptine.

BIBLIOGRAPHY

1. Adamopoulos DA, Lawrence DM, Vassilopoulos P, et al: Pituitary-testicular relationships in mumps orchitis and other viral infections. BMJ 1:1177, 1978.
2. Baker HWG, Burger HF, DeKretser DM, et al: Changes in the pituitary-testicular system with age. Clin Endocrinol 5:349, 1976.
3. Bannister P, Handley T, Chapman C, Losowsky MS: Hypogonadism in chronic liver disease: Impaired release of luteinising hormone. BMJ 293:1191, 1986.
4. Bhasin S: Androgen treatment of hypogonadal men. J Clin Endocrinol Metab 74:1221, 1992.
5. Carter JN, Tyson JE, Tolis G, et al: Prolactin-secreting tumors and hypogonadism in 22 men. N Engl J Med 299:847, 1978.
6. Castro-Magana M, Bronsther B, Angulo MA: Genetic forms of male hypogonadism. Urology 35:195, 1990.
7. Griffin JE, Wilson JD: The syndromes of androgen resistance. N Engl J Med 302:198, 1980.
8. Holdsworth S, Atkins RC, DeKretser DM: The pituitary-testicular axis in men with chronic renal failure. N Engl J Med 296:1245, 1977.
9. Hsueh WA, Hsu TH, Federman DD: Endocrine features of Klinefelter's syndrome. Medicine 57:447, 1978.

10. Lee PA, O'Dea LS: Primary and secondary testicular insufficiency. Pediatr Clin North Am 37:1359, 1990.
11. Lieblich JM, Rogol AD, White BJ, Rosen SW: Syndrome of anosmia with hypogonadotropic hypogonadism (Kallmann syndrome): Clinical and laboratory studies in 23 cases. Am J Med 73:506, 1982.
12. Matsumoto AM, Bremner WJ: Endocrinology of the hypothalamic-pituitary-testicular axis with particular reference to the hormonal control of spermatogenesis. Baillieres Clin Endocrinol Metab 1:71, 1987.
13. Schilsky RL, Lewis BJ, Sherins RJ, Young RC: Gonadal dysfunction in patients receiving chemotherapy for cancer. Ann Intern Med 93:109, 1980.
14. Schwartz ID, Root AW: The Klinefelter syndrome of testicular dysgenesis. Endocrinol Metab Clin North Am 20:153, 1991.
15. Wang C, Baker HWG, Burger HG, et al: Hormonal studies in Klinefelter's syndrome. Clin Endocrinol 4:399, 1975.
16. Whitcomb RW, Crowley WF: Male hypogonadotropic hypogonadism. Endocrinol Metab Clin North Am 22:125, 1993.

39. IMPOTENCE

John A. Merenich, M.D.

1. What is impotence?
Classically impotence has been defined as the inability to attain and maintain an erection of sufficient rigidity for sexual intercourse in 50% or more attempts. A more descriptive term for impotence is erectile dysfunction.

2. Do men with impotence have disturbances in other sexual function?
Most impotent men are able to ejaculate. Premature ejaculation may precede the development of impotence and is sometimes associated with drug therapy. Sexual desire (libido) is also usually preserved; loss of libido is suggestive of hypogonadism or severe systemic or psychiatric illness.

3. Is impotence common?
At least 10 million American men and perhaps as many as 20 million are impotent. Another 10 million may suffer from partial erectile dysfunction. The prevalence of impotence increases with age; about 2% of 40-year-old, 20% of 55-year-old, and 50–75% of 80-year-old men are impotent.

4. How does a normal erection occur?
Erection is primarily a vascular event that results from the complex interplay of the hormonal, vascular, peripheral nerve, and central nervous systems. Erection is usually initiated by various psychic and/or physiologic stimuli in the cerebral cortex. The stimuli are modulated in the limbic system and other areas of the brain, integrated in the hypothalamus, transmitted down the spinal cord, and carried to the penis via both autonomic and lower spinal nerves. Sensory nerves from the glans of the penis enhance the message and help to maintain erection during sexual activity via a reflex arc. The stimuli mediate the release of neurotransmitters that dilate blood vessels and relax penile smooth muscle, resulting in an erection.

5. How does increased blood flow to the penis result in an erection?
Within the two spongy corpora cavernosae of the penis are millions of tiny spaces called lacunae, each lined by a wall of trabecular smooth muscle. As neurotransmitters dilate cavernosal and helicine arteries to the penis and relax the trabecular smooth muscle, the lacunar spaces in the penis become engorged with blood. This results in entrapment of outflow vessels between the expanding trabecular walls and the rigid tunica albuginea that surround the corpora cavernosae, thereby greatly reducing venous outflow from the penis. This venoocclusive mechanism accounts for tumescence and rigidity.

6. What type of nerves and neurotransmitters play a role in penile erection?
At least 3 neuroeffector systems play a role in penile erection. Adrenergic nerves generally inhibit erection; cholinergic nerves and nonadrenergic, noncholinergic (NANC) substances enhance erection as follows:
- Sympathetic nerves (via alpha-adrenergic receptors)
  Constrict carvernosal and helicine arteries
  Contract trabecular smooth muscle
- Parasympathetic nerves (via cholinergic receptors)
  Inhibit adrenergic fibers
  Stimulate NANC fibers
- NANC messengers (nitric oxide, vasoactive intestinal polypeptide, prostaglandins, or other endothelium-derived factors)
  Dilate cavernosal and helicine arteries
  Relax trabecular smooth muscle

7. What are the common causes of impotence?

The frequency of the various causes of impotence is difficult to assess because of the large number of patients who do not report the problem, confusion regarding the diagnosis, and variability in the sophistication of the initial evaluation. Primary causes of impotence in men presenting to a medical outpatient clinic are approximated below:

Endocrine factors	30%
Diabetes mellitus	15%
Medications	20%
Systemic disease and alcoholism	10%
Primary vascular causes*	5%
Primary neurologic causes	5%
Psychogenic or unknown	15%

*Alterations of blood flow are thought to play a role in many causes of impotence, but specific lesions amenable to therapy are relatively rare.

8. Besides diabetes mellitus, what are the most common causes of endocrinologic impotence?

The three main endocrinologic disorders associated with impotence are the following:

- Hypogonadotropic hypogonadism (i.e., secondary hypogonadism; decreased luteinizing hormone (LH) and decreased testosterone).
- Hypergonadotropic hypogonadism (i.e., primary hypogonadism; increased LH and decreased testosterone).
- Hyperprolactinemia

Less common causes include hyperthyroidism, hypothyroidism, adrenal insufficiency, and Cushing's syndrome.

9. What are the most common drugs known to induce impotence?

Drugs most commonly associated with impotence include the following:

- Antihypertensive agents, especially methyldopa, clonidine, beta blockers, vasodilators (e.g., hydralazine), and diuretics
- Antipsychotic medications
- Antidepressants and tranquilizers
- Other (especially cimetidine, digoxin, phenytoin, carbamazepine, and metoclopramide)

10. Which antihypertensive agents should be used in patients with impotence?

Although virtually every blood pressure medication has been associated with impotence, the drugs least likely to effect erectile function are angiotensin-converting enzyme inhibitors and calcium channel-blocking agents. When beta blockade is required, selective beta-antagonists such as atenolol have the least impact on erectile function.

11. What is "stuttering" impotence? What is its significance?

Impotence alternating with periods of entirely normal sexual function is termed stuttering impotence. Multiple sclerosis is the most significant organic cause of stuttering impotence. It may be the initial manifestation of multiple sclerosis and may be present in up to 50% of men afflicted with the disease.

12. What historical information helps to separate organic from psychogenic impotence?

True psychogenic impotence is uncommon and should be a diagnosis of exclusion. Questions that may help to separate psychogenic from organic impotence are listed below:

	Organic	Psychogenic
Was onset abrupt?	No	Yes
Is impotence stress-dependent?	No	Yes
Is libido preserved?	Yes	No

	Organic	**Psychogenic**
Do you have morning erections?	No	Yes
Do you have orgasm?	Yes	No
Can you masturbate?	No	Yes
Does impotence occur with all partners?	Yes	No

13. Name the essential components of a physical exam in a man complaining of impotence.

Physical examination in an impotent man should specifically address the following:

- Measurement of standing and supine blood pressure and heart rate response to deep breathing (to evaluate autonomic nerve function)
- Secondary sexual characteristics, such as muscle development, hair pattern, and presence of breast tissue
- Vascular examination, especially of the femoral and lower extremity pulses
- Focused neurologic examination, including assessment of anal sphincter tone and bulbo-cavernous reflex
- Examination of the genitalia to determine penile size, shape, presence of plaque or fibrous tissue; size and consistency of the testes; prostate examination
- Thyroid examination

14. What is the appropriate laboratory assessment for men with impotence?

Laboratory assessment should be based on history and physical examination findings, but generally include the following:

- Complete blood count
- Urinalysis
- Fasting glucose
- Fasting lipid profile
- Serum creatinine
- Thyroid function tests
- Serum testosterone and luteinizing hormone

15. Should prolactin levels be measured in all impotent men?

Whether serum prolactin should be measured in all men with impotence is somewhat controversial. In general, patients with normal levels of testosterone and luteinizing hormone and a normal neurologic examination do not require measurement of prolactin. However, if testosterone is low and associated with low-to-normal luteinizing hormone or if history or examination suggests pituitary lesion, prolactin should be measured. Because prolactin interferes were the action of testosterone, prolactin status should be assessed in hypogonadal men unresponsive to testosterone replacement therapy. Hypothyroidism and renal failure also may elevate prolactin.

16. What is a penile brachial index?

Comparison of the penile and brachial systolic blood pressure allows a general assessment of the vascular integrity of the penis. This technique is not highly sensitive, but it is noninvasive and easy to perform and may help to identify men who require more extensive vascular studies. Penile systolic blood pressure obtained with Doppler ultrasound should be the same as brachial systolic pressure (i.e., ratio approximately = 1.0). An index <0.7 is highly suggestive of vasculogenic impotence. Diagnostic yield is increased if the brachial penile index is repeated after exercising the lower extremities for several minutes. This maneuver may uncover a pelvic steal syndrome that is characterized by a difference of more than 0.15 between the resting and exercise ratios.

17. What is nocturnal penile tumescence (NPT) monitoring?

Most men experience 3–6 erections during the night. By monitoring such events, one can assess the frequency, duration, and with some instruments even the rigidity of erection. This procedure helps to distinguish organic from psychogenic impotence. While helpful in some men, the cost, awkwardness, and lack of normative data preempt the routine use of NPT in the evaluation of impotent men at this time.

18. What are the therapeutic options in the treatment of impotence?

The many treatment options for men with impotence include the following:

- Medical treatments
    Remove offending drugs
    Treat underlying medical conditions
    Replace testosterone in hypogonadal men
    Reduce hyperprolactinemia with bromocriptine
    Prescribe adrenergic receptor blockers (e.g., yohimbine)
- Psychological therapy, especially for men who have no obvious organic cause of impotence
- Intracavernosal injection of vasoactive substances, especially prostaglandin E, papaverine, and phenotolamine
- External mechanical aids and vacuum/suction devices
- Surgical treatments
    Revascularization procedures
    Obliteration of venous shunts
    Surgical penile implants

19. Are medical treatments for impotence safe and effective?

Androgen replacement therapy for hypogonadal men is relatively safe, provided that liver enzymes, prostate size, and prostate-specific antigen are monitored. Androgen therapy should be given intramuscularly in the form of long-acting testosterone derivatives, such as enanthate or cypionate, 200–300 mg every 2–3 weeks. Bromocriptine is helpful in men with elevated levels of prolactin, even when levels of testosterone are normal. Many other oral and parenteral treatments for impotence are under investigation. Few have been proved effective in well-designed trials; thus routine use in men with erectile dysfunction cannot be recommended. The one exception may be yohimbine hydrochloride (6.5 mg orally 3x/day), which has shown promise in some, but not all, placebo-controlled studies.

20. What are the complications of intracavernosal injection?

Injection of vasodilitory substances directly into the corpora cavernosae of the penis results in erection satisfactory for intercourse in many men with impotence. Side effects, which depend on the type and quantity of substances injected, include hypotension, elevation of liver enzymes, and headache. Local complications include hematoma, swelling, inadvertent injection into the uretha, and local fibrosis with long-term use. The most serious local complication is priapism (a sustained erection) for more than 4 hours, which may necessitate injection of alpha-adrenergic agonists or corpora cavernosal aspiration.

BIBLIOGRAPHY

1. Krane RJ, Goldstein I, DeTejada IS: Impotence. N Engl J Med 321:1648–1659, 1989.
2. Lerner SF, Melman A, Christ GJ: A review of erectile dysfunction: New insights and more questions. J Urol 149 (5 Pt 2):1246–1252, 1993.
3. Morley JE, Kaiser FE: Impotence: The internists' approach to diagnosis and treatment. Adv Intern Med 38:151–168, 1993.
4. Morley JE: Impotence. Am J Med 80:897–905, 1986.
5. Neisler AW, Carey NP: A critical reeavaluation of nocturnal penile tumescence monitoring in a diagnosis of erectile dysfunction. J Nerv Ment Dis 178:78–89, 1990.
6. NIH Consensus Conference: Impotence. JAMA 270:83–90, 1993.
7. Sidi AA: Vasoactive intracavernous pharmacotherapy. Urol Clin North Am 15:95–101, 1988.
8. Wilson JD, Foster DW (eds): Williams' Textbook of Endocrinology. Philadelphia, W.B. Saunders, 1992.
9. Witherington R: Mechanical aids for treatment of impotence. Clin Diabetes 7:1–22, 1989.

40. GYNECOMASTIA

Brenda K. Bell, M.D.

1. What is the definition of gynecomastia?
Gynecomastia is defined as the presence of palpable breast tissue in a male.

2. How does gynecomastia present clinically?
Gynecomastia usually presents as a palpable discrete button of firm subareolar breast tissue (>2 cm) or as a diffuse collection of fibroadipose tissue. Physical examination can differentiate fibroadipose tissue from simple fat by pinching the fat tissue in the anterior axillary fold and comparing the texture and consistency with the breast tissue in question. Gynecomastia may be painful.

3. What is the significance of painful gynecomastia?
Pain or tenderness implies recent, rapid growth of breast tissue.

4. Is gynecomastia always bilateral?
The involvement tends to be bilateral, but asymmetry is common. Unilateral enlargement is present in 5–25% of patients.

5. Does gynecomastia have a racial predilection?
No.

6. What is the pathophysiology of gynecomastia?
Estrogens stimulate ductal proliferation. Androgens may inhibit breast development. Gynecomastia results from an increase in the ratio of estrogen to androgen, which may be due to increased production of estrogens, decreased production of testosterone, or increased conversion of androgens to estrogens in peripheral tissue.

7. Where are estrogens produced in the male?
Direct testicular production of estrogen accounts for less than 15%. The majority of estrogen comes from the conversion of adrenal and testicular androgen to estrogen in peripheral tissues, particularly adipose tissue and the liver.

8. What is the most common etiology of gynecomastia?
Asymptomatic palpable breast tissue is common in normal males, particularly in the neonate (60–90%), at puberty (60–70% between the ages of 12–15 years), and with increasing age (30–85% over age 45 years). Because of high prevalence, gynecomastia is considered a relatively normal finding during the above periods of life. Gynecomastia occurring at these ages is often called physiologic or idiopathic and accounts for 50% of cases.

9. Why does gynecomastia occur so commonly during these stages of life?
Neonatal gynecomastia occurs due to placental transfer of estrogen. During early puberty, production of estrogen rises sooner than production of testosterone, causing an imbalance in the ratio of estrogen to androgen. With aging, production of testosterone decreases, and peripheral conversion of androgen to estrogen often increases because of an age-associated increase in adipose tissue.

10. What are the other causes of gynecomastia?
Drugs account for 10–20% of cases; primary hypogonadism for 10%; and adrenal or testicular tumors for less than 3%. Other causes combined, including secondary hypogonadism, androgen-

resistant disorders, malnutrition, cirrhoisis, alcohol abuse, renal disease, congenital adrenal hyperplasia, extragonadal tumor, and hyperthyroidism, account for less than 10%.

11. What drugs cause gynecomastia?

Many drugs have been implicated, some with known steroid effects, others with no clear mechanism:

Anabolic steroids	Methyldopa	Theophylline
Estrogen creams	Metoclopramide	Amiodarone
Spironolactone	Reserpine	Nifedipine
Flutamide	Marijuana	Verapamil
Cimetidine	Heroin	Tricyclic antidepresants
Ranitidine	Methadone	Phenothiazines
Isoniazid	Phenytoin	Captopril
Digitoxin	Diazepam	Enalapril
Ketoconazole	Metronidazole	

12. How do testicular tumors cause gynecomastia?

The most common mechanism is increased production of human chorionic gonadotropin (hCG) by germ cell tumors. Like luteinizing hormone (LH), hCG increases testicular production of estradiol. Less commonly, Leydig cell tumors may directly secrete estradiol.

13. What extragondal tumors cause gynecomastia?

Pancreatic, gastric, and pulmonary tumors have been associated with production of hCG. Hepatomas may have increased aromatase activity that results in increased conversion of androgens to estrogens.

14. Who should undergo evaluation for gynecomastia?

Gynecomastia is so common that many experts recommend evaluation only when breast enlargement is symptomatic, progressive, or greater than 5 cm in diameter or has no simple explanation. A history and physical examination are indicated in all cases.

15. What information is significant in the history?

Age	Thyroid symptoms
Duration of enlargement	Nutritional status and recent changes in weight
Breast symptoms (tenderness, discharge)	Alcohol use
Other illnesses	Congenital abnormalities
Drugs	Pubertal progression
Impotence and libido	

16. What should be noted on the physical examination?

The most important features include characteristics of the breast tissue (irregular, firm, eccentric; nipple discharge), testes (size, asymmetry), abdomen (liver enlargement, palmar erythema, ascites, spider angioma), secondary sexual characteristics, thyroid status (goiter, tremor, reflexes), and any signs of excessive cortisol (buffalo hump, central obesity, hypertension, purple striae, moon facies).

17. Should laboratory tests be ordered?

When the diagnosis is not apparent after the history and physical examination, one should measure serum levels of testosterone, estradiol, luteinizing hormone (LH), follicle-stimulating hormone (FSH), prolactin, thyrotropin (TSH), human chorionic gonadotropin (hCG), liver-associated enzymes, blood urea nitrogen, and creatinine, and a chest radiograph should be obtained. If hCG or estradiol is elevated, a testicular ultrasound is indicated. For prepubertal patients, an adrenal computed tomographic (CT) scan should also be considered.

18. What findings raise the suspicion of breast cancer?

Breast cancer is rare in men (0.2%), and does not increase with gynecomastia, except in Klinefelter's syndrome (3–6%). Bloody discharge, ulceration, firmness, fixation to the underlying tissue, eccentric location (not subareolar), and adenopathy are suspicious findings. If doubt remains, biopsy should be considered.

19. Will gynecomastia spontaneously regress?

In most cases, yes. Neonatal gynecomastia usually resolves within 4 months. Pubertal gynecomastia tends to resolve within 6 months but may persist for 2–3 years. The tissue becomes more fibrous with time and less likely remit spontaneously. The more developed the breast tissue (Tanner stages III, IV, and V), the less likely it is to regress. Gynecomastia in older men is not likely to resolve spontaneously.

20. What is the treatment when gynecomastia does not regress?

If gynecomastia has been present for a long time and is greater than 3 cm, the treatment is surgery. Tamoxifen, clomiphene, danazol, dihydrotestosterone, and testolactone also have been used. Tamoxifen has the fewest side effects. Tenderness improves, but there is little decrease in size if the breasts are large.

BIBLIOGRAPHY

 1. Braunstein G: Gynecomastia: Current concepts. N Engl J Med 328:490–495, 1993.
 2. Carlson H: Gynecomastia: Pathogenesis and therapy. Endocrinologist 1:337–342, 1991.
 3. Carlson H: Gynecomastia. N Engl J Med 303:795–799, 1980.
 4. Leung A: Gynecomastia. Am Fam Physician 39:215–222, 1989.
 5. Longcope, C: Gynecomastia: Current Therapy in Endocrinology and Metabolism, 4th ed Philadelphia, B.C. Decker, 1991.
 6. Niewoehner C, Nuttall F: Gynecomastia in a hospitalized male population. Am J Med. 77:633–638, 1984.
 7. Nuttall F: Gynecomastia as a physical finding in normal men. J Clin Endocrinol Metab 48:338–340, 1979.
 8. Santon R: Gynecomastia: Endocrinology and Metabolism, 2nd Ed. New York, McGraw-Hill, 1987.
 9. Webster D: Benign disorders of the male breast. World J Surg 13:726–730, 1989.
10. Wilson J, Aiman J, MacDonald P: The Pathogenesis of Gynecomastia. Chicago, Year Book, 1980.

41. AMENORRHEA

Julie I. Rifkin, M.D.

1. Define amenorrhea.

Amenorrhea is the absence of menses. It is normal for a girl to be amenorrheic until she enters puberty. Physiologic amenorrhea also occurs during pregnancy and lactation and after the menopause. A girl who has not started to menstruate by 16–18 years of age has primary amenorrhea. A woman who has undergone menarche but fails to menstruate for 3–6 months has secondary amenorrhea.

2. How does puberty begin?

Between the ages of 6 and 9 years, long before secondary sexual characteristics appear, secretion of gonadotropins (luteinizing hormone [LH] and follicle-stimulating hormone [FSH]) gradually rises. The rise in gonadotropins occurs in response to pulses of hypothalamic gonadotropin-releasing hormone (GnRH). In young children, such pulses are inhibited by centers in the central nervous system (tracts routed through the posterior hypothalmamus) that constrain secretion of GnRH. As these centers mature, their inhibitory restraint decreases.

Specific pulse configurations of GnRH during sleep trigger the onset of puberty. Elevated levels of gonadotropins sensitize the female gonads (ovaries). The ovarian granulosa cells in turn secrete the sex hormones estrogen and progesterone. Sexual maturity is finally obtained when the levels of female hormones are able to stimulate the midcycle surge of pituitary gonadotropins (positive feedback). The midcycle surge of LH eventually triggers ovulation on a consistent basis. It is not uncommon for the first several menstrual cycles to be irregular, because ovulation may not occur with each cycle.

A prepubertal girl has *no* physical evidence of pubarche or thelarche. A pubertal girl usually has evidence of both. The overlap in serum levels of gonadotropins, estradiol, androstenedione, testosterone, and dehydroepiandrosterone sulfate ($DHEA-SO_4$) between prepubertal girls over the age of 8 years and pubertal girls is substantial. On average, pubertal changes occur between ages 10 and 11 years. The time from the onset of breast buds to menarche is about 2.3 years. Menstruation usually begins at about 12.7 years of age.

3. What important details need to be elicited when taking a history from a patient with primary amenorrhea?

It is useful to know how the patient's growth and development have proceeded to the present time. Has she noticed breast development (thelarche) or pubic or axillary hair (pubarche or adrenarche)? Does the patient have a history of abnormal or ambiguous genitalia noted at birth? An affirmative answer suggests the possibilities of maternal androgen ingestion, adrenogenital syndrome, or müllerian tract abnormalities.

Developmental milestones tend to occur near the same age in family members. It is useful to know when the patient's mother, aunts, and grandmother began menstruation. Does the family have a history of inherited disorders?

A thorough psychosocial assessment (often difficult to obtain during the first visit) is highly important in each evaluation. Fad dieting, bulimia, and anorexia nervosa are associated with amenorrhea. Prolonged psychological stress and emotional difficulties likewise may inhibit menstruation. Strenuous exercise as engaged in by gymnasts, dancers, and runners is also associated with amenorrhea.

Systemic diseases involving one or more organ systems are often linked with pubertal delay. Finally, the physician must never overlook the possibility of pregnancy when evaluating primary amenorrhea.

4. During the physical examination, what findings may suggest an etiology for primary amenorrhea?

The patient's height must be accurately measured. A stature of less than 60 inches, webbed neck, shield chest, and increased carrying angle at the elbows suggest Turner's syndrome (45 XO).

The presence of breasts without pubic and axillary hair and nonvisualization of a cervix raise the question of testicular feminization. Testicular feminization occurs when a child is born with a male (46 XY) karyotype, but bodily tissues cannot respond to the normal effects of testosterone (complete androgen insensitivity). The gonads (testes) in such patients may be intraabdominal but palpable as a hernia or labial mass.

The appearance of normal secondary sexual characteristics and the absence of menarche suggests an abnormality of the müllerian tract (congenital absence of the uterus), stress-associated amenorrhea (hypothalamic dysfunction), a tumor of the anterior pituitary, or unresponsive ovaries. The total absence of secondary sexual characteristics indicates constitutional delay of puberty or the possible presence of gonadotropin or GnRH deficiency.

A thorough genital examination must always be performed. It may be useful to perform this examination with an ultrasound study. An imperforate hymen or transverse vaginal septum is easily identified. Ambiguous genitalia may represent a masculinized female or an incompletely masculinized male; however, such patients are usually identified and evaluated at birth. A breast examination demonstrating galactorrhea may indicate an elevated level of prolactin as the cause of the amenorrhea.

5. What criteria suggest that primary amenorrhea is due to constitutional or physiologic delay of puberty?

Constitutional delay of puberty may be suspected in a 12- to 14-year-old girl without clinical evidence of puberty. Prospective observation of the patient's growth curve reveals a deceleration as puberty is delayed. The physiologic spurt in linear growth accompanies the onset of puberty, generally at a bone age of 11 years. Prepubertal and pubertal measurements of serum hormone levels display a wide degree of overlap. Constitutional delay of puberty is possible but less likely when the patient presents at 16 years or older.

6. When should a formal evaluation of primary amenorrhea be initiated?

Amenorrhea in a 16-year-old girl with or without normal growth or secondary sexual characteristics needs evaluation. Some authorities lower the age to 14 years when no secondary sexual characteristics are present.

7. What type of work-up is usually performed to evaluate primary amenorrhea?

If the physical examination and pelvic ultrasound disclose anomalies of the reproductive tract, an intravenous pyelogram should be performed because of the high incidence of concomitant urinary tract anomalies.

The initial laboratory evaluation includes measurement of serum prolactin, thyroid-stimulating hormone (TSH), FSH, and beta human chorionic gonadotropin (βhCG), if indicated. An elevated level of prolactin may be due to pituitary prolactinoma, hypothyroidism, or ingestion of phenothiazine. Elevated levels of prolactin are also found in long-distance runners. A serum TSH should be drawn to rule out hypothyroidism. The serum FSH should be performed on at least two samples; it may be normal or elevated.

Patients with primary ovarian failure, gonadal dysgenesis (Turner's syndrome), forms of congenital adrenal hyperplasia, or congenital ovarian resistance to gonadotropin action (defective receptor-adenylate cyclase coupling) have elevated levels of FSH and incomplete development of secondary sex characteristics.

Prepubertal patients aged 14–16 years with a nonelevated level of FSH are further evaluated with radiographs to determine bone age. If the bone age is below 11 years, all forms of hypogonadism, including constitutional delay, must be considered. A bone age between 11 and 13 years (menarche typically occurs at this bone age) in a prepubertal girl with a nonelevated level of FSH generally indicates a diagnosis of hypothalamic hypogonadism.

8. What is the progesterone challenge test?

The progesterone challenge test provides information about the physical reproductive tract. The test is performed by giving oral medroxyprogesterone acetate (Provera), 10 mg orally, for 7–10 days. A positive test, defined as menstrual-like bleeding 4–14 days after the last tablet, indicates an intact hypothalamic-pituitary-ovarian axis and patency of the reproductive tract. If the progesterone withdrawal test is negative, an estrogen and progesterone withdrawal test is performed. Conjugated estrogen (Premarin) is given orally as 1.25 mg tablets for 25 days, along with 10 mg of oral Provera on days 16–25. Withdrawal bleeding indicates that the uterine endometrium is capable of responding and thus eliminates the uterus as a cause of amenorrhea.

9. How are patients with primary hypothalamic amenorrhea and Turner's syndrome treated?

The goals of hormone replacement therapy are to develop secondary sexual characteristics, to allow normal sexual function, and to prevent osteoporosis. Treatment is best guided by a pediatric endocrinologist in conjunction with psychological counseling.

Patients with primary hypothalamic amenorrhea (termed Kallmann's syndrome if anosmia is present) may be treated with gradually increasing doses of estrogen every 3 months until vaginal bleeding occurs. A progestational agent may then be added. When pregnancy is desired, patients may be given subcutaneous GnRH in a pulsatile fashion and should be referred to centers with expertise in reproductive endocrinology.

For patients with Turner's syndrome, final adult height is a major concern. A 6-month course of an anabolic steroid (low-dose depot testosterone 30mg/m^2/month intramuscularly or oxandroline 0.1 mg/kg/day) augments the final height. Human growth hormone may also be useful, but it is costly. To induce secondary sexual characteristics, a regimen similar to that employed for hypogonadotropic hypogonadism may be used. In vitro fertilization (donor egg and partner's sperm) may allow patients to carry a pregnancy.

10. What are the frequently encountered causes of secondary amenorrhea in women of reproductive age?

Secondary amenorrhea occurs when a menstruating female ceases to have periods for 3–6 months. Polycystic ovarian syndrome, premature ovarian failure, and disturbances of hypothalamic function are frequently uncovered. Pregnancy must always be ruled out, along with thyroid dysfunction and hyperprolactinemia. Amenorrhea may occur for up to 6 months after an oral contraceptive is stopped. Less common causes of secondary amenorrhea include excessive postpartum curettage that damages the endometrium and masculinizing tumors, such as gonadoblastomas, dysgerminomas, or hilar cell tumors.

11. What disorders cause secondary hypothalamic amenorrhea?

Functional hypothalmic amenorrhea may occur when a woman is under physical or psychological stress. It is commonly encountered in women with eating disorders (anorexia nervosa, bulimia) and in women who are competitive athletes (runners, swimmers, gymnasts, dancers).

Stress-induced hyperactivity in the hypothalamic-pituitary-adrenal axis produces increased levels of corticotropin-releasing hormone (CRH), which in turn increases the activity of central opioid and serotonin pathways. The increased activity in these central pathways inhibits the normal pulsatile secretion of GnRH.

Structural hypothalamic amenorrhea may occur if the hypothalamus is damaged by head injury, tumor (craniopharyngioma), or an infiltrative process such as histiocytosis X.

Treatment of functional or structural hypothalamic amenorrhea consists of hormone replacement therapy (estrogen and progesterone) with or without supplemental multivitamins and calcium.

12. What complications are associated with the estrogen deficient state of untreated hypothalamic amenorrhea?

Patients with all causes of hypothalamic amenorrhea are at increased risk for osteopenia and bone fracture because of inadequate levels of circulating estrogen. A recent prospective study demonstrated that young amenorrheic athletes do not achieve a normal peak bone mass as adults. This health problem may be long-term. Low levels of circulating estrogen are also associated with unfavorable lipid profiles: a tendency toward higher levels of LDL cholesterol and lower levels of HDL cholesterol. Both amenorrheic and eumenorrheic female athletes have lower-than-average serum levels of aproprotein B (a major protein of LDL), and the amenorrheic athlete has a lower level of apo-A (a major protein of HDL). Exercise alone does not achieve a favorable atherosclerotic risk profile for such patients.

13. What are the causes of hyperprolactinemia?

The level of serum prolactin varies somewhat during the normal menstrual cycle. Levels of prolactin are higher in the mornings and may be elevated by stress, breast examinations, and food intake. It is best to measure prolactin in the late morning before an examination and at least 1 hour after a meal.

Prolactin may be elevated in patients with hypothyroidism, because thyrotropin-releasing hormone (TRH) also stimulates prolactin. Meningitis, herpes zoster, chest wall trauma, repetitive nipple stimulation, and systemic illness such as renal failure or cirrhosis may induce hyperprolactinemia. Drugs that commonly elevate prolactin include high-estrogen contraceptives, diazepam, opiates, tricyclic antidepressants, phenothiazines, and neuroleptics.

Prolactin-secreting pituitary adenomas may cause amenorrhea and galactorrhea. Hyperprolactinemia inhibits the pulsatile secretion of GnRH and also directly affects ovarian function (follicle atresia and progesterone synthesis dysfunction). Approximately 33% of patients with hyperprolactinemia have galactorrhea. Levels of prolactin greater than 100 ng/ml are frequently associated with pituitary prolactinoma. Levels above the laboratory's upper limit of normal but less than 100 ng/ml may be due to another cause.

14. How are patients with pituitary prolactinomas treated?

Patients with adenomas smaller than 10 mm (microadenomas) respond well to dopamine agonist therapy (bromocriptine). Transsphenoidal hypophysectomy is generally not performed. Patients with macroadenomas also respond well to dopamine agonist therapy but on occasion may require surgery. The patient can be expected to resume menses and ovulatory function when the level of prolactin normalizes.

15. Hyperandrogenic amenorrhea is commonly caused by which disorder?

Polycystic ovarian disease (PCOD) clinically presents in the peripubertal period with oligomenorrhea or amenorrhea and hyperandrogenism. The ovaries contain many small subcapsular cysts and may be normal-sized or enlarged. The neuroendocrine abnormality responsible for PCOD is not yet clearly identified, but hyperandrogenism is common to all subsets of the disorder.

Anovulation is the hallmark of PCOD; thus patients are frequently infertile. Approximately 55% of patients present with amenorrhea; 70% compliant of hirsutism. Genetic sensitivity of the hair follicle to androgen determines the degree of hirsutism. The patient may or may not be obese.

16. How is PCOD diagnosed?

Some authorities advocate that the diagnosis be made on clinical grounds alone. The usual patient presents with a combination of irregular menses or amenorrhea, hirsutism, and infertility. True virilization is uncommon but requires evaluation for the rare androgen-producing adrenal or gonadal neoplasm. Lab findings in PCOD include an elevated LH, low or low-normal FSH and a high-normal or slightly elevated serum testosterone. A progesterone challenge test induces withdrawal bleeding. There is significant overlap between hormone values in patients with PCOD and normal females. Lab tests must be interpreted in light of the patient's history and clinical exam.

17. How is PCOD treated?
Chronic absence of withdrawal bleeding is associated with adenomatous hyperplasia or neoplasia of the endometrium. An endometrial biopsy should be considered for the patient with long-standing anovulation. If prenancy is not desired, a combination oral contraceptive is commonly prescribed to induce regular menses and to improve hirsutism. Ovulation induction therapy may be successful if the patient wishes to become pregnant.

18. How is premature ovarian failure diagnosed?
Premature ovarian failure is suggested when a woman under the age of 40 years fails to menstruate for at least 3 months and has at least two FSH measurements greater than 40 mIμ/ml. The term premature ovarian failure does not accurately describe all women who meet the above criteria. Some women (<10%) actually ovulate and conceive after the diagnosis is made, even while they are on estrogen replacement therapy. There is currently no way to predict which patients will or will not be fertile.

19. Which disorders or conditions are associated with premature ovarian failure? How is it treated?
A portion of patients have recognized cytogenetic abnormalities such as 47 XXX and 45 XO mosaics. Previous chemotherapy or radiation therapy to the pelvis may cause permanent or temporary ovarian failure. Several autoimmune disorders are associated with premature ovarian failure, including diabetes mellitus, rheumatoid arthritis, Graves' disease and thyroiditis, myasthenia gravis, idiopthic thrombocytopenic purpura, systemic lupus erythematosus, Addison's disease, and primary biliary cirrhosis. In the majority of cases, no specific cause is identified.

The work-up includes a thorough history and physical examination, complete blood count and sedimentation rate; RA and ANA, and thyroid hormones including antimicrosomal antibodies, LH, FSH, and estradiol (on at least two occasions); and evaluation of bone density. A karyotype is usually recommended if the patient is under 30 years old to rule out the possibility of mosaicism with a Y chromosome. This condition requires a laparotomy for the excision of gonadal tissue. The presence of any testicular component carries a 25% chance of malignant tumor formation.

Treatment consists of hormone replacement therapy with estrogen and progesterone. In vitro fertilization (donor eggs and partner's sperm) may allow a patient to carry a pregnancy.

BIBLIOGRAPHY

1. Blackwell RE: Hyperprolactinemia. Endocrinol Metab Clin North Am 21:105, 1992.
2. Hall JE: Polycystic ovarian disease as a neuroendocrine disorder of the female reproductive axis. Endocrinol Metab Clin North Am 22:75, 1993.
3. Havens CS (ed): Manual of Outpatient Gynecology, 2nd ed. Boston, Little, Brown, 1991, p 92.
4. Lamon-Fava S, Fischer EC, et al: Effect of exercise and menstrual cycle status on plasma lipids, low density lipoprotein particle size, and apolipoproteins. J Clin Endocrinol Metab 68:17, 1989.
5. Nappi RE, Petraglia F, et al: Hypothalamic amenorrhea: Evidence for a central derangement of hypothalamic-pituitary-adrenal cortex axis activity. Fertil Steril 59:571, 1993.
6. Rebar RW, Connolly HV: Clinical features of young women with hypergonadotropic amenorrhea. Fertil Steril 53:804, 1990.
7. Rebar RW, Cedars MI: Hypergonadotropic forms of amenorrhea in young women. Endocrinol Metab Clin North Am 21:173, 1992.
8. Rosenfield RL: Puberty and its disorders in girls. Endocrinol Metab Clin North Am 20:15, 1991.
9. Speroff L (ed): Clinical Gynecologic Endocrinology and Infertility, 4th ed. Baltimore, Williams & Wilkins, 1989 p 165.
10. Wilson JD, Foster DW (eds): Williams' Textbook of Endocrinology, 8th ed. Philadelphia, W.B. Saunders, 1992, p 733.
11. Woodruff JD, Pickar JH: Incidence of endometrial hyperplasia in postmenopausal women taking conjugated estrogens (Premarin) with medroxyprogesterone acetate or conjugated estrogens alone. Am J Obstet Gynecol 170(5)Pt 1:1213–1223, 1994.
12. Yen S: Female hypogonadotropic hypogonadism. Endocrinol Metab Clin North Am 22:29, 1993.

42. GALACTORRHEA

William J. Georgitis, M.D., COL, MC

CAUSES

1. What hormones are essential for lactation?

Estrogen and prolactin are both necessary for milk production. Estrogens promote cellular proliferation and ductular development in the breast. Prolactin rises dramatically in pregnancy, stimulating differentiation of acini in preparation for the production of milk protein. Paradoxically the high levels of estrogen in pregnancy inhibit milk production, but 2 or 3 days after delivery, lactation begins as levels of estrogen decline. Growth hormone, insulin, and cortisol serve as necessary permissive factors for cell growth in cultures of breast tissue. Androgens inhibit growth and differentiation of the breast; thus galactorrhea is a rare finding in men.

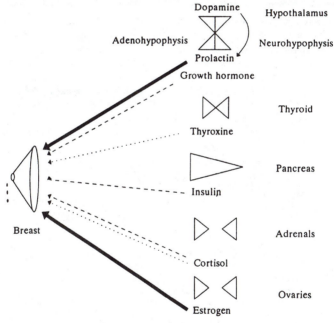

Hormones essential for lactation. Major stimulatory hormones are indicated by bold arrows. Permissive hormones are shown with dashed arrows. Hormones playing predominantly regulatory roles appear with dotted arrows.

2. Can failure to lactate and menstruate postpartum indicate a serious disorder?

The inability to lactate and menstruate after delivery may be clues to the diagnosis of Sheehan's syndrome. Postpartum pituitary necrosis is associated with difficult deliveries complicated by obstetrical hemorrhage and hypotension. In the United States, pituitary insufficiency is usually limited to the adenohypophysis, but countries where obstetrical care is lacking have reported cases of vasopressin deficiency, indicating neurohypophysial involvement.

3. How frequent is galactorrhea?

A milklike discharge from the breast of a nongravid woman or milk secretion persisting for 6 months after a nursing mother ceases breast feeding is fairly common. The lifelong frequency of galactorrhea in normal women has been reported to range from 2–20%. Milk should not be found in normal nulligravidas, postmenopausal women not receiving hormone replacement, or men.

4. Does galactorrhea always look like milk?
No. Breast milk is basically an emulsion of fat and water with over 100 known constituents. Because the quantity of fat varies, the gross appearance may vary from milky to opalescent or clear. Microscopic examination is helpful in classifying a breast secretion as galactorrhea by revealing fat globules. Special stains for fat or chemical analysis for lactose or specific milk proteins are rarely necessary.

5. Is galactorrhea always expressed from both breasts?
Galactorrhea may be unilateral or bilateral. Although many patients report frank leaking or staining of garments, some may not notice the discharge. Galactorrhea expressed from a single breast may be indicative of an important pathologic condition such as prolactinoma, but small amounts of serous fluid are expressed from the majority of normal women who have experienced pregnancy.

6. Is the differential diagnosis for galactorrhea simple or complex?
The differential diagnosis for galactorrhea is actually more complex than it appears at first glance. Causes for nonpuerperal galactorrhea are not easy to arrange in a logical and memorable list. Some lists categorize possible diagnoses by anatomic location, some by causality, and some by symptoms or signs such as amenorrhea or presence or absence of hyperprolactinemia. Careful scrutiny usually reveals that a logical approach somehow falls apart before the differential is complete. Even a shift in gender subtly creeps into many of the differentials listed in articles and textbooks. I apologize for another unsuccessful attempt in the table below and challenge imaginative medical students everywhere to devise an effective mnemonic for galactorrhea.

Causes of Nonpuerperal Galactorrhea

Idiopathic galactorrhea
Pituitary tumor
    Prolactinoma
    Somatotrophinoma
Hypothalamic disorders
    Tumor (craniopharyngioma, meningioma)
    Infiltrations (sarcoid, histiocytosis, metastases)
    Infundibular disruption (surgical, compression by tumor)
Medications
    Psychotropic (chlorpromazine)
    Antihypertensive (alpha-methyldopa)
    Cannabinoid (morphine)
    Estrogenic compound (oral contraceptives)
    Antiemetic (metoclopramide)
Extrapituitary endocrinopathies
    Primary hypothyroidism
    Hyperthyroidism
    Addison's disease
Endogenous estrogens
    Feminizing adrenal carcinoma
Reflex arc activation
    Suckling or mechanical breast stimulation
    Thoracic nerve stimulation (surgery, burns, herpes zoster, mastitis)
Miscellaneous disorders
    Stress
    Empty sella syndrome
    Renal or hepatic failure
    Polycystic ovary syndrome

7. Which medications cause galactorrhea?
Psychotropic medications are the leading culprits. The most common are phenothiazines, tricyclic antidepressants, haloperidol, benzodiazepines, butyrophenones, amphetamines, and inhibitors of monoamine oxidase (MAO). Other commonly prescribed drugs implicated as causes for galactorrhea include cimetidine, metoclopramide, verapamil, and estrogens in various formulations.

EVALUATION

8. Is the presence or absence of amenorrhea significant in a woman with galactorrhea?
A comprehensive menstrual history is an essential part of the evaluation of a woman with galactorrhea. A common physiologic cause for galactorrhea with amenorrhea is pregnancy. The galactorrheic woman with normal menses carries a 20% chance of having a pituitary tumor. When amenorrhea accompanies galactorrhea, the percentage increases to 34%, according to a widely cited series. Furthermore, when amenorrhea is present, the clinician should consider the additional problems of infertility and accelerated bone mineral loss from hyperprolactinemic hypogonadotropic hypogonadism.

9. What percentage of women with elevated levels of serum prolactin have galactorrhea?
Of women with elevated levels of prolactin, 50–80% have galactorrhea. The lack of correlation between the degree of elevation and amount of lactation is of interest. Nonetheless, absolute levels of prolactin may be used to categorize diagnostic possibilities.

10. How is the level of serum prolactin useful in determining the cause of galactorrhea?
Serum prolactin is a dynamic polypeptide that displays diurnal fluctuation and responds to various stimuli. Levels rise after meals, after stressors such as hypoglycemia and seizures, and after intercourse or vigorous nipple stimulation. Normal levels range as high as 20 ng/ml. Drug-induced galactorrhea is associated with normal or moderately elevated levels of prolactin; medications should not be assumed to explain elevations above 100 ng/ml. Mild hyperprolactinemia also may be seen with pituitary, hypothalamic, or parasellar processes. Many drugs cause galactorrhea by a common mechanism involving diminished dopaminergic inhibition of secretion of prolactin. Perhaps this mechanism explains why mass lesions that compress or disrupt the normal hypothalamic-pituitary portal connections result in hyperprolactinemia comparable in magnitude to the elevations found with drug-induced galactorrhea.

With prolactin elevations over 100 ng/ml, the odds of finding a pituitary tumor are proportionate to the extent of hyperprolactinemia. Levels above 300 ng/ml are strongly indicative of prolactinoma. Patients with levels ranging from 100–300 ng/ml should be investigated carefully. Even when sella imaging fails to detect a tumor, such patients, if left untreated, merit continued surveillance, because the majority probably harbor microprolactinomas.

11. Should any laboratory test other than measurement of prolactin be included in the evaluation?
Yes. Levels of thyroid-stimulating hormone (TSH) also should be measured. Primary hypothyroidism may present as an amenorrhea-galactorrhea syndrome with pituitary hyperplasia that mimics pituitary adenoma. Published reports include patients with massive hyperplasia who present with symptoms and signs of optic chiasmal compression; yet the hypothyroidism may be easily missed. Both pituitary hyperplasia and the amenorrhea-galactorrhea syndrome resolve with thyroxine therapy. Preoperative measurement of TSH level is thus a necessary component of the evaluation of every patient with a pituitary mass and galactorrhea.

12. Can galactorrhea be present in the absence of excessive prolactin?
Yes. About one-third of women with acromegaly have galactorrhea due to hyperprolactinemia from secretion of prolactin by the tumor or by stalk disruption. Some patients, however, have

normal levels of prolactin, and the galactorrhea results from activation of breast prolactin receptors by growth hormone, which shares structural homology with prolactin.

13. Is galactorrhea associated with an increased risk of breast cancer?
No. Even a nonmilky breast discharge is not commonly associated with cancer; when it is, there is usually a palpable mass. Even bloody breast secretions more often result from benign conditions than cancer. Some evidence suggests that the risk of breast cancer is reduced in premenopausal women who have lactated.

TREATMENT

14. What class of medication is most effective in reducing galactorrhea?
Dopamine agonists, such as bromocriptine, pergolide, and newer investigational agents, dramatically reduce secretion of prolactin and thereby decrease or abolish lactation.

15. How quickly does bromocriptine inhibit postpartum lactation?
If all available milk is removed with a breast pump before bromocriptine is administered, no further milk can be obtained 4–6 hours later. Postpartum treatment should be continued for 10–14 days to prevent rebound breast engorgement.

16. Are there other effective means of suppressing lactation?
Estrogens were used effectively in the 1930s. Before the 1930s, various relatively ineffective measures, including breast binders, diuretics, and laxatives, were tried. An alternative to bromocriptine is ethinyl estradiol, 2.5 mg 3 times/day for 5 days. Estrogens fail in about 10–20% of cases, and bromocriptine is clearly more effective in suppressing physiologic galactorrhea.

17. How common are side effects with bromocriptine treatment of physiological lactation?
One-third of treated patients have one or more side effects, usually mild or moderate in severity. The most frequent complaints are headache, dizziness, nausea, vomiting, fatigue, diarrhea, and cramps. Serious adverse events, such as stroke, seizures, and syncope, have been reported but fortunately are rare. A first-dose phenomenon occurs in about 1% of patients.

18. Bromocriptine is a member of which chemical family?
Bromocriptine is a semisynthetic ergot alkaloid that acts as a dopamine agonist to suppress prolactin. As anticipated from its action on the dopamine receptor, bromocriptine has applications in addition to the treatment of hyperprolactinemia or galactorrhea. Listed in diminishing order of efficacy, the drug is used to suppress growth hormone and prolactin in acromegaly, to shrink nonfunctional pituitary tumors, and to relieve the movement disorders associated with parkinsonism. The ergot alkaloid family of medications has a rich historical background.

Ergot alkaloids were isolated from the fungus *Claviceps purpurea,* a mold that infects a wide variety of grains. Collections of fungal spores on spoiled rye form a black smut. Exposure to the vasoactive ergot alkaloids can be harmful. A toxic manifestation of ergotism recognized in antiquity was ischemic gangrene. Some unfortunate victims who ingested foodstuffs prepared from moldy grain suffered bloodless autoamputation of blackened extremities, and infants of affected mothers sometimes died from a lack of breast milk. Limbs of afflicted persons appeared to turn into charcoal, as if ravaged by fire. Pilgrimages to the shrine of Saint Anthony permitted some victims to experience miraculous recoveries. Such recuperations undoubtedly resulted from elimination of the toxin, an unrecognized benefit stemming from the careful selection of wholesome provisions for the journey to the shrine. As a result, the affliction was labeled **Saint Anthony's fire**. The potential vasoactive properties of bromocriptine relative to its parent alkaloid were substantially reduced by structural modifications to confer specificity for dopamine receptors. As a result, vasospasm is a rarely reported side effect.

BIBLIOGRAPHY

1. Aragona C, Friesen HG: Lactation and galactorrhea. In DeGroot LJ (ed): Endocrinology, 2nd ed. Philadelphia, W. B. Saunders, 1989, pp 2074–2086.
2. Atchinson JA, Lee PA, Albright AL: Reversible suprasellar pituitary mass secondary to hypothyroidism. JAMA 262:3175–3177, 1989.
3. Devitt JE: Management of nipple discharge by clinical findings. Am J Surgery 149:789, 1985.
4. Edge DS, Segatore M: Assessment and management of galactorrhea. Nurse Pract 18:35–49, 1993.
5. Fradkin JE, Eastman RC, Lesniak MA, et al: Specificity spillover at the hormone receptor—exploring its role in human disease. N Engl J Med 320:640, 1989.
6. Frantz AG, Wilson JD: Endocrine disorders of the breast. In Wilson JD, Foster DW (eds): Williams' Textbook of Endocrinology, 8th ed. Philadelphia, W. B. Saunders, 1992, pp 954–961.
7. Gluskin LE, Strasberg B, Shah JH: Verapamil-induced hyperprolactinemia and galactorrhea. Ann Intern Med 95:66–67, 1981.
8. Kleinberg DL, Noel GL, Frantz AG: Galactorrhea: A study of 235 cases, including 48 with pituitary tumors. N Engl J Med 296:589–600, 1977.
9. Koppelman MCS, Jaffe MJ, Rieth KG, et al: Hyperprolactinemia, amenorrhea, and galactorrhea. Ann Intern Med 100:115–121, 1984.
10. Marchant DJ: Nonmalignant diseases of the breast. In Wyngaarden JB, Smith LH, Bennett JC (eds): Cecil's Textbook of Medicine, 19th ed. Philadelphia, W. B. Saunders, 1988, pp 1378–1381.
11. Molitch ME: Manifestations, epidemiology, and pathogenesis of prolactinomas in women. In Olefsky JM, Robbins RJ (eds): Prolactinomas. New York, Churchill Livingstone, 1986, pp 67–95.
12. Newcomb PA, Storer BE, Longnecker MP, et al: Lactation and a reduced risk of premenopausal breast cancer. N Engl J Med 330:81–87, 1994.
13. Potetsky L, Garber J, Kleefield J: Primary amenorrhea and pseudoprolactinoma in a patient with primary hypothyroidism: Reversal of clinical, biochemical and radiologic abnormalities with levothyroxine. Am J Med 81:180, 1986.

43. HIRSUTISM AND VIRILIZATION

Nadine H. Alex, M.D.

1. What is the definition of hirsutism?

Hirsutism refers to excessive terminal hair growth on a woman, occurring in a male pattern. Although terminal hair is not unusual on the arms, legs, upper lip, periareolar areas, and linea alba of women, it is abnormal on the chin, sternum, upper abdomen, and upper back. Hirsutism occurs in up to 5% of women and is usually benign.

2. What is the definition of virilization?

Virilization refers to signs of masculinization, which may include hirsutism, temporal balding, acne, deepened voice, increased muscle mass with a male physique, clitoromegaly, and increased libido. Unlike simple hirsutism, virilization is uncommon and much more suggestive of a serious underlying disorder.

3. What are the general etiologic categories of hirsutism?

Excessive androgen
Drugs
Familial patterns
Idiopathic hirsutism

4. What are the causes of excessive androgen in women?

The two sources of androgens in women are the ovaries and the adrenals. The following disorders may result in excessive androgens:

Ovarian disorders
  Hormonal disturbances
    Polycystic ovarian disease (PCOD)
    Hilus cell hyperplasia (hyperthecosis)—excessive number of
      thecal cells in the ovarian stroma
    Insulin resistance
  Neoplasms
    Arrhenoblastoma (Sertoli-Leydig cell tumor)
    Hilus cell tumor
    Granulosa-theca cell tumor
Adrenal disorders
  Congenital adrenal hyperplasia (CAH)
    21-hydroxylase deficiency
    11-hydroxylase deficiency
    3-beta-hydroxysteroid dehydrogenase deficiency
  Neoplasms
    Adrenal adenoma
    Adrenal carcinoma
  ACTH-dependent Cushing's syndrome (pituitary tumor or
    ectopic adrenocorticotropic hormone [ACTH])

5. What is the pathophysiology of a polycystic ovarian disease (PCOD)?

PCOD is believed to be due to an abnormality of the gonadotropin-releasing hormone (GnRH) pulse generator in the hypothalamus. An increased GnRH pulse frequency favors secretion of luteinizing hormone (LH) over secretion of follicle-stimulating hormone (FSH). The end result is thecal cell hyperplasia within the ovary, leading to increased synthesis of androgen and anovulation with irregular menses. Because follicles cannot mature, multiple follicular cysts develop, contributing to the enlarged ovaries.

6. What is the pathophysiology of a late-onset congenital adrenal hyperplasia (CAH)?
Late-onset CAH is characterized by partial deficiency of a cortisol-producing enzyme and thus results in a relative deficiency of cortisol. This causes increased release of ACTH with resultant excessive stimulation of the adrenal glands. The glands become hypertrophied and produce an excess of precursor hormones, including the androgen pathway hormones, dehydroepiandrosterone sulfate (DHEA-S) and androstenedione, which are converted to testosterone in the peripheral tissues. The excessive androgen accounts for hirsutism and masculinization. The best characterized and most common cause of CAH is 21-hydroxylase deficiency.

7. What drugs cause hirsutism?

Minoxidil	Diazoxide	Metyrapone
Phenytoin	Cyclosporine	Androgenic progestins
Phenothiazines	Danazol	Androgenic steroids

8. Describe the excessive hair growth that occurs with the above drugs other than the androgenic progestins and steroids.
These drugs cause an increase in *vellus* hair growth, which is distinctly different from androgen-sensitive *terminal* hair. Vellus hair is diffuse, fine lanugo hair over most body parts (not solely in androgen-dependent areas). In addition, such drugs do not cause other signs and symptoms of masculinization.

9. What is familial hirsutism?
Familial hirsutism refers to the occurrence of hirsutism within families (genetic) and certain ethnicities; it is due to an increased density of hair follicles per unit area of skin. This form of hirsutism is common among women of Mediterranean backgrounds. Northern European women have a much lower prevalence, and Asian women rarely have excessive hair growth. Generally, no other masculinizing features are present.

10. What is the presumed pathophysiology of idiopathic hirsutism?
Because some of the biochemical findings are similar to those in PCOD, one theory is that idiopathic hirsutism may actually be a subtle form of PCOD, which spares the development of anovulation and ovarian cysts. **Together, PCOD and idiopathic hirsutism account for about 90% of all causes of hirsutism.** Other abnormalities that may be etiologic in this condition include the following:
1. Increased sensitivity of the hair follicle to androgens
2. Increased androgen receptors in the skin; and
3. Increased activity in the hair unit of 5-alpha-reductase (the enzyme that increases the conversion of testosterone to dihydrotestosterone).

11. What aspects of the history are important in the evaluation of hirsutism?
The history is the most important component in the work-up. The etiology often is ascertained by focusing on the following aspects of the history:
1. Onset, duration, progression, and severity of hirsutism and of virilizing features, if present;
2. Menstrual history—age of menarche, regularity and normality of menses, fertility, and libido;
3. Ethnic background;
4. Family history of hirsutism;
5. Drug and medication history; and
6. Measures the patient has taken to manage hirsutism

12. What aspects of the physical examination are important in the evaluation of hirsutism?
- Pattern and severity of hirsutism
- Signs of virilization (acne, deep voice, temporal balding, clitoromegaly, loss of female contours, increased musculature and male physique)
- Palpation to detect abdominal and ovarian masses and enlarged ovaries
- Features of Cushing's syndrome

13. What laboratory tests should be ordered in the evaluation of hirsutism?
The one essential test is measurement of serum levels of total testosterone (normal = 20–70 ng/dl) or free testosterone:

    1. If testosterone is < 60 ng/dl, no further evaluation is necessary.

    2. If testosterone is 60–200 ng/dl, levels of 17-hydroxyprogesterone should be measured before and after stimulation with ACTH (Cortrosyn).

    3. If testosterone is > 200 ng/dl, the ovaries and adrenal glands should be imaged.

    4. If cushingoid features are present, 24-hour urinary excretion of cortisol should be measured.

    5. Although not strictly necessary, some experts recommend measuring levels of LH, FSH, prolactin, and DHEA-S in most hirsute patients; however, the cost-effectiveness of these tests is controversial.

14. What findings suggest PCOD?
Typically patients with PCOD present with oligomenorrhea since menarche (and occasionally with secondary amenorrhea), infertility, stable hirsutism that started at puberty, acne, and other features of mild androgen excess, and sometimes obesity. They may have large ovaries on examination, and a pelvic or vaginal ultrasound reveals bilateral cystic ovaries. The diagnosis is made most often on the basis of these clinical features. Suggestive laboratory abnormalities include the following:

    1. Mildly elevated levels of total and free testosterone
    2. Normal to high levels of LH
    3. Normal to low levels of FSH
    4. LH:FSH ratio greater than 2:1
    5. Mildly elevated levels of prolactin

15. What other disorders may be associated with PCOD?
If PCOD is diagnosed, the patient should be screened for diabetes mellitus and hyperlipidemia, both of which may be concurrent diseases. The patient also should have an annual pelvic examination because of the higher risk of endometrial and ovarian carcinomas. A subset of patients with PCOD has a constellation of findings referred to as **HAIR-AN syndrome:** hirsutism, androgen excess, insulin resistance, and acanthosis nigricans.

16. What findings are characteristic of late-onset CAH?
Slowly progressive hirsutism and oligomenorrhea since puberty, infertility, acne, and fatigue are common features of late-onset CAH; fatigue is due to a partial deficiency of cortisol. This autosomal recessive disorder has a much higher prevalence among Ashkenazi Jews, Hispanics, and Yugoslavians. Laboratory abnormalities generally include the following:

    1. Mildly elevated testosterone
    2. Mildly elevated DHEAS
    3. Elevated 17-hydroxyprogesterone (17-OH PROG)

    17-OH PROG, a precursor of cortisol, is elevated in deficiencies of 21-hydroxylase and 11-beta-hydroxylase. An elevated morning level greater than 800 ng/dl (normal = less than 200 ng/dl) is consistent with CAH. If levels are between 200–800 ng/dl, then an ACTH (Cortrosyn) stimulation test should be done to unmask the enzyme deficiency. If CAH exists, the 1-hour stimulated 17-OH PROG is high. Baseline and 1-hour stimulated values are plotted on standard nomograms to determine if CAH is present.

17. What findings are characteristic of androgen-producing neoplasms?

An abrupt onset of rapidly progressive hirsutism (particularly among prepubertal girls and postmenopausal women), virilization, and recent onset of amenorrhea or oligomenorrhea in a woman with previously normal menses and fertility are highly suggestive of an adrenal or ovarian neoplasm. A significantly elevated level of serum testosterone (> 200 ng/dl) is highly suggestive of a tumor and should prompt imaging studies of the ovaries and adrenals. A very high serum level of DHEA-S is characteristic of adrenal tumors.

18. What findings suggest familial hirsutism?

A positive family history of hirsutism or an ethnic background in which hirsutism is common, a stable pattern of hirsutism, no signs or symptoms of virilization, normal menses, fertility, and normal laboratory values are consistent with familial hirsutism.

19. What findings are most consistent with idiopathic hirsutism?

This common form of hirsutism is a diagnosis of exclusion. As in familial hirsutism, a stable pattern of hirsutism, no other signs and symptoms of virilization, normal menses and fertility, and no other complaints is the typical presentation. Laboratory values may be normal, or mildly elevated levels of total and free testosterone may be present. The ovaries are of normal size and without cysts.

20. What treatment options are available for PCOD and idiopathic hirsutism?

Treatment revolves around three objectives:
    1. Reduction of androgens from the ovaries and/or adrenals;
    2. Androgen receptor blockade to prevent terminal hair growth; and
    3. Cosmetic hair removal by mechanical (shaving, plucking); bleaching; depilatories (products that remove surface hair); and epilatories (products that remove hair at the root).

Treatment with the following medications often requires 6 months to 1 year for appreciable results:

    1. **Birth control pills** (BCPs) are the first-line medication. By turning off LH and FSH, BCPs decrease ovarian production of androgen and increase sex hormone-binding globulin, thereby decreasing free testosterone. They also serve to regulate menses.

    2. **Spironolactone** (Aldactone) blocks androgen receptors and inhibits synthesis of testosterone. It has additive effects in combination with BCPs. Birth control is needed, because treatment may interfere with the masculinization of the male fetus.

    3. **GnRH analogs** turn off LH and FSH but also cause estrogen deficiency. Therefore, estrogen should be replaced during its use.

    4. **Clomiphene citrate** (Clomid) often induces ovulation if pregnancy is desired.

21. What is the treatment for CAH?

Cortisol replacement breaks the cycle of precursor overproduction in addition to providing the patient with adequate cortisol.

22. What is the treatment for familial hirsutism?

The treatment for familial hirsutism is cosmetic removal of hair (see question 20).

BIBLIOGRAPHY

1. Aiman J: Virilizing ovarian tumors. Clin Obstet Gynecol 34:835–847, 1991.
2. Ehrmann DA, Rosenfield RL: An endocrinologic approach to the patient with hirsutism. J Clin Endocrinol Metab 71:1–4, 1990.

3. Hirschner M: Hirsutism. Current Therapy in Endocrine and Metabolism, 4th ed. Philadelphia, B. C. Decker, 1991.
4. Kessel B, Liu J: Clinical and lab evaluation of hirsutism. Clin Obstet Gynecol 34:805–816, 1991.
5. Lobo RA: Hirsutism in polycystic ovary syndrome: Current concepts. Clin Obstet Gynecol 34:817–826, 1991.
6. Rittmaster RS, Loriaux DL: Hirsutism. Ann Intern Med 106:95–107, 1987.
7. Rittmaster RS: Treating hirsutism. Endocrinologist 3:211–218, 1993.
8. Wilson JD, Foster DW (eds): Williams' Textbook of Endocrinology, 8th ed. Philadelphia, W. B. Saunders, 1992.
9. Wilson JD (ed): Harrison's Principles of Internal Medicine, 12th ed. New York, McGraw-Hill, 1991.
10. Wilson JR, Carrington ER: Obstetrics and Gynecology, 8th ed. St. Louis, C. V. Mosby, 1987.

44. INFERTILITY

Barrett L. Chapin, M.D., and Robert E. Jones, M.D.

1. What is the definition of infertility?

Infertility is defined as unprotected sexual intercourse without conception for at least 1 year. One-half of normally fertile couples conceive by 3 months, three-quarters by 6 months, and 90% by 1 year. Thus the normal fecundity rate (frequency of pregnancy in 1 month) is 20%, in other words, the chance of fertility with each ovulation is at best 20%.

2. How common is infertility?

Approximately 10–15% of married couples are unable to conceive. The contributions of male and female factors are roughly equal. Population studies have documented that 8–9% of women of childbearing age are unable to become pregnant, and a similar percentage of men are unable to father a child. Roughly one-half of the infertile women have primary infertility (no previous delivery), and one-half have secondary infertility (previous delivery).

3. Describe the initial evaluation of the infertile couple.

The initial evaluation for the woman should consist of a history, physical examination, and laboratory evaluation, including a blood count, urinalysis, fasting glucose level, and Papanicolaou smear. The man should have several semen analyses. Ovulation may be documented by serial measurement of basal body temperatures or by measurement of serum or urine levels of progesterone 7–8 days after the midcycle (ovulation) temperature rise or 21 days after the cessation of menstrual flow. A postcoital test (PCT) is performed at the expected time of ovulation to look for possible cervical or immunologic causes of infertility. A PCT entails the evaluation of a specimen of cervical mucus obtained from the fornix within 2 hours of sexual intercourse. Any abnormality identified at this point must be pursued before more invasive tests are performed. If the above evaluation is normal, hysterosalpingography should be performed to determine tubal patency and to visualize uterine anatomy. Laparoscopy may be required to evaluate other pelvic causes. Further evaluation of the man is discussed in questions 11–18.

Infertility Tests

TEST	EVALUATES
CBC, UA, FBS, Pap smear	Maternal health
Semen analysis	Male factor
Menstrual history	Ovulation
Postcoital test	Cervical factor
Hysterosalpingogram	Tubal patency, anatomy of uterus
Laparoscopy	Pelvic factor

CBC = complete blood count, UA = urinalysis; FBS = fasting blood sugar.

4. What are the common causes of infertility?

Common Causes of Infertility

CAUSE OF INFERTILITY	FREQUENCY (%)
Male factor	30–40
Pelvic factor	30–40
Anovulation	10–15
Cervical factor	10–15

5. What is the initial laboratory evaluation for the patient with secondary amenorrhea or oligomenorrhea?

The most common cause of secondary amenorrhea in a woman of reproductive age is pregnancy. A timely serum or urine pregnancy test may prevent embarrassment on the physician's part. Hyperprolactinemia and hypothyroidism are relatively common, potentially remediable causes of menstrual dysfunction; therefore, assessment of basal levels of thyroid-stimulating hormone (TSH) and prolactin is essential. Follicle-stimulating hormone (FSH) provides a prognosis for future fertility, because levels greater than 40 mIU/ml indicate probable menopause. If the above laboratory values are normal, it is reasonable to continue the evaluation by obtaining serum levels of testosterone, dehydroepiandrosterone sulfate (DHEA-S), and luteinizing hormone (LH) to evaluate the patient for congenital adrenal hyperplasia, polycystic ovarian disease, or neoplasm. Such conditions, of course, may be suspected earlier in the evaluation on the basis of historical facts or evidence of androgenization on physical examination.

6. How does clomiphene stimulate ovulation?

Clomiphene citrate (Clomid) is usually considered an estrogen antagonist, but it also has weak estrogenic activity. By competing with estrogen for receptor sites in the hypothalamus, clomiphene prevents the normal feedback inhibition of estrogen on release of gonadotropin-releasing hormone (GnRH). The resulting increase in GnRH pulses stimulates an increase in LH and FSH pulses, which in turn stimulates recruitment of ovarian follicles and ovulation.

7. How are human menopausal gonadotropin and human chorionic gonadotropin used to stimulate ovulation?

Human menopausal gonadotropin (hMG) is purified LH and FSH extracted from the urine of postmenopausal women. An individualized injection schedule is given to stimulate follicle development. The dose and frequency are based on close monitoring of either serum or urine levels of estrogen and ovarian ultrasound. When a mature follicle is visualized ultrasonically, hMG injections are halted, and human chorionic gonadotropin (hCG) is used to stimulate ovulation. An additional injection of hCG is usually given in approximately 7 days to maintain the corpus luteum.

8. Are twins more common with ovulation stimulation?

The normal frequency of multiple pregnancies is about 1%. Ovulation stimulation with either hMG or clomiphene results in similar frequencies of multiple gestations. The data for multiple gestations in over 2,000 pregnancies with clomiphene are 92% singleton, 7% twins, 0.5% triplets, 0.3% quadruplets, and 0.1% quintuplets. The frequency of birth defects, spontaneous abortion, and ectopic pregnancy with clomiphene is the same as in the normal population. The frequency of spontaneous abortion after use of hMG is about 20–30% compared with 19% in the general population.

9. Are complications other than multiple gestations associated with the use of gonadotropins?

On rare occasions patients who receive gonadotropins develop ascites, multiple ovarian cysts, and shock. To prevent this condition, called ovarian hyperstimulation syndrome, close monitoring is required in all patients.

10. Define in vitro fertilization and gamete intrafallopian transfer.

In vitro fertilization (IVF) involves the harvesting of mature ova from the woman and a semen sample from the man. After incubation of the sperm in capacitation media, fertilization is accomplished outside the body. After fertilization, the embryo is implanted into the uterus. Gamete intrafallopian transfer (GIFT) is somewhat similar to IVF. The difference is that fertilization occurs in vivo—the harvested eggs and sperm are injected into the fallopian tubes and fertilization occurs in situ. GIFT obviously requires intact fallopian tubes, whereas IVF does not. Both have a fecundity rate of approximately 20% (the same as normal couples); however, the procedures are invasive, expensive, and uncomfortable. Moreover, the rate of successful pregnancy varies significantly among groups offering assisted reproduction services.

11. How many semen samples are adequate to assess a man for fertility potential?

Semen quality may vary widely on a day-to-day as well as a seasonal basis. Consequently, a minimum of two samples obtained within a 3-month interval is required. If the results are disparate, additional samples should be collected.

12. How should a semen sample be obtained?

A period of sexual abstinence of 48–72 hours but no longer than 7 days is necessary to ensure a representative volume of ejaculate without the complicating factor of necrospermia from autolysis. Masturbation is the preferred method for collection, but nonspermicidal condoms are available. No matter how it is obtained, the entire sample must be submitted for analysis. Incomplete ejaculates should be discarded.

13. What may cause a transient reduction in semen quality?

Dramatic reductions in sperm concentration or motility may be observed during any febrile illness or during times of intense physiological stress (e.g., strenuous physical exercise and high environmental temperatures). It may take as long as 3 months after resolution of the condition before semen parameters return to baseline.

14. What are the normal parameters for a semen analysis?

Many different ranges have been proposed to predict fertility potential on the basis of semen variables. The World Health Organization offers the following criteria as representative of a normal ejaculate:

Criteria for Normal Semen Ejaculate

CRITERIA	VALUE
Sperm concentration	$> 20 \times 10^6$ spermatozoa/ml
Total sperm in ejaculate	$> 40 \times 10^6$ spermatozoa/ejaculate
Motility	$> 50\%$ of sperm with forward progression
Morphology	$> 30\%$ with normal, oval forms
White blood cells	$< 1 \times 10^6$ WBC/ml

15. List the common causes of falsely low motility.

Asthenospermia or reduced sperm motility may result either from primary disorder, such as Kartagener syndrome and the presence of immobilizing sperm antibodies, or from improper collection and handling of the specimen. An excessive delay in delivery of the sample to the laboratory or a delay in examination may result in a loss of sperm viability. The time between ejaculation and delivery must be as short as possible (< 1 hour), and the sample must be analyzed within 30 minutes of liquefaction. Standard condoms are coated with spermicidal lubricants designed to immobilize sperm. Coitus interruptus is also unacceptable, because incomplete collections are common and the sample is frequently contaminated with vaginal secretions or bacteria that may impair motility. Soaps or other lubricants may also be spermicidal and must be avoided. Lastly, care must be taken in the selection of the container. Because some plastics are spermicidal, a wide-mouthed sterile glass container is usually preferred.

16. What are the common causes of male infertility?

In an infertile but otherwise healthy man the cause of infertility is usually not identified. Approximately one-third of infertile men have a varicocele. A history of cryptorchidism, orchitis, or significant trauma is obtained in less than 15% of infertile men, and ductal obstruction occurs in less than 5%. Less common causes include Klinefelter syndrome (see chapter 38), Kallmann syndrome (see chapter 38), or a history of prior chemotherapy or radiation therapy. Any systemic illness may temporarily reduce a man's fertility potential.

17. What are the reproductive consequences of a varicocele?

A varicocele is a palpable dilation or venous engorgement of the pampiniform plexus. It is the most frequent cause of potentially remediable infertility in men; however, not all men with varicoceles have primary infertility or any evidence of testicular dysfunction. The relationship between the presence of a varicocele and infertility is poorly understood. Recent studies have suggested that varicoceles may be implicated in secondary infertility. The clinical manifestations of a varicocele are reduced sperm number, diminished motility, and reduction in the percentage of normal oval spermatozoa. On occasion, a significant number of large, immature spermatozoa may be observed. This constellation of findings is sometimes called a "stress pattern" and usually portends a poorer prognosis for fertility. Men with varicoceles have other evidence of Sertoli cell impairment, including lower inhibin levels, higher basal FSH values and an enhanced FSH response to GnRH.

18. How is azoospermia evaluated?

If the patient lacks the features of Klinefelter syndrome, levels of seminal fluid fructose and serum FSH should be assessed. The finding of normal fructose levels verifies the presence of the seminal vesicles and excludes congenital absence of the vasa deferentia or the rare phenomenon of ejaculatory duct obstruction. If the FSH level is >1.5 times the upper limit of normal, further evaluation is not warranted because of the high likelihood of severe, irreparable damage to seminiferous tubules. Otherwise, a vasogram to assess patency of the ejaculatory mechanism and a testicular biopsy to evaluate spermatogenesis are indicated.

19. How is male infertility treated?

Various regimens, including testosterone rebound, clomiphene, and bromocriptine, have been used to treat male infertility. Unfortunately, such empirical forms of therapy have not been demonstrated to be any more effective than nontreatment. As a result, the management of male infertility is frustrating for both physician and patient. Assisted reproduction techniques (such as IVF, GIFT, and intrauterine insemination) yield occasional spectacular results but are disappointing for the majority of couples with male factor infertility. Two conditions, hypogonadotropic hypogonadism (Kallmann syndrome) and varicocele, merit special discussion, because treatment may enhance fertility potential in afflicted men. The use of pulsatile GnRH analogs or gonadotropins has been demonstrated to restore spermatogenesis in men with Kallmann syndrome. The effectiveness of varicocele repair by high ligation of the spermatic vein is more controversial, but most andrologists recommend the procedure because of its low morbidity and potential for great reward.

20. What is the prognosis for conception in a couple seeking medical intervention?

Successful pregnancy varies with the reason for infertility. If anovulation is the cause, medical induction of ovulation results in an 80–90% chance of conception. If the female factor is not anovulation, a 30% chance of pregnancy is expected. Male factor infertility carries a poorer prognosis, but approximately 40% of men classified as infertile can ultimately father a child.

BIBLIOGRAPHY

1. Aksel S: Immunologic aspects of reproductive diseases. JAMA 268:2930–2934, 1992.
2. Bronson R, Cooper G, Rosenfeld D: Sperm antibodies: Their role in infertility. Fertil Steril 42:171–183, 1984.
3. Corsan GH, Kemmann E: The role of superovulation with menotropins in ovulatory infertility: A review. Fertil Steril 55:468–477, 1991.
4. D'Amico JF, Gambone JC: Advances in the management of the infertile couple. Am Fam Physician 39:257–264, 1989.
5. Gorelick JI, Goldstein M: Loss of fertility in men with varicocele. Fertil Steril 59:613–616, 1993.
6. Jaffe SB, Jewelewicz R: The basic infertility investigation. Fertil Steril 56:599–613, 1991.
7. Jones HW, Toner JP: The infertile couple. N Engl J Med 329:1710–1715, 1993.

8. Levine RJ, Mathew RM, Chenault CB, et al: Differences in the quality of semen in outdoor workers during summer and winter. N Engl J Med 323:12–16, 1990.
9. Lobo RA: Unexplained infertility. J Reprod Med 38:241–249, 1993.
10. Winfield AC, Fleischer AC, Moore DE: Diagnostic imaging of fertility disorders. Curr Probl Diagn Radiol 19:9–38, 1990.
11. World Health Organization: WHO Laboratory Manual for the Examination of Human Semen and Sperm-Cervical Mucous Interaction, 3rd ed. Cambridge, Cambridge University Press, 1992.

45. MENOPAUSE

William J. Georgitis, M.D., COL, MC

CLINICAL FEATURES

1. Define menopause.
The climacteric or menopause is characterized by cessation of cyclic ovarian function. It spans approximately one-third of a woman's life, encompassing the transition from the fertile reproductive years to the final menstruation and extending beyond for the remainder of life. For individual women, the final menstruation is commonly used to define the onset of menopause.

2. When do ovulatory cycles decrease in frequency?
Ovulatory cycles decrease in frequency around age 38–42 years.

3. When does menopause usually occur?
The median age for the last menses is 51.4 years.

4. What determines the timing of the menopause?
Menses stop when the supply of oocytes is exhausted. The number of oocytes peaks in utero, and 80% of the maximal population has already disappeared by birth. It is also a curious fact that vastly more follicles end their existence through atresia than by achieving ovulation.

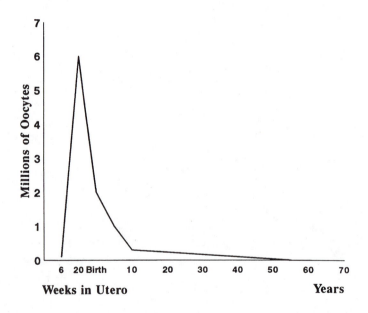

5. What is premature ovarian failure? What causes it?
Cessation of cyclic ovarian function before age 30 or 35 years is attributed to either an inadequate complement of follicles from birth or accelerated attrition of follicles due to mumps oophoritis, irradiation, chemotherapy, autoimmune destruction, or genetic defects.

6. Does the age of menopause vary with race, parity, body size, age of menarche, geography, or socioeconomic conditions?
No. But menopause does occur earlier in cigarette smokers.

7. Does the appearance of the ovary change with menopause?
The menopausal ovary shrinks in size to less than 2.5 grams, and its surface becomes wrinkled. Cortical width diminishes, whereas interstitial and hilar cells become more prominent, giving the appearance of hyperplastic stroma.

8. What is the predominant circulating estrogen in menopause?
Estradiol is the major estrogen during the reproductive years; during menopause, however, the weaker hormone, estrone, becomes the principal estrogen. Estrone is derived by conversion of the adrenal androgen, androstenedione, in adipose tissue.

9. What is a hot flash? Or should it be called a flush?
Menopausal spells last seconds to minutes, rarely as long as an hour. Symptoms include a sudden reddening of the skin accompanied by a warm sensation that is some women is followed by profuse sweating. Body surface temperature rises, whereas core temperature falls because of hypothalamic-directed, vasomotor-mediated dilation of surface blood vessels. Pathophysiology is complex and involves changes in catecholamines, prostaglandins, endorphins, and other neuropeptides.

Both expressions, flash and flush, appear in the medical literature, and each is appropriately descriptive. Flush aptly emphasizes vasodilation, whereas flash signifies abrupt onset and brief duration. Many menopausal women also describe prodromal auras.

10. Hot flushes are accompanied by surges in levels of luteinizing hormone. Do the increases in LH cause the spells?
No. The LH surge is an epiphenomenon. Hypophysectomized women who have no associated LH pulses still may have menopausal hot flushes. Patients with gonadal dysgenesis, who have highly elevated levels of gonadotropins, nonetheless fail to manifest hot flushes until after estrogen treatment and subsequent withdrawal. The hypothalamus appears to require priming with estrogens for later supervision of the body's reaction to falling levels of estrogen.

11. Do all women develop menopausal vasomotor hot flushes? Do they last indefinitely?
About 85% of women experience vasomotor symptoms. The rate of change in estrogen levels in part determines their severity. Women experiencing abrupt declines in estrogen levels after ovariectomy are often bothered the most. Left untreated, hot flushes tend to diminish after 2–5 years.

12. Do any menopausal symptoms have an uncertain relation to estrogen?
Yes. A partial list of symptoms includes fatigue, nervousness, headaches, insomnia, depression, irritability, joint pain, muscle pain, dizziness, palpitations, and formication, which is a form of paresthesia that resembles the sensation of ants crawling over the skin.

13. What important physiologic changes accompany menopause?
Hot flushes, urogenital atrophy, loss of bone calcium, increased rates of coronary heart disease, and alterations in serum lipids, including rises in LDL cholesterol and triglycerides with declines in HDL cholesterol, occur during menopause.

14. What is the principal cause of death in postmenopausal women?
Cardiovascular disease.

15. Does male menopause exist?
Not really. Hypogonadal men may also suffer spells and accelerated loss of bone mineral. In a man complaining of hot flushes, a pathologic diagnosis should be suspected, because, unlike the

hot flushes of menopause, such symptoms in men do not represent a physiologically programmed event.

16. Historical records indicate that the age of menarche has decreased over the centuries, perhaps as a result of improved nutrition and general health. Is this also true for the timing of menopause?
No. A shift in the average age of menopause has not been recorded.

MANAGEMENT AND ESTROGEN REPLACEMENT THERAPY

17. How does one establish a diagnosis of menopause?
In a woman older than 45 years with secondary amenorrhea of 6–12 months' duration, a diagnosis of menopause based on historical evidence alone is reasonable. Pelvic examination may be confirmatory by revealing atrophic vaginal changes.

Toward the end of the fertile years, serum levels of follicle-stimulating hormone (FSH) gradually rise. Anovulatory periods ensue and lead to heavier endometrial bleeding and menorrhagia. Once amenorrhea occurs, gonadotropins become tonically elevated, FSH more dramatically so (10–20-fold) than LH (3-fold). Levels of FSH above 40 IU/L are considered diagnostic of ovarian failure. However, elevated gonadotropin levels alone can be misleading, because FSH and LH frequently rise into the menopausal range during the midcycle surge in premenopausal women.

18. What regimens of menopausal hormone replacement are in common use?
Continuous daily replacement with estrogen alone is appropriate for women who lack an endometrium because of hysterectomy. Such women are usually given conjugated equine estrogens, 0.625–1.25 mg daily. Combination therapy should be used for women who require the addition of progesterone to prevent endometrial hyperplasia or neoplasia. Such therapy frequently consists of conjugated estrogens, 0.625–1.25 mg daily on days 1–25 of each month, and medroxyprogesterone acetate, 5–10 mg daily on days 13 through 25; neither hormone is given the last 5 days of the month. Withdrawal bleeding is common with sequential therapy. An alternative regimen uses a combination of conjugated estrogens, 0.625–1.25 mg, and medroxyprogesterone acetate, 2.5–5.0 mg, on every day of the month. Spotting may occur with any therapy, but persistent bleeding, especially early in the cycle of sequential therapy, may warrant an endometrial biopsy.

19. What is the most common indication for menopausal hormone replacement therapy?
The most common indication is the relief of vasomotor symptoms or urogenital atrophy.

20. What are the benefits?
Vasomotor symptoms improve, dyspareunia is reduced, and the frequency of cystitis may be decreased by restoration of a normal vaginal flora. Other benefits include favorable alterations in serum lipids (reduced LDL and increased HDL cholesterol levels), decreased risk of stroke and coronary heart disease, and prevention of bone loss and associated osteoporotic fractures.

21. What are the potential detrimental effects?
Estrogen administration without progesterone increases the risk of endometrial hyperplasia or carcinoma by 6- to 8-fold. Whether menopausal replacement therapy increases the prevalence of hypertension, thromboembolic events, or breast cancer is still unclear. Certainly estrogens should not be prescribed to a woman with breast cancer. However, a recent study has shown that adjuvant tamoxifen therapy diminishes the rate of bone mineral loss in patients with breast cancer.

Progesterone, which markedly decreases the risk of endometrial carcinoma, may cause fluid retention as well as lower HDL and higher LDL cholesterol levels.

22. Insomnia is a troublesome symptom. Does hormone replacement alter sleep?
Evidence from objective sleep laboratory studies suggests that estrogen replacement improves sleep quality, decreases the time to onset of sleep, and increases rapid eye movement (REM) sleep.

23. What levels of estradiol and estrone are achieved with replacement?
Oral conjugated equine estrogens (0.625 mg), micronized estradiol (1.0 mg), and estrone sulfate (1.25 mg) deliver peak estradiol levels of 30–40 pg/ml and peak estrone levels of 150–250 pg/ml. Intravaginal estrogens yield levels about one-fourth those achieved with oral regimens.

24. Can gonadotropin levels of estradiol levels be used to monitor adequacy of replacement?
No. Unlike primary hypothyroidism, in which TSH can be used to individualize requirements of thyroxine replacement, gonadotropin levels remain elevated during sex steroid replacement in many postmenopausal women. This elevation may result from a deficiency in inhibin, a polypeptide hormone normally produced by ovarian granulosa cells to inhibit secretion of FSH. Menopausal hormone replacement therapy must be guided by the patient's symptoms and signs, not by gonadotropin levels.

25. What alternative therapies may be used for the menopausal woman with contraindications for estrogen replacement?
Clonidine may be tried at bedtime for the relief of hot flushes, but hypotensive side effects may limit its use. Medroxyprogesterone in a daily pill or as a depot injection every 3 months also may relieve hot flushes.

BIBLIOGRAPHY

1. Amundsen DW, Diers CJ: The age of menopause in medieval Europe. Hum Biol 45:605–612, 1973.
2. Daly E, Gray A, Barlow D, et al: Measuring the impact of menopausal symptoms on quality of life. BMJ 307:836–840, 1993.
3. Felson DT, Zhang Y, Hannan MT, et al: The effect of postmenopausal estrogen therapy on bone density in elderly women. N Engl J Med 329:1141–1146, 1993.
4. Finuncane FF, Madans JH, Bush TL, et al: Decreased risk of stroke among postmenopausal hormone users. Arch Intern Med 153:73–79, 1993.
5. Grady D, Rubin AM, Petitti DB, et al: Hormone therapy to prevent disease and prolong life in postmenopausal women. Ann Intern Med 117:1016–1041, 1992.
6. Love RR, Mazess RB, Barden HS, et al: Effect of tamoxifen on bone mineral density in postmenopausal women with breast cancer. N Engl J Med 326:852–856, 1992.
7. Nabulsi AA, Folsom AR, White A, et al: Association of hormone replacement therapy with various cardiovascular risk factors in postmenopausal women. N Engl J Med 328:1069–1075, 1993.
8. Schiff I, Regestein Q, Tulchinsky D, Ryan KJ: Effect of estrogens on sleep and psychological state of hypogonadal women. JAMA 242:2405–2407, 1979.
9. Walsh BW, Schiff I, Rosner B, et al: Effects of postmenopausal estrogen replacement on the concentrations and metabolism of plasma lipoproteins. N Engl J Med 323:1196–1204.

VII. Miscellaneous

46. MULTIPLE ENDOCRINE NEOPLASIA

Arnold A. Asp, M.D.

1. Name and define the multiple endocrine neoplasia (MEN) syndromes.

There are three well-characterized, inherited pluriglandular disorders in which several endocrine glands simultaneously undergo neoplastic transformation and become hyperfunctional. The three disorders, which are genetically transmitted in an autosomal dominant fashion, are characterized below:

MEN 1: Hyperplasia or neoplastic transformation of the parathyroids, pancreatic islets, and pituitary.

MEN 2A: Hyperplasia or neoplastic transformation of the thyroid parafollicular cells (medullary carcinoma of the thyroid), parathyroid glands, and adrenal medulla (pheochromocytoma).

MEN 2B: Hyperplasia or neoplastic transformation of the thyroid parafollicular cells (medullary carcinoma of the thyroid) and adrenal medulla (pheochromocytoma) with concomitant development of mucosal neuromas.

2. How can so many endocrine organs be affected in the MEN syndromes?

This question is a matter of controversy and ongoing research. The cells that comprise many endocrine organs are able to decarboxylate various amino acids and to convert the molecules to amines or peptides that act as hormones or neurotransmitters. Such cells have been classified as APUD (amine precursor uptake and decarboxylation) cells and are believed to be embryologically of neuroectodermal origin. APUD cells type contain markers of their common neuroendocrine origin, including neuron-specific enolase and chromogranin A. Neoplastic transformation of APUD cells long after organogenesis is complete may be due to the heritable loss of a tumor suppressor gene and/or mutation of a protooncogene before the neuroectodermal cells migrate to their respective tissues. This genetic alteration, early in embryologic development, may explain the later simultaneous neoplastic changes in so many diverse tissues. This hypothesis, labelled the APUD theory, is still tentative but gaining wider acceptance.

3. What is Wermer's syndrome?

Wermer's syndrome is the eponym for MEN 1. In 1954 Wermer first described the association of parathyroid hyperplasia, multicentric pituitary tumors, and pancreatic islet cell tumors in several kindreds. Wermer's syndrome, the most common form of MEN, is characterized by a high degree of penetrance; expression increases with age. Prevalence is estimated to vary between 0.02 and 0.2/1000. Although neoplastic transformation occurs most commonly in the parathyroids, pituitary, and pancreas, hyperplastic adrenal cortical and nodular thyroid disorders have been described. Carcinoid tumors, especially involving the foregut (thymus, lung, stomach, and duodenum), are uncommon but have been reported in the MEN 1 syndrome.

4. Is hyperparathyroidism in MEN 1 similar to sporadic primary hyperparathyroidism?

No. Hyperparathyroidism associated with MEN 1 results from hyperplasia of all four glands, whereas sporadic primary hyperparathyroidism usually is characterized by adenomatous change in a single gland. Hyperparathyroidism is the most common and earliest manifestation of MEN 1, occurring in 80–95% of cases. It has been described in patients as young as 17 years of age and develops in nearly all patients with MEN 1 by the age of 40 years.

Hyperplasia of glands affected by MEN 1 occurs as a result of expansion of multiple-cell clones, whereas sporadic parathyroid adenomas result from activation of a single-cell clone. Several groups have described a mitogenic factor (possibly transforming growth factor) in the sera of patients with MEN 1. This factor potentiates neoplastic transformation of parathyroid tissue. Production of parathyroid hormone by hyperplastic glands, though supranormal, is more easily suppressed by elevated serum calcium than production by sporadic adenomas; the set points are different. Complications of MEN 1 hyperparathyroidism are similar to those of sporadic hyperparathyroidism, including nephrolithiasis, osteoporosis, mental status changes and muscular weakness.

Therapy of both sporadic adenomas and MEN 1–associated hyperplastic glands depends on surgical resection. In sporadic primary hyperparathyroidism, removal of the solitary adenoma is curative in 95% of cases. In MEN 1-associated hyperplasia, at least $3\frac{1}{2}$ hyperplastic glands must be resected to restore normocalcemia. Only 75% of patients are normocalcemic postoperatively; 10–25% are rendered hypoparathyroid. Unfortunately, the parathyroid remnants in the patient with MEN 1 have a great propensity to regenerate; 50% of cases become hypercalcemic within 10 years of surgery. This recurrence rate dictates that surgery be delayed until complications of hypercalcemia are imminent or gastrin levels are elevated, as discussed below.

5. What type of pancreatic tumors are found in MEN 1 syndrome?

Neoplastic transformation of the pancreatic islet cells is the second most common manifestation of MEN 1, occurring in approximately 80% of cases. Such tumors are usually multicentric and often capable of elaborating several peptides and biogenic amines. They are, by convention, identified on the basis of the clinical syndrome produced by the predominant secretory product. This group of tumors characteristically progresses from hyperplasia to malignancy with metastases, making curative resection unlikely. Tumors of the pancreas may arise from normal islet cells (eutopic) or cells that are not normal constituents of the adult pancreas (ectopic).

Gastrinomas, the most common pancreatic neoplasms in the MEN 1 syndrome (58–78% of cases), are ectopic tumors; G-cells are normally present in the fetal pancreas only. The most common endocrine pancreatic tumor, gastrinomas may occur independently of MEN 1 (only 15–48% of all patients with gastrinoma are later found to have MEN 1). Excessive secretion of gastrin by these tumors causes production of gastric acid with resultant duodenal and jejunal ulcers and diarrhea. Basal acid output exceeds 15 mmol/hr, and basal fasting levels of gastrin usually exceed 300 pg/ml. Any condition or agent that stimulates normal secretion of gastrin (hypercalcemia) or interferes with normal secretion of gastric acid and feedback to the G-cells will elevate serum levels of gastrin including: achlorhydria, gastric outlet obstruction, retained antrum with Billroth II procedure, vagotomy, histamine$_2$ blockers, and proton pump inhibitors (omeprazole). Hyperparathyroidism (see question 4) may falsely elevate serum levels of gastrin. A secretin stimulation test may aid in differentiation of gastrinoma from other hypergastrinemic states; levels of gastrin in patients with gastrinoma increase by at least 200 pg/ml. Curative surgical resection is possible in only 10–15% of cases. Therapy is usually based on histamine$_2$ blockers or omeprazole. More information on gastrinomas is included in chapter 48.

Insulinomas are the second most common pancreatic islet cell tumor in the MEN 1 syndrome (20–36% of islet cell tumors) as well as the most common eutopic type. Insulinomas associated with MEN 1 syndrome are more frequently multicentric and malignant than the sporadic tumors. Approximately 1–5% of all patients with insulinoma are eventually discovered to have MEN 1. An excellent discussion of the diagnosis and therapy of insulinomas is found in chapter 48.

Pancreatic tumors less frequently associated with MEN 1 include glucagonomas, somatostatinomas, and vasoacitive intestinal polypeptide-secreting tumors (VIPomas). Associated syndromes and therapy are also described in chapter 48.

6. Which pituitary tumors are associated with MEN 1?

Pituitary tumors occur in 50–71% of cases of MEN 1. They may result either from neoplastic transformation of anterior pituitary cells with clonal expansion to a tumor or from excessive stimulation of the pituitary by ectopically-produced hypothalamic releasing factors elaborated by carcinoids or pancreatic islet cells.

Prolactinomas are the most common pituitary tumor associated with MEN 1, constituting 60% of the total. The symptoms of hyperprolactinemia are the third most common manifestation of MEN 1. The tumors are typically multicentric and large but respond to dopamine agonists such as bromocriptine. In earlier series, many pituitary tumors described as chromophobe adenomas were, in reality, prolactinomas that contained sparse poorly staining secretory granules. Prolactinomas are also discussed in chapter 17.

The second most commonly encountered pituitary tumor type is the growth-hormone producing tumor, which is reported in 10–25% of patients. Overproduction of growth hormone results in features of acromegaly. The tumors are often multicentric and may result from secretion of growth hormone-releasing hormone by pancreatic or carcinoid tumors. Diagnosis and therapy are described in chapter 18.

Finally, corticotropin (ACTH)-producing tumors that cause Cushing's syndrome may be associated with MEN 1. Such tumors result from neoplastic transformation of the pituitary or elaboration of corticotropin-releasing hormone by pancreatic or carcinoid tumors. Diagnosis and therapy are described in chapter 20.

7. What causes MEN 1?

Combined tumor-deletion mapping and linkage studies have implicated a genomic locus on the long arm of chromosome 11 (11q13) as the genetic abnormality that causes the MEN 1 syndrome. This locus may encode a tumor suppressor gene that normally coordinates cellular reproduction in the involved organs. The proband inherits an allele prediposing to MEN 1 from the affected parent, whereas a normal allele is passed down from the unaffected parent. When a somatic mutation later inactivates the normal allele, suppressor function is lost, permitting hyperplasia to occur. This locus is referred to as the MEN 1 gene.

8. How should kindreds be screened after the proband is identified?

Asymptomatic carriers of the genetic defect must be identified first; then the extent of organ involvement must be determined. As mentioned above, deletions at 11q13 are apparent in patients with MEN 1 and may be used to identify carriers of the disorder in the near future. Until this technique becomes widely available, periodic measurement of associated hormones is the best alternative to detect disease within affected kindreds. Manifestations of MEN 1 syndrome rarely occur before the age of 15 years; therefore, individuals at risk should not undergo endocrine screening before that time. Nearly all individuals at risk develop the disorder by the age of 40 years; screening may be unnecessary in members older than 50 years who are proved to be disease-free.

Because hyperparathyroidism is temporally the first manifestation of MEN 1 syndrome, concentrations of serum calcium and levels of parathyroid hormone constitute the best screening tests to identify asymptomatic carriers. Biochemical evidence of hyperparathyroidism in a member of an affected kindred establishes a presumptive carrier state. Evaluation then should focus on delineation of pancreatic and pituitary involvement. Serum levels of gastrin disclose the presence of a gastrinoma, whereas levels of prolactin reveal the presence of pituitary disease (especially in women). The latter two tests are cost-effective only in established disease, and should not be used for preliminary screening of the kindred (unless symptoms of hypergastrinemia or prolactinoma are present). The frequency of screening has not been prospectively studied, but recommended intervals range from 2 to 5 years.

9. What is Sipple's syndrome?

Sipple's syndrome is the eponym for MEN 2A. In 1961 Sipple recognized and described kindreds with medullary carcinoma of the thyroid (MCT), pheochromocytomas, and hyperparathyroidism. The disorder is inherited in an autosomal dominant fashion and exhibits a high degree of penetrance and variable expressivity. It is less common than MEN 1 syndrome.

10. Is the form of medullary carcinoma of the thyroid (MCT) associated with MEN 2A similar to the sporadic form of MCT?

No. Medullary carcinoma of the thyroid results from malignant transformation of the parafollicular cells (or C-cells) that normally elaborate calcitonin and are scattered throughout the gland. MCT comprises <5% of all thyroid malignancies. The sporadic form of MCT, as described in chapter 33, is more common (75% of all MCT), occurs in a solitary form (<20% multicentric), and metastasizes to local lymphatics, liver, bone, and lung early in the course of disease (metastasis may occur with primary tumors less than 1 cm in diameter). Sporadic MCT occurs more commonly in an older population (peak age; 40–60 years) and is usually located in the upper two-thirds of the gland.

MCT associated with MEN 2A, on the other hand, is multicentric (90% at the time of diagnosis) and occurs at a younger age (as young as 2 years) but generally has a better prognosis than the sporadic form. MCT occurs in nearly 95% of all cases of MEN 2A and is usually the first tumor to appear. Calcitonin or other peptides elaborated by the tumor may cause a secretory diarrhea that is present in 4–7% of patients at the time of diagnosis, but which will develop in 25–30% during the course of their disease. Parafollicular cells in MEN 2A patients characteristically progress through a state of C-cell hyperplasia to nodular hyperplasia to malignant degeneration over a variable period of time. It is imperative that patients at risk be diagnosed while still in the C-cell hyperplasia stage; total thyroidectomy will preclude malignant degeneration and metastases. Detection of C-cell hyperplasia is facilitated by the pentagastrin stimulation test. MCT also expresses peptides and hormones not commonly elaborated by parafollicular cells, including somatostatin, thyrotropin-releasing hormone, vasoactive intestinal peptide, proopiomelanocortin, carcinoembryonic antigen and neurotensin.

11. If MCT is the most common neoplasm associated with MEN 2A, what is the second most common neoplasm?

Pheochromocytoma occurs in 50–70% of cases of MEN 2A and is bilateral in as many as 84% of patients. Unlike the sporadic form, pheochromocytomas associated with MEN 2A secrete greater amounts of epinephrine. Hypertension is therefore less common, and urinary excretion of catecholamines may become supranormal later in the course of the disease. Surgical resection is indicated, but controversy surrounds the need for prophylactic resection of contralateral uninvolved adrenals, 50% of which develop pheochromocytomas within 10 years of the original surgery. The diagnosis and management of pheochromocytomas is discussed in chapter 24.

12. Is hyperparathyroidism associated with MEN 2A similar to that found in MEN 1?

Yes. But it is encountered much less commonly, involving only 40% of cases. No mitogenic factor (as in MEN 1) has been described in the sera of patients.

13. What is the genetic basis for the MEN 2A syndrome?

The genetic basis of the MEN 2A syndrome is more tentative than that proposed for the MEN 1 syndrome. Linkage analysis initially indicated a deletion in chromosome 20 that did not appear in all kindreds. These studies were followed by research that indicated linkage to a locus on chromosome 10; however, a deletion at that point has not been demonstrated. Most recently, point mutations in the RET protooncogene coding for a transmembrane tyrosine kinase were described in several kindreds with MEN 2A and may explain neoplastic activity. These findings await confirmation.

14. How should a kindred be screened after the proband with MEN 2A is identified?

As explained in question 8, a screening initially entails the differentiation of gene carriers from uninvolved family members and subsequently the delineation of organ involvement in the affected members. When the genetic basis of MEN 2A is determined and genomic analysis becomes available, initial screening will be relatively simple. At the present time, hormonal markers of the earliest components of the syndrome must be assessed to establish gene carriage.

Because MCT is usually the first manifestation of MEN 2A and because C-cell hyperplasia has been described in infancy and on rare occasions after the age of 35 years, all members of a kindred should be screened with a pentagastrin stimulation test on an annual basis until 35–50 years of age. Because MEN 2A-associated pheochromocytoma may produce large amounts of epinephrine that do not cause hypertension, annual timed urine collections for catecholamines should be obtained for a similar duration. Serum levels of calcium should be assessed every 2 years. Once the presence of the syndrome is established, screening for adrenal and parathyroid involvement should continue through life.

15. What comprises the MEN 2B syndrome?

MEN 2B syndrome is the association of MCT and pheochromocytoma with multiple mucosal neuromas in an effected individual or kindred. Hyperparathyroidism is not associated with MEN 2B. This syndrome is less common than MEN 2A and occurs more often in a sporadic rather than a familial form, but if inherited, it is transmitted in an autosomal dominant fashion. The occurrence of multiple mucosal neuromas on the distal tongue, lips, and along the gastrointestinal tract should always raise the possibility of MEN 2B. Other manifestations include marfanoid habitus without ectopia lentis or aortic aneurysms, hypertrophic corneal nerves, and slipped femoral epiphysis.

The MCT associated with this syndrome is more aggressive than other forms; metastastic lesions have been described in infancy. Because of the propensity toward early metastasis, many advocate that provocative tests be waived in children with the syndrome and that they undergo total thyroidectomy as soon as surgery can be tolerated. Pheochromocytomas occur in nearly one-half of all patients and follow a clinical course similar to those in the MEN 2A syndrome. Overall morality in MEN 2B is more severe; the average age of death for patients with MEN 2A is 60 years, whereas in patients with MEN 2B the average age of death is 30 years.

The genetic basis of MEN 2B is largely unknown, but linkage studies have implicated the same site on chromosome 10 that has been reported in MEN 2A. Screening with pentagastrin stimulation for MCT should occur from birth and continue through life if thyroidectomy is deferred. Screening for pheochromocytoma should begin at 5 years and continue for life.

16. Have the clinical presentations and prognoses of the MEN syndromes changed since the time of their original descriptions?

Yes. When the MEN syndromes were initially described, most patients presented with involvement of all the aforementioned organ systems, because diagnostic capabilities were limited. In the present day, early diagnosis of the proband and aggressive screening of the kindred may permit detection of hyperplasia and prompt prophylactic surgery or medical therapy that limits morbidity.

BIBLIOGRAPHY

1. Brandi ML, Auerbach GD, Fitzpatrick LA, et al: Parathyroid mitogenic activity in plasma from patients with familial multiple endocrine neoplasia type 1. N Engl J Med 314:1287–1293, 1986.
2. Benson L, Ljunghall S, Akerstrom G, Oberg K: Hyperparathyroidism presenting as the first lesion in multiple endocrine neoplasia type 1. Am J Med 82:731–737, 1987.
3. Cadiot G, Laurent-Piug P, Thuille B, et al: Is the multiple endocrine neoplasia type 1 gene a suppressor for fundic argyrophil tumors in Zollinger-Ellison syndrome? Gastroenterology 105:579–582, 1993.
4. Donis-Keller H, Dou S, Chi D, et al: Mutations in the RET proto-oncogene are associated with MEN 2A and FMTC. Hum Mol Genet 2:851–856, 1993.
5. Gagel RF: Multiple endocrine neoplasia. In Wilson JD, Foster DW (eds): Williams' Textbook of Endocrinology. Philadelphia, W. B. Saunders, 1992, pp 1537–1553.
6. Grauer A, Raue F, Gagel RF: Changing concepts in the management of hereditary and sporadic medullary thyroid carcinoma. Endocrinol Metab Clin North Am 19:613–635, 1990.
7. Herman V, Draznin NZ, Gonsky R, Melmed S: Molecular screening of pituitary adenomas for gene mutations and rearrangements. J Clin Endocrinol Metab 77:50–55, 1993.
8. Marx SJ, Vinik AI, Santen RJ, et al: Multiple endocrine neoplasia type 1: Assessment of laboratory tests to screen for the gene in a large kindred. Medicine 65:2226–2241, 1986.
9. Pont A: Multiple endocrine neoplasia syndromes. West J Med 132:301–312, 1980.
10. Saad MF, Ordenez NG, Rashid RK, et al: Medullary carcinoma of the thyroid. Medicine 63:319–342, 1964.

47. AUTOIMMUNE POLYGLANDULAR ENDOCRINOPATHIES

Arnold A. *Asp*, M.D.

1. Define the autoimmune polyglandular endocrinopathies. How many clinical forms are there?

The polyglandular endocrinopathies (PGE) are disorders in which two or more endocrine glands are simultaneously hypo- or hyperfunctional as the result of autoimmune dysfunction. It is theorized that a defect in the T-suppressor cell subset inadvertently permits activation of the cellular and humoral arms of the immune system. The nature of this dysfunction is unknown. The two widely recognized clinical forms are appropriately designated PGE I and PGE II. The common clinical link between the syndromes is adrenal insufficiency.

2. Is evidence of nonendocrine autoimmune dysfunction associated with PGEs?

Yes. Connective tissue diseases and hematologic and gastrointestinal autoimmune disorders are commonly associated with the PGEs.

3. What constitutes PGE I?

PGE I is a pediatric disorder manifested by the presence in a sibship of two of the following three disorders: hypoparathyroidism, adrenal insufficiency, and chronic mucocutaneous candidiasis. Usually hypoparathyroidism and candidiasis present by the age of 5 years. Adrenal insufficiency occurs by the age of 12 years, and all manifestations are present by the age of 15 years. Some members of the sibship develop only one manifestation. Other endocrine conditions may also occur; the largest series of patients have noted the following endocrine manifestations:

Hypoparathyroidism	89 %
Adrenal insufficiency	60 %
Gonadal failure	45 %
Thyroid disease	12 %
Diabetes mellitus, type I	1–4 %

4. Are nonendocrine manifestations associated with PGE I?

Yes. Chronic mucocutaneous candidiasis occurs in 75% of patients, malabsorption in 25%, alopecia in 20%, pernicious anemia in 16%, and chronic active hepatitis in 9%.

5. What is the etiology of PGE I?

The etiology is largely unknown. The clustering of disease among equal numbers of boys and girls within a single sibship (not multiple generations) raises the possibility of autosomal recessive inheritance. There appears to be no HLA association. The cause of the candidiasis is not known, although delayed hypersensitivity is defective in affected patients. Antibodies to poorly characterized adrenal and parathyroid antigens have been described by some groups.

6. What therapy can be offered?

Annual screening of levels of serum calcium, cosyntropin-stimulated cortisol, and liver-associated enzymes is performed in affected sibships until the age of 15 years. Adrenal insufficiency and hypoparathyroidism are treated with glucocorticoids and oral calcium supplementation, respectively. Mucocutaneous candidiasis is treated with ketoconazole. Use of prophylactic immunosuppressives, such as cyclosporine, is not recommended.

7. What disorders are associated with PGE II?

PGE II occurs in adulthood and consists of autoimmune adrenal insufficiency with autoimmune thyroid disease and/or diabetes mellitus, type I. The age of onset is between 20 and 30 years; one-half of the cases are spontaneous, and one-half are familial. Endocrine organ involvement is as follows:

Adrenal insufficiency	100 %
Autoimmune thyroid disease	70 %
Diabetes mellitus, type I	50%
Gonadal failure	5–50%

Adrenal insufficiency is the presenting disorder in one-half of cases, whereas adrenal insufficiency with diabetes mellitus or thyroid disease is present at the time of diagnosis in 20% of cases. In the remaining 20%, adrenal insufficiency occurs after other endocrine dysfunction. Between 60–90% of patients have circulating antibodies to an adrenal 32 kd protein.

Thyroid disorders associated with PGE II include Graves' disease (50%) and Hashimoto's disease or atrophic thyroiditis (50%). As expected, thyroid-stimulating immunoglobulins (TSI) are present in cases of hyperthyroidism, whereas antibodies to thyroid peroxidase or thyroglobulin are present in cases of hypothyroidism.

Cytoplasmic islet cell antibodies (ICA) are present in individuals with PGE II and diabetes mellitus; however, the significance of these antibodies is questionable. Nondiabetic patients with PGE II and ICA may have no compromise of beta-cell function and develop diabetes at the rate of 2% per year, whereas ICA-positive first-degree relatives of non-PGE II, type 1 diabetics develop diabetes at the rate of 8% per year.

Gonadal failure is more common in women than men and is associated with antibodies to gonadal tissue. Very rarely geriatric hypoparathyroidism may be encountered in elderly patients with PGE II.

8. Are nonendocrine abnormalities described in PGE II?
Yes. In about 5% of cases other autoimmune disorders are found, including vitiligo, pernicious anemia, alopecia, myasthenia gravis, celiac disease, Sjögren's syndrome, and rheumatoid arthritis.

9. How should kindreds with suspected PGE II be screened?
Because PGE II appears in multiple generations and because 20 years may lapse between the development of various endocrine organ failures, affected patients should be screened by assessing levels of serum glucose, thyrotropin (TSH), and vitamin B12 every 3–5 years. Symptoms of adrenal insufficiency should be investigated by assessing levels of cosyntropin-stimulated cortisol. First-degree relatives of the proband should be educated about the syndrome and advised to undergo screening every 3–5 years. Antibodies to thyroid peroxidase or thyroglobulin are so common in the general population as to preclude their use as a screening test.

10. What is the etiology of PGE II?
The genetic basis of PGE II is uncertain, although it appears to be associated with an HLA-DR3 phenotype that may be permissive for the development of autoimmunity. Organ-specific antibodies may cause organ dysfunction—for example, TSI may cause Graves' disease and antiacetylcholine receptor antibodies may cause myasthenia gravis—or they may be epiphenomena of disease, such as antithyroglobulin antibodies. The only consistent abnormality noted in affected patients is decreased function of T-suppressor cells.

BIBLIOGRAPHY

1. Ahonen P, Myllarniemi S, Sipila I, Perheentupa J: Clinical variation of autoimmune polyendocrinopathy-candidiasis-ectodermal dystrophy (APECED) in a series of 68 patients. N Engl J Med 322:1829–1836, 1990.
2. Eisenbarth GS, Jackson RA: The immunoendocrinopathy syndromes. In Wilson JD, Foster DW (eds): Williams' Textbook of Endocrinology. Philadelphia, W. B. Saunders, 1992; pp 1555–1566.
3. Leshin M: Polyglandular autoimmune syndromes. Am J Med Sci 290:77–88, 1985.
4. Neufeld M, Maclaren NK, Blizzard RM: Two types of autoimmune Addison's disease associated with different polyglandular autoimmune (PGA) syndromes. Medicine 60:355–362, 1981.
5. Trence DL, Morley JE, Handwerger BS: Polyglandular autoimmune syndromes. Am J Med 77:107–116, 1984.

48. PANCREATIC ISLET CELL TUMORS

Michael T. McDermott, M.D.

1. What are the pancreatic islet cell tumors?

These tumors arise from the islet cells of the pancreas. They often cause syndromes due to overproduction of insulin, gastrin, glucagon, somatostatin, or vasoactive intestinal polypeptide (VIP).

2. Are the pancreatic islet cell tumors usually benign or malignant?

Insulinomas are usually benign (80–90%), but the other islet cell tumors are frequently malignant (40–60%).

3. What are the clinical manifestations of insulinomas?

Insulinomas cause hypoglycemia, usually in the fasting state or after exercise. Common symptoms include confusion, slurred speech, blurred vision, seizures, and coma due to neuroglycopenia (reduced delivery of cerebral glucose). Less often tremors, sweating, palpitations, headache, and nausea may result from a catecholamine discharge.

4. How is the diagnosis of insulinoma made?

Hypoglycemia (glucose < 55 mg/dl in men, < 40 mg/dl in women) with simultaneous hyperinsulinemia (insulin-to-glucose ratio > 0.33) occurring spontaneously or during a supervised 12–72 hr-fast is diagnostic.

5. What other disorders cause hyperinsulinemic hypoglycemia?

The other major causes of hyperinsulinemic hypoglycemia are administration of insulin, ingestion of sulfonylurea, and treatment with pentamidine, which damages beta cells and thus causes leakage of insulin into the circulation.

6. What tests are useful in the differential diagnosis of hyperinsulinemic hypoglycemia?

Measurement of serum C-peptide, which is co-secreted with insulin, helps to distinguish an insulinoma (high) from surreptitious administration of insulin (low). Serum proinsulin also tends to be elevated in insulinomas and normal otherwise. The urine should also be screened for sulfonylureas, and inquiries should be made into a history of pentamidine treatment.

7. How is an insulinoma localized?

Imaging procedures such as computed tomographic (CT) scan, ultrasonography, transhepatic portal vein sampling, and splanchnic arteriography may give the correct location, but some tumors cannot be found before surgery. Palpation and ultrasonography during surgery usually provide correct localization in such cases.

8. What is the treatment for an insulinoma?

Solitary benign insulinomas should be removed surgically. Patients with unresectable malignant tumors should be treated with frequent feedings and inhibitors of insulin secretion, such as diazoxide, verapamil, propranolol, phenytoin, and octreotide. Chemotherapy with streptozotocin and doxorubicin or 5-fluorouracil increases survival and improves symptoms.

9. What are the clinical manifestations of gastrinomas?

Gastrinomas secrete excessive gastrin, which stimulates prolific secretion of gastric acid. Patients develop severe peptic ulcer disease, often associated with diarrhea. This disorder is also known as the Zollinger-Ellison syndrome.

10. Do gastrinomas always arise from pancreatic islet cells?
No. Gastrinomas usually arise from the pancreatic islets but also may occur in the duodenum and stomach.

11. How is the diagnosis of gastrinoma made?
The diagnosis is made by demonstrating the presence of high gastric acidity (pH < 3.0) in association with a fasting serum gastrin level > 1000 pg/ml or a moderately elevated gastrin that increases by more than 200 pg/ml within 15 minutes after the intravenous administration of secretin.

12. What is the best way to localize a gastrinoma?
Localization of the tumor may be pursued with various techniques, including CT scan, magnetic resonance imaging (MRI), ultrasonography, endoscopic ultrasonography, transhepatic portal venous sampling, selective arterial secretin infusions, and radioactive octreotide scanning.

13. What is the treatment for gastrinoma?
Most benign and some malignant gastrinomas can be cured by surgery. Otherwise, attention should be directed toward reduction of gastric acid overproduction. High-dose histamine-receptor antagonists, omeprazole, and octreotide effectively decrease acid secretion and symptoms in most patients. Refractory patients may require total gastrectomy for symptomatic relief.

14. What are the characteristics of glucagonomas?
Glucagon antagonizes the effects of insulin in the liver by stimulating glycogenolysis and gluconeogenesis. Glucagonomas, which secrete excessive glucagon, cause diabetes mellitus, weight loss, anemia and a skin rash, necrolytic migratory erythema. The diagnosis depends on finding an elevated level of serum glucagon (> 500 pg/ml).

15. How are glucagonomas treated?
Treatment options include surgery for localized disease, octreotide to reduce glucagon secretion, and chemotherapy with streptozotocin, 5-fluorouracil, and dacarbazine.

16. What are the characteristics of somatostatinomas?
Among its multiple systemic effects, somatostatin inhibits secretion of insulin and pancreatic enzymes, production of gastric acid, and gallbladder contraction. Somatostatinomas secrete excess somatostatin, causing diabetes mellitus, weight loss, steatorrhea, hypochlorhydria, and cholelithiasis. The diagnosis is made by finding an elevated level of serum somatostatin.

17. What is the treatment for somatostatinoma?
Surgery is the treatment of choice. When surgery is not possible, streptozotocin may reduce secretion of somatostatin and tumor size.

18. What are the characteristics of vasoactive intestinal polypeptide-secreting tumors (VIPomas)?
VIPomas cause watery diarrhea, hypokalemia, and achlorhydria (WDHA syndrome, pancreatic cholera). The diagnosis is made by finding an elevated level of serum VIP.

19. How are VIPomas treated?
Surgery is the treatment of choice. Octreotide effectively reduces diarrhea in most patients. Radiation therapy, streptozotocin, and alpha interferon also may reduce diarrhea and tumor size.

20. What syndromes may be caused by pancreatic carcinoid tumors?
In addition to the carcinoid syndrome, pancreatic carcinoids may cause Cushing's syndrome due to ectopic secretion of corticotropin (ACTH) and acromegaly due to ectopic production of growth hormone-releasing hormone (GHRH).

BIBLIOGRAPHY

1. Friesen SR: Tumors of the endocrine pancreas. N Engl J Med 306:580–590, 1982.
2. Krejs GJ, Orci L, Conlon M, et al: Somatostatinoma syndrome: Biochemical, morphologic and clinical features. N Engl J Med 301:285–292, 1979.
3. Leichter SB: Clinical and metabolic aspects of glucagonoma. Medicine 59:100–113, 1980.
4. Moertel CG, Lefkopoulo M, Lipsitz S, et al: Streptozocin-doxorubicin, streptozocin-fluorouracil, or chlorozotocin in the treatment of advanced islet-cell carcinoma. N Engl J Med 326:519–523, 1992.
5. Service FJ, McMahon MM, O'Brien PC, Ballard DJ: Functioning insulinomas—incidence, recurrence, and long-term survival of patients: A 60-year study. Mayo Clin Proc 66:711–719, 1991.
6. Wolfe MM, Jensen RT: Zollinger-Ellison syndrome: Current concepts in diagnosis and management. N Engl J Med 317:1200–1209, 1987.

49. CARCINOID SYNDROME

Michael T. McDermott, M.D.

1. What are carcinoid tumors?

Carcinoid tumors are neoplasms that arise from enterochromaffin or Kulchitsky cells.

2. How are carcinoid tumors classified anatomically?

Carcinoid tumors are classified as originating in the foregut (bronchus, stomach, duodenum, bile ducts, pancreas), midgut (jejunum, ileum, appendix, ascending colon), or hindgut (transverse colon, descending and sigmoid colon, rectum). They also occasionally occur in the gonads, prostate, kidney, breast, thymus, or skin.

3. What is the carcinoid syndrome?

The carcinoid syndrome is a humorally mediated disorder that consists of cutaneous flushing (90%), diarrhea (75%), wheezing (20%), endocardial fibrosis (33%), right-heart valvular lesions, and occasionally pleural, peritoneal, or retroperitoneal fibrosis.

4. Why does pellagra sometimes accompany the carcinoid syndrome?

Pellagra is due to niacin deficiency that results when the tumor diverts tryptophan from synthesis of niacin to synthesis of serotonin.

5. What are the biochemical mediators of the carcinoid syndrome?

Carcinoid tumors produce a variety of humoral mediators, including serotonin, bradykinin, tachykinins, histamine, prostaglandins, neurotensin, and substance P. Diarrhea and formation of fibrous tissue may be caused by serotonin, whereas flushing and wheezing are likely due to kinins, histamine, or prostaglandins.

6. Why do intestinal carcinoid tumors so infrequently cause carcinoid syndrome?

Humoral mediators must reach the systemic circulation to cause carcinoid syndrome. Mediators secreted by intestinal carcinoids are almost totally metabolized in the liver. Thus carcinoid syndrome does not usually occur unless hepatic metastases impair metabolism of the mediators or secrete mediators directly into the hepatic vein. Extraintestinal carcinoids may cause carcinoid syndrome in the absence of metastases.

7. Do carcinoid tumors cause any other humoral syndromes?

Yes. Carcinoids, particularly bronchial carcinoids, may secrete corticotropin (ACTH), which causes Cushing's syndrome, or growth hormone-releasing hormone (GHRH), which causes acromegaly.

8. How is the diagnosis of carcinoid syndrome made?

The diagnosis depends on the demonstration of increased serum concentrations of serotonin, neurotensin, or substance P or increased urinary excretion of 5-hydroxyindoleacetic acid (5-HIAA).

9. Can surgery cure the carcinoid syndrome?

Benign extraintestinal tumors causing carcinoid syndrome may be cured by surgery. Malignant carcinoids with metastases are usually incurable but are slow-growing and allow prolonged survival. Extensive debulking is risky and rarely helpful. Chemotherapy and radiation are relatively ineffective.

10. What is the medical treatment for carcinoid syndrome?

Niacin should be given to prevent pellagra. Flushing may decrease with histamine antagonists, phenoxybenzamine, phenothiazines, or glucocorticoids. Diarrhea may respond to methysergide, cyproheptadine, diphenoxylate, loperamide, or codeine. Octreotide, a somatostatin analog, often controls both flushing and diarrhea.

BIBLIOGRAPHY

1. Feldman JM: The carcinoid syndrome. Endocrinologist 3:129–135, 1993.
2. Godwin JD II: Carcinoid tumors: An analysis of 2837 cases. Cancer 36:560–569, 1975.
3. Kvols LK, Moertel CG, O'Connell MJ, et al: Treatment of the malignant carcinoid syndrome: Evaluation of a long-acting somatostatin analogue. N Engl J Med 315:663–666, 1986.
4. Scully RE, Galdabini JJ, McNeely BU: Case records of the Massachusetts General Hospital: Case 22-1981. N Engl J Med 304:1350–1356, 1981.

50. CUTANEOUS MANIFESTATIONS OF DIABETES MELLITUS AND THYROID DISEASE

James E. Fitzpatrick, M.D., COL, MC

1. How often do patients with diabetes mellitus demonstrate an associated skin disorder?
Most published studies report that 30–50% of patients with diabetes mellitus ultimately develop a skin disorder attributable to their primary disease. However, if one includes subtle findings such as nail changes, vascular changes, and alteration of the cutaneous connective tissue, the incidence approaches 100%. Skin disorders most often present in patients with known diabetes mellitus, but cutaneous manifestations also may be an early sign of undiagnosed diabetes.

2. Are any skin disorders pathognomonic of diabetes mellitus?
Yes. Bullous diabeticorum (bullous eruption of diabetes, diabetic bullae) is specific for diabetes mellitus, but it is uncommon. Bullous diabeticorum most often occurs in patients with severe diabetes, particularly those with associated peripheral neuropathy. Clinically it presents as blisters, usually of the lower extremity, that arise without a history of preceding trauma. The pathogenesis is unknown, but electron microscopy studies suggest that it is a due to structural abnormalities at the junction of the epidermis and dermis. In general, all other reported skin findings may be found to some extent in normal individuals. However, some cutaneous conditions (e.g., necrobiosis lipoidica diabeticorum) demonstrate strong associations with diabetes.

3. What are the skin disorders most likely to be encountered in diabetics?
The most common skin disorders are finger pebbles, nail bed telangiectasia, red face, skin tags (acrochordons), diabetic dermopathy, yellow skin, yellow nails, and pedal petechial purpura. Less common cutaneous disorders that are closely associated with diabetes mellitus include necrobiosis lipoidica diabeticorum, bullous eruption of diabetes, acanthosis nigricans, and scleredema adultorum.

Common Cutaneous Findings in Diabetes Mellitus

CUTANEOUS FINDING	INCIDENCE IN CONTROLS (%)	INCIDENCE IN DIABETICS (%)
Finger pebbles	21	75
Nail bed telangiectasia	12	65
Rubeosis (red face)	18	59
Skin tags	3	55
Diabetic dermopathy	Uncommon	54
Yellow skin	24	51
Yellow nails	Uncommon	50
Erythrasma	Uncommon	47
Diabetic thick skin	Uncommon	30

4. What are finger pebbles?
Finger pebbles are multiple, grouped minute papules that tend to affect the extensor surfaces of the fingers, particularly near the knuckles. They are asymptomatic and may be extremely subtle in appearance. Histologically finger pebbles are due to increased collagen in the dermal papillae.

5. What is acanthosis nigricans?
Acanthosis nigricans is a skin condition due to papillomatous (wartlike) hyperplasia of the skin. It is associated with various conditions, including diabetes mellitus, obesity, acromegaly, Cushing's

syndrome, certain medications, and underlying malignancies. Acanthosis nigricans has been specifically linked to diabetics with insulin resistance.

6. What does acanthosis nigricans look like?

It is most noticeable in axillary, inframammary, and neck creases where it appears as hyperpigmented velvety skin that has the appearance of being "dirty." The tops of knuckles may also demonstrate small papules that resemble finger pebbles except that they are more pronounced.

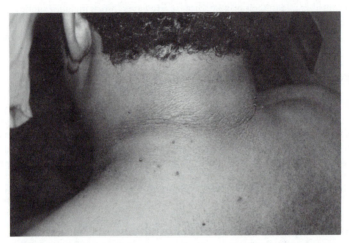

Acanthosis nigricans. Characteristic velvety hyperpigmentation of flexural areas.

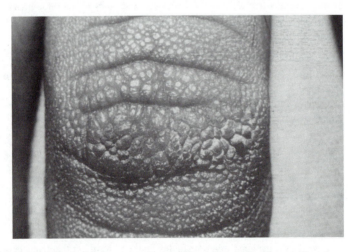

Acanthosis nigricans. Typical lesions over the knuckles demonstrating the papillomatous nature of this cutaneous finding.

7. What is diabetic dermopathy? What is the pathogenesis?

Diabetic dermopathy (shin spots or pretibial pigmented patches) is a common affliction of diabetics that initially presents as erythematous papules or macules with variable scale that heal with atropic, scarred hyperpigmented areas on the pretibial surface.

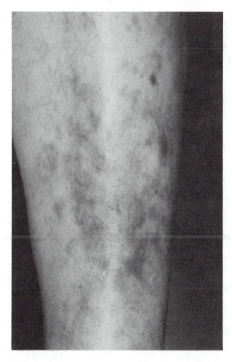

Diabetic dermopathy. Characteristic brown macules of pretibial areas.

Similar lesions are less commonly seen in nondiabetics. Skin biopsies from the lesions demonstrate microangiopathy characterized by a proliferation of endothelial cells and thickening of the basement membranes of arterioles, capillaries, and venules. It is not clear whether the lesions are attributable entirely to vascular changes or whether other secondary factors, such as trauma or venous stasis, are required. There is no known effective treatment. Individual lesions often resolve within 1–2 years, although new lesions will frequently develop.

8. What is necrobiosis lipoidica diabeticorum?

Necrobiosis lipoidica diabeticorum is a disease that most commonly occurs on the pretibial areas, although it may occur at other sites. Early lesions present as nondiagnostic erythematous papules or plaques that evolve into annular lesions characterized by a yellowish color, dilated blood vessels, and central epidermal atrophy. Developed lesions are characteristic and usually can be diagnosed by clinical appearance. Less commonly, ulcers may develop.

Biopsies demonstrate palisaded granulomas that surround large zones of necrotic and sclerotic collagen. Additional findings include dilated vascular spaces, plasma cells, and increased neutral fat. Biopsies of developed lesions are usually diagnostic, although some cases may be difficult to separate from granuloma annulare. The pathogenesis is now known, but proposed causes include an immune complex vasculitis and a platelet aggregation defect.

9. What is the relationship of necrobiosis lipoidica diabeticorum to diabetes mellitus?

In a major study of patients with necrobiosis lipoidica diabeticorum, 62% had diabetes. Approximately one-half of the nondiabetic patients had abnormal glucose tolerance tests, and almost one-half of the nondiabetics gave a family history of diabetes. However, necrobiosis lipoidica diabeticorum is present in only 0.3% of patients with diabetes. Some dermatologists prefer the term ''necrobiosis lipoidica'' for patients who have the disorder without associated

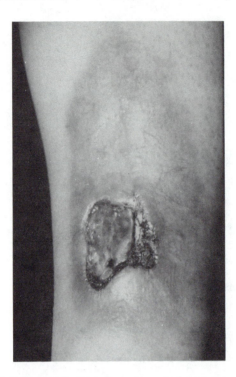

Necrobiosis lipoidica diabeticorum. Pretibial plaque demonstrating atrophic center with ulceration and mildly raised annular edge.

diabetes. Because of the strong association between these conditions, patients who present with necrobiosis lipoidica should be screened for diabetes; patients who test negative should be reevaluated periodically.

10. How should necrobiosis lipoidica diabeticorum be treated?
Necrobiosis lipoidica occasionally may resolve without treatment. It does not seem to respond to treatment of diabetes in new cases or to tighter control of established diabetes. Early lesions may respond to treatment with potent topical or intralesional corticosteroids. More severe cases may respond to oral treatment with acetylsalicyclic acid and dipyridamole, although some cases show no response. Severe cases with recalcitrant ulcers may require surgical grafting.

11. Are skin infections more common in diabetics than in control populations?
Yes. But skin infections are probably not as common as most medical personnel believe. Studies show that an increased incidence of skin infections strongly correlates with elevated levels of mean plasma glucose.

12. What are the most common bacterial skin infections associated with diabetes mellitus?
The most common serious skin infections associated with diabetes mellitus are diabetic foot and amputation ulcers. One autopsy study revealed that 2.4% of all diabetics had infectious skin ulcerations of the extremities compared with 0.5% of a control population. Staphylococcal skin infections, including furunculosis and staphylococcal wound infections, are usually described in textbooks as more common and more serious in diabetics than in the normal population. Although it is universally accepted that staphylococcal infections are more serious and difficult to manage in diabetics, no well-controlled studies prove that the incidence is higher in diabetics. This controversial issue remains to be resolved. Erythrasma, a benign superficial bacterial infection

caused by *Corynebacterium minutissimum,* was present in 47% of adult diabetics in one study. Clinically it presents as tan to reddish-brown macular lesions with slight scale in intertriginous areas, usually of the groin; however, the axilla and toe web spaces also may be affected. Because the organisms produce porphyrin, the diagnosis can be made by demonstrating a spectacular coral red fluorescence with a Wood's lamp.

13. What are the most common fungal skin infections associated with diabetes mellitus?
The most common mucocutaneous fungal infection associated with diabetes is candidiasis, usually caused by *Candida albicans.* Women are particularly prone to get vulvovaginitis. One study demonstrated that two-thirds of all diabetics have positive cultures for *Candida albicans.* In women with signs and symptoms of vulvitis, the incidence of positive cultures approaches 99%. Similarly, positive cultures are extremely common in diabetic men and women who complain of anal pruritus. Other mucocutaneous forms of candidiasis include thrush, perleche (angular cheilitis), intertrigo, erosio interdigitalis blastomycetica chronica (see figure below), paronychia (infection of the soft tissue around the nail plate), and onychomycosis (infection of the nail). The mechanism appears to be due to increased levels of glucose that serve as a substrate for *Candida* species to proliferate. Patients with recurrent cutaneous candidiasis of any form should be screened for diabetes. Diabetics in ketoacidosis are particularly prone to develop mucormycosis (zygomycosis) caused by various zygomycetes, including *Mucor, Mortierella, Rhizopus,* and *Absidia* species. Fortunately, such fulminant and often fatal infections are rare. Although early studies had suggested that dermatophyte infections were more common in diabetics than in controls, more recent epidemiologic data do not support this association.

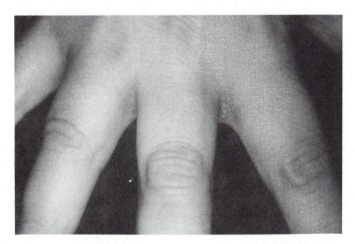

Erosio interdigitalis blastomycetica chronica. *Candida* infection in the interdigital spaces in a diabetic patient. A very long name for a very small infection!

14. Why are diabetics in ketoacidosis especially prone to mucormycosis?
The fungi are thermotolerant, prefer an acid pH, grow rapidly in the presence of high levels of glucose, and are one of the few fungi that utilize ketones as a growth substrate. Thus, diabetics in ketoacidosis provide an ideal environment for the proliferation of these fungi.

15. Are any skin complications associated with the treatment of diabetes mellitus?
Yes. Adverse reactions to injected insulin are relatively common. The reported incidence varies from 10–56%, depending on the study. In general these complications may be divided into three categories: reactions due to faulty injections (e.g., intradermal injection), idiosyncratic reactions, and allergic reactions. Several types of allergic reactions have been described, including localized and generalized urticaria, Arthus reactions, and localized delayed hypersensitivity. Oral hypogly-

cemic agents occasionally may produce adverse cutaneous reactions, including photosensitivity, urticaria, erythema multiforme, and erythema nodosum. Chlorpropamide in particular may produce a flushing reaction when consumed with alcohol.

16. What are the most important cutaneous manifestations of the hypothyroid state?
Generalized myxedema is the most characteristic cutaneous sign of hypothyroidism. Other skin findings include xerosis (dry skin), follicular hyperkeratosis, diffuse hair loss, dry brittle nails, yellowish discoloration of the skin, and thyroid acropachy.

17. Why do hypothyroid patients often have yellow skin?
The yellow color is due to the accumulation of carotene (carotenoderma) in the top layer of the epidermis (stratum corneum). Carotene is excreted by both the sweat glands and sebaceous glands and tends to concentrate on the palms, soles, and face. The increased levels of carotene are probably secondary to impaired hepatic conversion of beta-carotene to vitamin A.

18. What are the clinical findings in generalized myxedema?
Generalized myxedema is characterized by pale, waxy, edematous skin that does not demonstrate pitting. These changes are most noticeable in the periorbital area but may also be observed in the distal extremities, lips, and tongue.

19. What is the pathogenesis of generalized myxedema?
The skin demonstrates an increased accumulation of dermal acid mucopolysaccharides, of which hyaluronic acid (ground substance) is the most important. Studies also have demonstrated that an increased transcapillary escape of serum albumin into the dermis adds to the endematous appearance. Neither of these changes are permanent; both are reversible with replacement therapy.

20. What is the difference between generalized myxedema and pretibial myxedema?
Generalized myxedema is associated only with the hypothyroid state, whereas pretibial myxedema is characteristically associated with Graves' disease. Patients with pretibial myxedema may be hypothyroid, hyperthyroid, or euthyroid. Thus this change appears to be due to some unknown factor other than alteration of the thyroid hormones.

21. What are the clinical manifestations of pretibial myxedema?
Pretibial myxedema occurs in about 3–5% of patients with Graves' disease. The majority of patient have associated exophthalmos. Clinically pretibial myxedema is characterized by edematous, indurated plaques over the pretibial areas, although other sites of the body also may be involved. The plaques are usually sharply demarcated, but diffuse variants are also reported. The overlying skin surface is usually normal, although it may be studded with smaller papules. The color varies from skin-colored to brownish-red (see figure, next page). Overlying hypertrichosis may be present on rare occasions. Histologically, pretibial myxedema demonstrates massive accumulation of dermal hyaluronic acid.

22. How is pretibial myxedema treated?
Studies comparing different treatment modalities have not been performed. Because the condition is not harmful to patients, treatment is not always indicated. Many cases respond to potent topical corticosteroids under occlusion or intralesional corticosteroids. More extensive cases may be treated with oral systemic corticosteroids. Treatment of the thyroid disease does not affect the cutaneous findings.

23. What are the skin manifestations of hyperthyroidism?
Studies have shown that as many as 97% of all patients with hyperthyroidism develop skin manifestations. Common cutaneous findings include cutaneous erythema, excoriations, smooth skin, hyperpigmentation, moist skin (due to increased sweating), pretibial myxedema, pruritus (itching), and warm skin. Nails are often brittle and may separate from the underlying bed (onycholysis). The hair also may be thinner than normal.

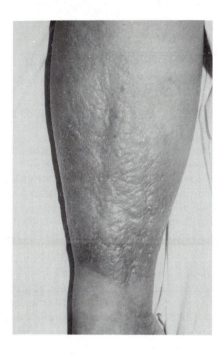

Pretibial myxedema. Indurated plaques of pretibial area. This case demonstrated a brownish-red color, but lesions may be skin-colored.

BIBLIOGRAPHY

1. Bernstein JE, Medanica M, Soltani K, Griem SF: Bullous eruption of diabetes mellitus. Arch Dermatol 115:324–325, 1979.
2. Danowski TS, Sabeh G, Sarver ME, et al: Skin spots and diabetes mellitus. Am J Med Sci 251:570–575, 1966.
3. Feingold KR, Elias PM: Endocrine-skin interactions. J Am Acad Dermatol 17:921–940, 1987.
4. Freinkel RK, Freinkel N: Hair growth and alopecia in hypothyroidism. Arch Dermatol 106:349–352, 1972.
5. Huntley AC: The cutaneous manifestations of diabetes mellitus. J Am Acad Dermatol 7:427–455, 1982.
6. Huntley AC: Finger pebbles: A common finding in diabetes mellitus. J Am Acad Dermatol 14:612–617, 1986.
7. Lang PG, Jr, Sisson JC, Lynch PJ: Intralesional triamcinolone therapy for pretibial myxedema. Arch Dermatol 110:197–202, 1975.
8. Montes LF, Dobson H, Dodge BG, Knowles WR: Erythrasma and diabetes mellitus. Arch Dermatol 99:674–680, 1969.
9. Muller SA, Winkelmann RK: Necrobiosis lipoidica diabeticorm: A clinical and pathological investigation of 171 cases. Arch Dermatol 93:272–281, 1966.
10. Mullin GE, Eastern JS: Cutaneous consequences of accelerated thyroid function. Cutis 37:109–112, 1986.
11. Quimby SR, Muller SA, Schroeter AL, et al: Necrobiosis lipoidica diabeticorum: Platelet survival and response to platelet inhibitors. Cutis 43:231–216, 1989.
12. Parving HH, Hansen JM, Nielsen SL, et al: Mechanism of edema formation in myxedema: Increased protein extravasation and relatively slow lymphatic drainage. N Engl J Med 301:460–465, 1979.
13. Plourde PV, Marks JG, Hammond JM: Acanthosis nigricans and insulin resistance. J Am Acad Dermatol 10:887–891, 1984.

51. INHERITED HORMONE RESISTANCE SYNDROMES

Michael T. McDermott, M.D.

1. What are the well-characterized genetic hormone resistance syndromes?

There are well-described syndromes caused by inherited resistance to insulin, thyroid hormone, parathyroid hormone (PTH), vitamin D, androgens, cortisol, vasopressin, and growth hormone.

2. What are the causes of inherited insulin resistance?

Inherited insulin resistance may result from a variety of abnormalities. Prereceptor disorders include genetic mutations involving the proinsulin and insulin molecule and autoantibodies directed against circulating insulin or insulin receptors. Receptor disorders are due to a multitude of genetic mutations affecting the insulin receptor. Postreceptor disorders may include mutations involving insulin-receptor substrate 1 (IRS-1), glucose transporters, and the enzymes involved in intracellular glucose metabolism.

3. What are the manifestations of insulin resistance?

Insulin resistance is characterized by normal or elevated levels of plasma glucose in the presence of moderate-to-extreme elevations of the serum insulin concentration. Patients may be asymptomatic or may have diabetes mellitus. Obesity, acanthosis nigricans, and excessive secretion of androgen may coexist.

4. What role does insulin resistance play in the development of atherosclerosis?

Mild-to-moderate insulin resistance, which appears to be hereditary, is commonly associated with essential hypertension, elevated serum triglycerides, low serum HDL cholesterol, and small, dense LDL particles. Referred to as syndrome X, this combination of coronary artery disease risk factors appears to be particularly atherogenic.

5. What causes the thyroid hormone resistance syndromes?

Generalized resistance to thyroid hormone (GRTH) is most often due to genetic mutations that involve the T_3-binding region of the thyroid hormone receptor and cause reduced T_3-binding affinity. Pituitary resistance to thyroid hormone feedback results in hypersecretion of thyroid-stimulating hormone (TSH), which in turn stimulates excessive production of thyroid hormone. Symptomatic thyrotoxicosis does not occur, however, because of peripheral tissue resistance.

6. What are the clinical manifestations of thyroid hormone resistance?

Patients with GRTH are clinically euthyroid or hypothyroid but have elevated levels of T_4 and T_3 and an inappropriately normal or elevated level of TSH. Hyperactivity–attention deficit disorder, low IQ, hearing impairment, and heart disease are sometimes associated.

7. What causes the parathyroid hormone resistance syndromes?

PTH receptors are normal but postreceptor signaling is defective, most often because of a genetic mutation affecting the Gs protein, which couples the PTH receptor to its cyclic adenosine monophosphate (cAMP) response cascade. Some cases are due to abnormalities at other sites in the signal pathways. Lack of PTH effect causes hypocalcemia and hyperphosphatemia despite an increased serum level of PTH. This disorder is also termed pseudohypoparathyroidism.

8. What are the clinical manifestations of parathyroid hormone resistance?

Affected patients often have short stature, short fourth and fifth metacarpals, mental retardation, and calcification of basal ganglia. Biochemically the serum calcium is low, phosphorus is high and PTH is moderately to greatly elevated.

9. What causes the vitamin D resistance syndromes?
The two major disorders are congenital 1-alpha-hydroxylase deficiency (C1HD) and congenital resistance to 1, 25-dihydroxyvitamin D (CRVD). C1HD is caused by genetic mutations affecting the renal enzyme that converts 25-hydroxyvitamin D to 1,25-dihydroxyvitamin D. CRVD is due to mutations involving vitamin D receptors. A third condition, congenital hypophosphatemic rickets, was initially termed "vitamin D resistant rickets," but the predominant cause is renal phosphate wasting.

10. What are the manifestations of vitamin D resistance?
Both C1HD and CRVD cause short stature, rickets, and muscle weakness; patients with CRVD also may have alopecia. Biochemically both disorders exhibit hypocalcemia, hypophosphatemia, and elevated levels of serum PTH. However, levels of 1,25-dihydroxyvitamin D are low in C1HD and elevated in CRVD.

11. What causes the androgen resistance syndromes?
There are two main categories of androgen resistance syndromes. Genetic mutations affecting the androgen receptors cause partial or complete androgen resistance in all tissues; complete androgen resistance is termed testicular feminization. Deficiency of 5-alpha-reductase, the enzyme that converts testosterone to dihydrotestosterone (DHT), causes androgen resistance only in DHT-dependent tissues, such as the external genitalia.

12. What are the clinical manifestations of androgen resistance?
Depending on their severity, androgen receptor abnormalities produce a spectrum of disorders ranging from simple oligospermia to ambiguous genitalia to a phenotypically normal-appearing female who fails to develop menses (testicular feminization). Hormone testing reveals normal or elevated male-range levels of testosterone and elevated levels of serum luteinizing hormone (LH). Deficiency of 5-alpha-reductase produces phenotypically female or ambiguous genitalia, which undergo significant masculinization at puberty when secretion of testosterone greatly increases.

13. What causes the cortisol resistance syndromes?
Cortisol resistance syndromes are due to genetic mutations involving cortisol receptors. Lack of normal cortisol receptors in the central nervous system results in ineffective suppression of ACTH by cortisol. Hypersecretion of ACTH stimulates increased adrenal production of cortisol, aldosterone, and androgens. Because of defective function of cortisol receptors, however, the body responds only to the excess of aldosterone and androgens.

14. What are the clinical manifestations of cortisol resistance?
Affected men often develop hypertension, whereas women may develop hypertension and hirsutism with or without virilization. Serum levels of cortisol, aldosterone, and testosterone are elevated, whereas ACTH is inappropriately normal or high.

15. What causes congenital resistance to vasopressin?
Congenital resistance to vasopressin has been found to be due to genetic mutations affecting renal vasopressin receptors, although some patients may have abnormalities in the Gs protein that couples the receptors to cAMP activation. In either case, the result is an inability of the renal collecting ducts to conserve water in response to vasopressin. The condition also has been termed congenital nephrogenic diabetes insipidus.

16. What are the clinical manifestations of vasopressin resistance?
Affected patients develop polyuria soon after birth. The increased urinary output does not respond to water deprivation or administration of vasopressin. When testing is available, levels of vasopressin should be elevated. If fluid intake is not adequate, severe volume depletion may result.

17. What causes the growth hormone resistance syndromes?
The best studied disorder, Laron dwarfism, is due to genetic mutations involving the growth hormone receptor. The result is an inability of growth hormone to stimulate hepatic production of insulin-like growth factor 1 (IGF-1), which is the major factor that stimulates peripheral growth.

18. What are the clinical manifestations of growth hormone resistance?
Affected patients have moderate-to-severe growth retardation. Serum levels of growth hormone are elevated but serum levels of IGF-1 are low.

BIBLIOGRAPHY

1. Amselem S, Duquesnoy P, Attree O, et al: Laron dwarfism and mutations of the growth hormone-receptor gene. N Engl J Med 321:989–995, 1989.
2. Amselem S, Sobrier M-L, Duquesnoy P, et al: Recurrent nonsense mutations in the growth hormone receptor from patients with Laron dwarfism. J Clin Invest 87:1098–1102, 1991.
3. Breslau NA: Pseudohypoparathyroidism: Current concepts. Am J Med Sci 298(2):130–140, 1989.
4. Farfel Z, Brickman AS, Kaslow HR, et al: Defect of receptor-cyclase coupling protein in pseudohypoparathyroidism. N Engl J Med 303:237–242, 1980.
5. Flier JS: Lilly lecture: Syndromes of insulin resistance; from patient to gene and back again. Diabetes 41:1207–1219, 1992.
6. Griffin JE: Androgen resistance—The clinical and molecular spectrum. N Engl J Med 326:611–618, 1992.
7. Holtzman EJ, Harris HW Jr, Kolakowski LF Jr, et al: Brief report: A molecular defect in the vasopressin V2-receptor gene causing nephrogenic diabetes insipidus. N Engl J Med 238:1534–1537, 1993.
8. Javier EC, Reardon GE, Malchoff CD: Glucocorticoid resistance and its clinical presentations. Endocrinologist 1:141–148, 1991.
9. Kristjansson K, Rut AR, Hewison M, et al: Two mutations in the hormone binding domain of the vitamin D receptor cause tissue resistance to 1,25 dihydroxyvitamin D_3. J Clin Invest 92:12–16, 1993.
10. Malchoff DM, Brufsky A, Reardon G, et al: A mutation of the glucocorticoid receptor in primary cortisol resistance. J Clin Invest 91:1918–1925, 1993.
11. McDermott MT, Ridgway EC: Thyroid hormone resistance syndromes. Am J Med 94:424–432, 1993.
12. McPhaul MJ, Marcelli M, Zoppi S, et al: Genetic basis of endocrine disease 4: The spectrum of mutations in the androgen receptor gene that causes androgen resistance. J Clin Endocrinol Metab 76:17–23, 1993.
13. Merendino JJ Jr, Spiegel AM, Crawford JD, et al: Brief report: A mutation in the vasopressin V2-receptor gene in a kindred with X-linked nephrogenic diabetes insipidus. N Engl J Med 238:1538–1543, 1993.
14. Moller DE, Flier JS: Insulin resistance—Mechanisms, syndromes, and implications. N Engl J Med 325:938–948, 1991.
15. Taylor SI: Lilly lecture: Molecular mechanisms of insulin resistance; lessons from patients with mutations in the insulin-receptor gene. Diabetes 41:1473–1490, 1992.
16. Yagi H, Ozono K, Miyake N, et al: A new point mutation in the deoxyribonucleic acid-binding domain of the vitamin D receptor in a kindred with hereditary 1,25-dihydroxyvitamin D-resistant rickets. J Clin Endocrinol Metab 76:509–512, 1993.

52. ENDOCRINE CASE STUDIES

Michael T. McDermott, M.D.

1. A 34-year-old woman has new-onset hypertension, a serum potassium level of 2.7 mmol/L, and the following results with hormone testing: supine plasma aldosterone = 55 ng/dl (normal = 1–16), supine plasma renin = 0.1 ng/ml/hr (normal = 0.15–2.33), plasma aldosterone after a saline infusion = 54 ng/dl (normal = 1–8), 4-hour upright plasma aldosterone = 32 ng/dl (normal = 4–31), 4-hour upright plasma renin = 0.1 ng/ml/hr (normal = 1.31–3.95), and serum 18-hydroxycorticosterone = 108 ng/dl (normal < 30). What is the probable diagnosis?

Hypertension, hypokalemia, elevated level of supine plasma aldosterone that does not suppress with volume expansion, and low plasma renin confirm the diagnosis of primary hyperaldosteronism. The etiology is usually an aldosterone-producing adrenal adenoma or bilateral adrenal hyperplasia. The very low basal serum potassium, the significant drop in plasma aldosterone during the 4-hour posture test, and the elevated level of 18-hydroxycorticosterone are most consistent with an adrenal adenoma.

2. A 32-year-old female business executive develops amenorrhea and has the following laboratory results: serum estradiol = 14 pg/ml (normal = 23–45), luteinizing hormone (LH) = 1.2 mIU/ml (normal = 2–15), follicle-stimulating hormone (FSH) = 1.5 mIU/ml (normal = 2–20), prolactin = 6.2 ng/ml (normal = 2–25), negative test for beta human chorionic gondadotropin (hCG), and normal pituitary with magnetic resonance imaging (MRI) scan. What is the probable diagnosis?

The patient has secondary amenorrhea with low levels of estradiol and gonadotropins. The clinical picture is most consistent with hypothalamic amenorrhea, which sometimes occurs in women who exercise excessively or who have stressful jobs. The disorder is due to reduced frequency of hypothalamic pulses of gonadotropin-releasing hormone (GnRH).

3. A clinically thyrotoxic nulliparous 48-year-old woman has a modest, nontender goiter, no exophthalmos and the following results on thyroid evaluation: T_4 = 16.2 ug/dl (normal = 4.5–12), T_3 = 245 ng/dl (normal = 90–200), T_3 uptake = 45% (normal = 35–45%), thyroid-stimulating hormone (TSH) < 0.1 µU/ml, 24-hour radioactive iodine uptake (RAIU) = 1% (normal = 20–35%), thyroglobulin = 25 ng/ml (normal = 2–20), and sedimentation rate = 10 mm/hr. What is the probable diagnosis?

The patient has clinical and biochemical hyperthyroidism with a low RAIU. The differential diagnosis includes subacute thyroiditis, painless thyroiditis, factitious thyrotoxicosis, and iodine-induced thyrotoxicosis. The elevated level of serum thyroglobulin suggests thyroiditis, whereas the nontender gland and normal sedimentation rate are most consistent with painless thyroiditis.

4. A 38-year-old man has coronary artery disease, xanthomas of the Achilles tendons, and the following serum lipid profile: cholesterol = 482 mg/dl, triglycerides = 152 mg/dl, HDL cholesterol = 42 mg/dl, and LDL cholesterol = 410 mg/dl. What is the probable diagnosis?

Significant elevations of total cholesterol and LDL cholesterol, normal triglycerides, tendon xanthomas, and premature coronary artery disease are most consistent with the diagnosis of familial hypercholesterolemia. This disorder is due to deficient or abnormal LDL receptors.

5. A 26-year-old man presents with infertility and is found to have small, firm testes, gynecomastia, and the following serum hormone abnormalities: testosterone = 2.6 ng/ml (normal = 3.0–10.0), LH = 88 mIU/ml (normal = 2–12), and FSH = 95 mIU/ml (normal = 2–12). What is the probable diagnosis?

The patient has hypergonadotropic hypogonadism with small firm testes and gynecomastia, which is most consistent with Klinefelter's syndrome. Such patients have a 47 XXY karyotype.

6. A 38-year-old nurse presents in a stuporous state. Significant laboratory abnormalities are as follows: blood glucose = 14 mg/dl, serum insulin = 85 μU/ml (normal < 22), C-peptide = 5.2 ng/ml (normal = 0.5–2.0), and proinsulin = 0.6 ng/ml (normal = 0–0.2). What is the probable diagnosis?
The patient has hyperinsulinemic hypoglycemia. The differential diagnosis includes insulinoma, surreptitious insulin injection, oral sulfonylurea ingestion or pentamidine use. The elevated serum C-peptide and proinsulin levels are most consistent with an insulinoma.

7. A 28-year-old woman with type I diabetes develops amenorrhea and has the following serum hormone values: estradiol = 15 pg/ml (normal = 23–145), LH = 78 mIU/ml (normal = 2–15), FSH = 92 mIU/ml (normal = 2–20), prolactin = 12 ng/ml (normal = 2–25), and negative test for beta hCG. What is the probable diagnosis?
The patient has secondary amenorrhea with low levels of estradiol and elevated levels of gonadotropins. The differential diagnosis includes premature ovarian failure and the resistant ovary syndrome. In a patient with another autoimmune disease (type I diabetes mellitus) the most likely diagnosis is premature ovarian failure.

8. A 34-year-old woman presents with headaches, amenorrhea, and weight gain. Laboratory evaluation reveals the following: prolactin = 55 ng/ml (normal = 2–25), T_4 = 1.8 μg/dl (normal = 4.5–12), T_3 = 85 ng/dl (normal = 90–200), T_3 resin uptake = 34% (normal = 35–45%), TSH > 60 μU/ml, and an enlarged pituitary gland on MRI scan. What is the probable diagnosis?
The patient has pituitary enlargement, increased serum prolactin, and primary hypothyroidism. The clinical picture is most consistent with primary hypothyroidism that causes secondary pituitary hyperplasia and hypersecretion of prolactin. All abnormalities should resolve after thyroid hormone replacement is begun.

9. A 6-year-old girl develops breast enlargement, pubic hair, and monthly vaginal bleeding. Laboratory tests produce the following results: estradiol = 42 pg/ml (normal = 23–145), LH = 12 mIU/ml (normal = 2–15), FSH = 14 mIU/ml (normal = 2–20), prolactin = 8 ng/ml (normal = 2–25), TSH = 1.9 μU/ml (normal = 0.1–4.5), and a normal pituitary MRI scan. What is the probable diagnosis?
The patient has gonadotropin-dependent true precocious puberty. The etiology includes pituitary and hypothalamic tumors, but most cases in girls are idiopathic. The normal pituitary MRI indicates that the primary diagnosis is idiopathic precocious puberty.

10. A 19-year-old man presents with excessive thirst and urination. Laboratory evaluation is as follows: urine volume = 8,800 ml/24 hr, serum sodium = 145 mmol/L, serum osmolality = 298 mOsm/kg, urine osmolality = 90 mOsm/kg with no response to a water deprivation test, but an increase in urine osmolality to 180 mOsm/kg after the administration of subcutaneous vasopressin. What is the probable diagnosis?
The patient has polyuria and polydipsia with maximally dilute urine. The differential diagnosis includes central diabetes insipidus, nephrogenic diabetes insipidus, and primary polydipsia. The lack of response to water deprivation and the more than 50% increase in urine osmolality after administration of vasopressin are most consistent with central diabetes insipidus.

11. A 25-year-old woman presents with a cushingoid appearance. The results of hormone testing are as follows: 24-hour urine cortisol = 218 μg (normal = 20–90), morning serum cortisol = 28 μg/dl (normal = 5–25), and morning plasma ACTH = 65 pg/ml (normal = 10–80). After an 8-mg oral bedtime dose of dexamethasone, the morning serum cortisol = 6 μg/dl. What is the probable diagnosis?

Cushingoid features and elevated urinary excretion of cortisol confirm the diagnosis of Cushing's syndrome. The etiology is usually an ACTH-secreting pituitary adenoma (65–80%), ectopic production of ACTH (10–15%), or cortisol-producing adrenal adenoma (10–15%). The normal plasma level of ACTH, which is inappropriate for the elevated level of serum cortisol, and suppression of plasma cortisol with high-dose dexamethasone are most consistent with pituitary adenoma.

12. An 8-year-old boy with known adrenal insufficiency complains of hand and leg cramps, and has carpopedal spasm on examination. Results of blood testing are as follows: calcium = 6.2 mg/dl (normal = 8.5–10.2), phosphorous = 5.8 mg/dl (normal = 2.5–4.5), intact PTH = 10 pg/ml (normal = 10–65), and 25-hydroxyvitamin D = 42 ng/ml (normal = 16–74). What is the probable diagnosis?

Hypocalcemia, hyperphosphatemia, and a low level of PTH are most consistent with primary hypoparathyroidism. This disorder, which is probably autoimmune in nature, may occur in association with adrenal insufficiency as part of the polyendocrine failure type I syndrome.

13. A 52-year-old man has a personal and family history of coronary artery disease, minimal alcohol consumption, no xanthomas, and the following results on serum testing: cholesterol = 328 mg/dl, triglycerides = 322 mg/dl, HDL = 35 mg/dl, LDL = 229 mg/dl, apoprotein B = 145 mg/dl (normal = 60–130), apoprotein E phenotype = E3/E3, TSH = 2.1 µg/ml (normal = 0.1–4.5), and glucose = 85 mg/dl. What is the probable diagnosis?

The patient has elevations of both cholesterol and triglycerides and no detected disorders that cause secondary dyslipidemia. The differential diagnosis of this profile includes familial combined hyperlipidemia and familial dysbetalipoproteinemia. The elevated level of apoprotein B and the normal apoprotein E phenotype are most consistent with familial combined hyperlipidemia.

14. A 58-year-old man has recent-onset diabetes mellitus, weight loss, and a skin rash that is most prominent on the buttocks and that a dermatologist diagnoses as necrolytic migratory erythema. What is the probable underlying diagnosis?

Diabetes mellitus, weight loss, and necrolytic migratory erythema are virtually diagnostic of a glucagon-secreting pancreatic islet cell tumor (glucagonoma).

15. A 29-year-old woman has hypercalcemia, a family history of hypercalcemia and failed parathyroidectomies, and the following laboratory results: serum calcium = 11.0 mg/dl (normal = 8.5–10.2), phosphorous = 3.0 mg/dl (normal = 2.4–4.5), intact PTH = 66 pg/ml (normal = 10–65), 25-hydroxyvitamin D = 42 ng/ml (normal = 16–74), and 24-hour urinary excretion of calcium = 23 mg (normal = 100–250). What is the probable diagnosis?

Although the vast majority of patients with hypercalcemia and a mildly elevated level of serum PTH have hyperparathyroidism, the presence of very low urinary excretion of calcium and a family history of unsuccessful parathyroidectomies points to a diagnosis of familial hypocalciuric hypercalcemia. This autosomal dominant disorder of transcellular calcium transport impairs renal excretion of calcium and calcium suppression of PTH secretion.

16. A 39-year-old HIV-positive man with *Pneumocystis carinii* pneumonia has the following values of serum thyroid hormones: T_4 = 4.0 µg/dl (normal = 4.5–12.0), T_3 = 22 ng/dl (normal = 90–200), T_3 resin uptake = 48% (normal = 35–45%), TSH = 4.3 µU/ml (normal = 0.1–4.5), and cortisol = 28 µg/dl (normal = 5–25). What is the most likely endocrine diagnosis?

A very low T_3, a mildly low T_4, an elevated T_3 resin uptake, and normal TSH are most consistent with the euthyroid sick syndrome. Serum cortisol also may be elevated in stressed patients.

17. An 18-year-old girl has not yet begun menstruation and has a height of 56 inches, a small uterus, and no breast development. The results of hormone tests are as follows: estradiol = 8 pg/ml (normal = 23–145), LH = 105 mIU/ml (normal = 2–15), FSH = 120 mIU/ml (normal = 2–20), prolactin = 14 ng/ml (normal = 2–15), and TSH = 1.8 µU/ml (normal = 0.1–4.5). What is the probable diagnosis?

Primary amenorrhea, short stature, a low level of estradiol, and an elevated level of gonadotropins are most consistent with the diagnosis of Turner's syndrome. This disorder, which results from a 45 XO karyotype, is characterized by ovarian dysgenesis.

18. A 28-year-old woman has infertility, regular menses, and normal findings on laparoscopy. Analysis of the husband's semen is normal. On day 25 of the menstrual cycle laboratory results are as follows: prolactin = 12 ng/ml (normal = 2–25), TSH = 2.2 uU/ml (normal = 0.1–4.5), and progesterone = 2.8 ng/ml (normal = 2.5–28). An endometrial biopsy is read as consistent with a day 20 endometrium. What is the probable diagnosis?

The patient has infertility despite evidence of ovulation and patent fallopian tubes. The low serum progesterone and significantly delayed endometrial development are most consistent with the diagnosis of luteal phase defect. In this disorder, the corpus luteum makes insufficient progesterone to promote normal endometrial development. Fertilization and implantation may occur, but the endometrium is inadequate to support continued pregnancy.

19. A 25-year-old man presents with a 3-cm thyroid mass, watery diarrhea, and a family history of thyroid cancer in his father and brother. What is the probable diagnosis?

The only type of thyroid cancer that occurs in a familial form with significant frequency is medullary thyroid carcinoma. This tumor secretes calcitonin and several other humoral factors; 33% of affected patients develop diarrhea. The patient probably has medullary thyroid carcinoma.

20. A 20-year-old man presents for failure to enter puberty and has small, soft testes, no gynecomastia, normal visual fields, and decreased sense of smell. Laboratory evaluation is as follows: serum testosterone = 0.7 ng/ml (normal = 3.0–10.0), LH = 2.0 mIU/ml (normal = 2–12), FSH = 1.6 mIU/ml (normal = 2–12), prolactin = 7 ng/ml (normal = 2–20), and a normal pituitary MRI study. What is the probable diagnosis?

Hypogonadotropic hypogonadism associated with anosmia is most consistent with idiopathic hypogonadotropic hypogonadism, also known as Kallman's syndrome. This disorder is due to a deficiency of gonadotropin-releasing hormone (GnRH) resulting from failure of fetal migration of the hypothalamic neurons that secrete GnRH. Maldevelopment of the olfactory lobes causes the associated anosmia.

53. FAMOUS PEOPLE WITH ENDOCRINE DISORDERS

Kenneth J. Simcic, M.D.

1. What former National Hockey League star led the Philadelphia Flyers to back-to-back Stanley Cup championships in 1973–74 and 1974–75, despite his insulin-dependent diabetes?
Bobby Clarke.

2. What female track star recovered from Graves' disease and went on to win the title of "Fastest Woman in the World" at the 1992 Summer Olympics in Barcelona, Spain?
Gail Devers.

3. Actor Gary Coleman starred in the television series *Different Strokes*. His short stature was caused by what medical illness?
Kidney failure.

4. Composer Ludwig van Beethoven (1770–1827) began to lose his hearing before he reached the age of 30 years. What bone disorder may have been the cause of his hearing loss?
Paget's disease of bone.

5. Name the dwarf actor who gained fame for his role as Tattoo on the television series *Fantasy Island*.
Hervé Villechaize (1943–1993).

6. Television actress Mary Tyler Moore has what endocrine disorder?
Insulin-dependent diabetes.

7. What famous male singer has a skin disorder that is often associated with autoimmune gland diseases?
Michael Jackson (vitiligo).

8. George Bush and his wife Barbara were both diagnosed with Graves' disease during the Bush Presidency (1988–1992). How did the President's disease present clinically?
Atrial fibrillation.

9. What mythical lumberjack is probably the most famous giant in American folklore?
Paul Bunyan.

10. At the 1988 Summer Olympics in Seoul, Korea, what Canadian sprinter was stripped of his gold medal after testing positive for anabolic steroids.
Ben Johnson.

11. What former television actor from *Rowan & Martin's Laugh-In* had obvious Graves' ophthalmopathy?
Marty Feldman.

12. Ancient Egyptian sculptures and paintings suggest that Tutankhamen (1357–1339 B.C.) and other pharaohs had what endocrine disorder?
Gynecomastia.

13. Elected to Baseball's Hall of Fame in 1987, pitcher Jim "Catfish" Hunter was undefeated in three World Series with the Oakland Athletics. With what endocrine disorder was he diagnosed?
Non–insulin-dependent diabetes.

14. What male ice-skater overcame growth failure related to a childhood illness to win the gold medal at the 1984 Winter Olympics in Sarajevo, Yugoslavia?
Scott Hamilton.

15. Despite a diagnosis of diabetes at age 26 years, which National Football League quarterback played for 10 seasons with the Minnesota Vikings and appeared in the Pro Bowl in 1988?
Wade Wilson.

16. Name the late professional wrestler who was well known for his acromegalic features.
Andre the Giant (1947–1993).

17. What former National Football League star developed a fatal brain tumor after using anabolic steroids?
Lyle Alzado (1949–1992).

18. Charles Sherwood Stratton (1838–1883) reached an adult height of only 3 feet, 4 inches. What was his "circus" name?
General Tom Thumb.

19. Ed Kranepool played first base for the New York Mets from 1962–1979. What endocrine disorder did he develop after his retirement from baseball?
Non–insulin-dependent diabetes.

20. Comedian and talk-show host Jay Leno has facial features suggestive of what benign endocrine disorder?
Benign prognathism.

54. INTERESTING ENDOCRINE FACTS AND FIGURES

Michael T. McDermott, M.D.

1. Who is the tallest man on record?

The man with the greatest medically documented height was Robert Wadlow of Alton, Illinois. He was 7 feet 1 3/4 inches at age 13 years and 8 feet, 11.1 inches when he died in 1940, at the age of 22 years. He weighed 439 lbs. His condition was the result of a growth hormone-secreting pituitary tumor that developed before closure of the skeletal epiphyseal plates (gigantism).

2. Name the tallest woman on record.

Zeng Jinlian of Hunan Province, China, is the tallest woman on record. She was 7 feet, 1 1/2 inches tall at age 13 years and reached 8 feet, 1 3/4 inches just before her death at age 17 in 1982. She also had a growth hormone-secreting tumor that developed during childhood.

3. How tall was the shortest man on record?

Calvin Phillips of Bridgewater, Massachusetts was 26 1/2 inches tall and weighed 12 pounds at the age of 19 years. He died at age 22 in 1812. He had progeria, which is characterized by dwarfism and premature senility.

4. Who is the shortest woman on record?

The shortest adult woman on record was Pauline Musters of the Netherlands. She was 23.2 inches tall and weighed 9 pounds shortly before her death at age 19 years in 1895. Because of her relatively normal proportions, she is believed to have had pituitary growth hormone deficiency, although growth hormone measurements were clearly not available in 1895.

5. Who had the most variable adult stature?

Adam Rainer of Austria was a 3-foot, 10.45-inch dwarf at the age of 21 years but rapidly grew into a 7-foot, 1 3/4-inch giant at age 32 years in 1931.

6. What is the tallest tribe in Africa?

The Watusi (or Tutsi) tribe of Sudan, Rwanda, Burundi, and Central African Republic are the tallest in the world. The men average 6 feet, 5 inches, and the women average 5 feet, 10 inches. Their tall stature is believed to be a genetic adaptation.

7. What is the shortest tribe?

The Mbuti pygmies of Zaire and Central African Republic have the lowest mean height. The men average 4 feet, 6 inches, and the women 4 feet, 5 inches. Their short stature is thought to result from genetic resistance to growth hormone, possibly due to deficient growth hormone receptors.

8. Who was the heaviest man on record?

Jon Brower Minnoch of Bainbridge Island, Washington was 6 feet, 1 inch tall and weighed approximately 1,400 pounds when he was admitted to the hospital at age 37 years in congestive heart failure. He remained in the hospital for 2 years on a 1,200-calorie diet and was discharged at 476 lbs. He weighed 798 lbs when he died at age 42 years in 1983. His wife weighed 110 lbs.

9. How much did the heaviest woman on record weigh?

The heaviest woman on record was Mrs. Percy Pearl Washington of Milwaukee, Wisconsin, who was 6 feet tall and weighed 880 pounds. She died in 1972.

10. What is the largest recorded waist size?

Walter Hudson of New York, who stood 5 feet, 10 inches, had a peak weight of 1,197 pounds and a waist size of 119 inches.

11. Who are the heaviest twins on record?
Billy and Benny McCrary of Hendersonville, North Carolina weighed 743 pounds and 723 pounds, respectively. Both had 84-inch waists. One brother died in a motorcycle accident, but the other is alive at the time of this printing.

12. What is the greatest known number of children born to one woman in a lifetime?
A peasant woman from Shuya, east of Moscow, Russia, gave birth to 69 children from 1725 to 1765. She had 27 pregnancies, producing 16 pairs of twins, 7 sets of triplets, and 4 sets of quadruplets. Sixty-seven of the children survived infancy.

13. Who is the oldest known woman to give birth?
In 1956 Ruth Alice Kistlen of California gave birth to a daughter at the age of 57 years, 129 days. She is the oldest medically verified mother to have become pregnant and delivered a child without a medically assisted reproductive method. Newer reproductive technologies have allowed this record to be eclipsed.

14. What is the highest reported number of multiple births for a single gestation?
Ten births (decaplets) were reported in Brazil (1946), China (1936), and Spain (1924). Nine births (nonuplets) were recorded in Australia (1971), Philadelphia (1972), and Bangladesh (1977).

15. What is the largest tumor ever reported?
In 1905 a 328-pound ovarian cyst was removed from a woman in Texas.

16. What is the longest hair ever recorded?
In 1780 a 52-year-old peasant woman from Poland was recorded to have hair 12 feet long. Because hair grows at approximately 1/2 inch per month, this would have required at least 24 years of continuous growth. Most hairs fall out and are replaced before they are 3 feet long.

17. Who has the largest chest and arm muscles on record?
Isaac ''Dr. Size'' Nesser of Greensburg, Pennsylvania, has a 68.06-inch chest and 26 1/8-inch biceps. He is 5 feet, 10 inches tall and weighs 351 pounds.

18. Did King David of Israel have an endocrine disorder?
''When King David was old and advanced in years, though they spread covers over him, he could not keep warm. His servants therefore said to him, 'Let a young virgin be sought to attend you, lord king, and to nurse you. If she sleeps with your royal majesty, you will be kept warm.' . . . The maiden, who was very beautiful, nursed the king and cared for him, but the king did not have relations with her'' (I Kings 1:1–4). Some speculate King David was afflicted with hypothyroidism.

19. What endocrine disorder might Goliath of Gath have had?
Goliath of Gath, who was killed by a stone from David's sling (I Samuel 17:1–51), probably stood about 6 feet, 10 inches. His tall stature may have resulted from a growth hormone-secreting pituitary tumor. Others add that the ease with which David's stone became embedded in Goliath's skull may have been due to hyperparathyroidism and his bizarre behavior may have resulted from hypoglycemia due to an insulinoma. He may thus be the earliest known case of MEN I syndrome.

20. What endocrine disorder did President John F. Kennedy have?
Kennedy had primary adrenal insufficiency—Addison's disease. He was sustained throughout the later years of his life and his presidency by therapy with oral glucocorticoids.

SOURCES

1. McFarlan D (ed): The Guiness Book of World Records. New York, Bantam Books, 1991.
2. Baumann G, Shaw MN, Merimee TJ: Low levels of high affinity growth hormone-binding protein in African Pygmies. N Engl J Med 320:1705–1709, 1989.
3. The New American Bible, Catholic Publishers, Inc., 1971.

INDEX

Page numbers in **boldface** type indicate complete chapters.